Handbook of Pediatric Retinal Disease

Handbook of Pediatric Retinal Disease

Edited by

Kenneth W. Wright, MD
Director, Wright Foundation for Pediatric Ophthalmology
Director, Pediatric Ophthalmology, Cedars-Sinai Medical Center, Clinical Professor of Ophthalmology, University of Southern California—Keck School of Medicine, Los Angeles, California

Peter H. Spiegel, MD
Focus On You, Inc., Palm Desert, California
Inland Eye Clinic, Murrieta, California
Children's Eye Institute, Upland, California

Lisa S. Thompson, MD
Attending Physician, Stroger Hospital of Cook County, Chicago, Illinois

Illustrators
Timothy C. Hengst, CMI
Susan Gilbert, CMI
Faith Cogswell

Springer

Kenneth W. Wright, MD
Director, Wright Foundation for Pediatric Ophthalmology
Director, Pediatric Ophthalmology, Cedars-Sinai Medical Center,
Clinical Professor of Ophthalmology, University of Southern California—Keck School of Medicine
Los Angeles, CA
USA

Peter H. Spiegel, MD
Focus On You, Inc.
Palm Desert, CA
Inland Eye Clinic,
Murrieta, CA
Children's Eye Institute
Upland, CA
USA

Lisa S. Thompson, MD
Attending Physician
Stroger Hospital of Cook County
Chicago, IL
USA

Library of Congress Control Number: 9005932935

ISBN 10: 0-387-27932-6 e-ISBN 0-387-27933-4
ISBN 13: 978-0387-27932-0

Printed on acid-free paper.

Printed in China. (BS/EVB)

9 8 7 6 5 4 3 2 1

springer.com

Preface

Pediatric ophthalmology is a broad field encompassing many diverse topics including embryology, chromosomal abnormalities, neurology, craniofacial abnormalities, systemic diseases, retina disease, and strabismus. This variety makes pediatric ophthalmology interesting and intellectually stimulating, but at the time somewhat daunting. The handbook series is designed to give the practitioner an easy to understand, succinct yet detailed reference on various subjects related to pediatric ophthalmology.

The *Handbook of Pediatric Retinal Disease* is a practical resource on the diagnosis and management of both the most common and more esoteric retinal disorders. An in-depth chapter on electrophysiology of the eye (with an emphasis on hereditary retinal disease) is included. This chapter provides important information for deciding which tests to order and how to interrupt electrophysiology results. Children with retinal disorders often are faced with irreversible visual loss and even blindness. In these cases, even a seasoned physician often feels uncomfortable when speaking with the family. A beautifully sensitive chapter, "Breaking the News," provides practical points to help the physician communicate both clearly and empathetically with the family.

A broad range of retinal disorders are covered in this volume, with many color photographs to demonstrate the ophthalmoscopic findings. Chapters in the handbook are reader friendly and are organized with clear sub-headings to guide the reader to their areas of interest quickly. Excellent color photographs and diagrams illustrate the clinical points and help establish firm diagnosis parameters. Extensive use of tables and information boxes simplify and summarize complex topics. Each chapter is fully referenced to provide evidence-based practice guidelines and further in-depth reading.

Another important use for the *Handbook of Pediatric Retinal Disease* is to serve as a basis for patient and family education. Information including diagrams and photographs from the handbook about their child's specific retinal disease can be shared with the families. This important information is often lacking in general texts on ophthalmology and pediatrics.

I hope you will find the *Handbook of Pediatric Retinal Disease* to be an invaluable adjunct to your pediatric practice.

Kenneth W. Wright, MD

Contents

Contributors

Christopher F. Blodi, MD

David M. Brown, MD

Nancy Chernus-Mansfield

Laurie E. Christensen, MD

Arlene V. Drack, MD

Richard M. Feist, MD

William L. Haynes, MD

Alan E. Kimura, MD

Anthony Kriss, PhD (Posthumous)

A. Linn Murphree, MD

Richard R. Ober, MD

Earl A. Palmer, MD

Jose S. Pulido, MD

Chittaranjan V. Reddy, MD

Peter H. Spiegel, MD

Dorothy Thompson, PhD

Anne Frances Walonker

Thomas A. Weingeist, MD, PhD

Kenneth W. Wright, MD

1

Pediatric Visual Electrophysiology

Anthony Kriss* and Dorothy Thompson

Visual electrodiagnostic tests can contribute significantly to pediatric ophthalmology. The tests are objective, safe, relatively swift, and easy to administer. They can give unique insight into the functional integrity of different levels of the visual pathway. The *electroretinogram* (*ERG*) indicates retinal function, the *electro-oculogram* (*EOG*) expresses pigment epithelium function, and the *visual evoked potential* (*VEP*) reflects optic pathway function beyond the eye to the visual cortex. These tests complement, and supplement, other visual methods of assessment. Thus, depending on the clinical context, an abnormal ERG may suggest the necessity for metabolic screening, and an abnormal VEP in association with a normal ERG can indicate the need for structural imaging studies.

There are advantages to being able to use visual electrodiagnostic tests in preliminary disease stages in young infants. This practice enhances the chances of successful surgical or clinical intervention and allows genetic counseling when it is most pertinent to young parents. It can also ease emotional acceptance and allow for more opportune implementation of

---

**In Memoriam:* On October 5, 2001, Dr. Kriss passed away after a long illness. Despite the gravity of his ill health, Dr. Kriss worked hard to finish this chapter and submitted it one week before his death. His tenacity in completing this definitive work on Pediatric Electrophysiology is a testament to his passion for this field. I have known Dr. Kriss professionally for almost 20 years and have the highest respect for his research, teaching, and clinical abilities. This chapter exemplifies Dr. Kriss' commitment to excellence, attention to detail, and his world-class expertise in the field of Pediatric Electrophysiology. It is my honor and privilege to include his chapter in this second edition by Kenneth W. Wright, MD.

educational programs. In many ways, the functional sensitivity of electrodiagnostic tests is not yet rivaled by functional imaging techniques. Despite advances in statistical manipulation and faster resolution, the application of imaging methods to young children is still a daunting challenge.

When ERG and VEP are tested together, they can help determine whether a baby's nystagmus or failure to fix and follow are a result of dysfunction of the anterior visual pathway. Together, they can help distinguish if the basis of the clinical problem lies with cones, rods, the inner retinal layer, optic nerve, or at the chiasm or postchiasmal pathway. In older infants, testing can help establish if there is an underlying reason why an eye is not responding to patching and can provide an objective indicator of the presence of posterior hemisphere dysfunction with an associated visual field loss. In older children, visual *electrophysiology* can be a useful complement in investigating headaches, malingering, or possible functional visual loss. Pattern VEP findings can also provide a helpful measure of the level of visual acuity, especially in preverbal children. Visual electrophysiology in the future will offer a key measure of the functional outcome of human gene therapy.

The results of visual electrophysiological tests are usually displayed as graphs of voltage (in microvolts) plotted against time (in milliseconds). These graphs have characteristic waveforms, and the constituent positive and negative peaks are quantified by their latency (called implicit time by some), relative to the onset of stimulus delivery, and their size (amplitude) relative to the previous peak or an estimated baseline. Formal identification usually recognizes the polarity and latency of a component; for example, P100 of the pattern reversal response refers to the positive component that peaks 100 milliseconds (ms) after the pattern reverses. Response measures are also altered by technical and physiological factors, which can mimic response changes associated with pathology. Therefore, it is important to be aware also of the effects of nonpathological factors, as they could lead to misinterpretation of recordings by the unwary. To reduce the possibilities of these types of error, international professional bodies have prescribed standards [e.g., ISCEV (International Society for the Electrophysiology of Vision) or International Federation of Clinical Neurophysiology].[35,36]

This chapter is a distillation of visual electrophysiology [ERG, EOG, pattern electroretinogram (PERG), and VEP]. It describes the physiological basis of responses with emphases on responses used clinically and on the application of visual electrophysiology to pediatrics. Details of the ISCEV recording standards are given also. These standards relate mainly to the testing of older children and adults; pediatric standards are being discussed at present. The authors have described testing protocols for young children that they found to be valuable in a pediatric practice dealing with both ophthalmologic and neuro-ophthalmologic problems (to about equal extents), testing approximately 1500 children per year.

THE ELECTRORETINOGRAM

Types of Electroretinograms

FLASH ERG, PATTERN ERG, AND MULTIFOCAL ERG

Some retinal cells hyperpolarize, others depolarize in response to changes in retinal illumination. The gross effect of these summed biopotentials is recordable at the front surface of the eye as a series of negative and positive voltage changes (peaks) in the first 200 ms after the light stimulation. These series of peaks are the ERG. The form and timing of the ERG is related to the eye's state of light adaptation and to the intensity, spatial, chromatic, and temporal characteristics of the stimulus. The *flash electroretinogram* (*F.ERG*) is generated by a uniform flash of light (e.g., from a strobe light flashed in a Ganzfeld or by LEDs) that reflects electrical activity from most of the retina. A *pattern electroretinogram* (*PERG*) is recorded when structured stimuli are used; for example, checkerboards or gratings. Usually, PERGs are recorded using stimuli localized to the macular and paramacular areas. Pattern stimuli contain equal numbers of black and white elements (usually checks) that counterphase, or appear from a background of uniform gray field of equal mean luminance (pattern onset). With these stimuli, there is no overall change in mean retinal luminance, and light scatter within the eye is minimized. A localized flash ERG can be applied if a bright stimulus surround is used to reduce the effect of scattered light (called focal ERG).

Multifocal ERGs (mfERGs) are obtained by stimulating the central 30° to 50° of the retina with a contiguous array of flickering hexagons. Each element is independently alternated between black (off) and white (illuminated) according to a pseudorandom binary order called the m-sequence. Multiple hexagons are simultaneously alternated, but the m-sequence determines that no pattern of simultaneous hexagon stimulation is repeated twice in the sequence. Cross-correlation techniques associate ERG activity with localized retinal areas and provide a topology (map) of the test field's retinal sensitivity.[150]

SEPARATING ROD AND CONE ACTIVITY

There are important clinical advantages in separately assessing rod and cone activity. Rods and cones can function separately or interactively, depending on the level of overall illumination. During light adaptation, the retinal circuitry alters to cater for a million-fold change in visual sensitivity (6 $\log_{10}$ unit). The cone pathways are preferentially stimulated by high-intensity white light and longer-wavelength (red) flashes presented under photopic conditions, as well as by fast flash rates delivered above 15/s. The rod pathway is preferentially activated by dim, short-wavelength (blue-green) light stimuli or by very dim white flashes presented at less than 10/s under fully darkened (scotopic) laboratory conditions.

Rods can detect single light quanta in dark backgrounds. Rod ERGs are slower responses than cone ERGs, as they are reflecting a longer pathway through the retina. Rods contact one bipolar type only: the "On" rod bipolar, which directly links to a rod amacrine cell that, in turn, feeds back to contact cone "On" bipolars. Cones are involved in analysis of spatial contrast discrimination mechanisms and detect decrements ("Off" changes), as well as increments ("On" changes) of light against an illuminated background. Cones directly contact both cone "On" and "Off" bipolars.[190] Other more direct rod-to-cone gap junction pathways and also an "Off" bipolar pathway have been described.[187] Electroretinography can help dissect these pathways and improve our understanding of retinal dysfunction.

Origins of the ERG

RETINAL RESPONSE TO LIGHT

Light stimulation of both rods and cones causes transient and sustained changes in the extracellular ion composition, particularly of potassium ions (K^+ ions). Müller cells, which are of glial origin and span the depth of the retina, have variations in their surface conductivity for K^+ ions. This variation causes localized buffering of K^+ ions and induces radial currents involving the length of the Müller cell. The movement of these ionic currents through the membrane and interstitial resistance of Müller cells give rise to an associated voltage change [V = current (I) × resistance (R)], and this mass dipolar response is detectable at the front surface of the eye as the ERG.

Component Origins

Granit, in 1933, suggested that three processes are involved in generating the flash ERG: process I (PI) is the main contributor to the c-wave (EOG), PII to the b-wave, and PIII to the a-wave.[70] Granit surmised that the ERG is an algebraic summation of these positive- and negative-going processes with different timing and size and that the processes are generated by different retinal structures. ERG analysis continues to be a lively area of research some 70 years later. A variety of neurotransmitter analogues, and antagonists, are now available to pharmacologically dissect out the various contributions of the different retinal networks whose function also contribute to the resultant ERG.[191] New components (e.g., the scotopic threshold response elicited by markedly dim flashes) have been discovered.[193] New analysis techniques (algorithms) have been applied to studying phototransduction,[171] and methods of assessing the different contributions of On and Off pathways have been elaborated.[193] Paired-flash ERGs have been used to study inactivation mechanisms and recovery rates of rhodopsin via the dynamics of the rod a-wave.[92] The lifetime of activated rhodopsin in normal human rods has been estimated to be 2.3 s.[167]

Three main features of the flash ERG are usually analyzed for clinical purposes:

- Size or amplitude of the negative and positive peaks (a- and b-waves)
- Latency or implicit time of these peaks
- Waveform, in particular, the relative size of each wave that determines the shape of the ERG (e.g., as when describing the "negative" ERG)

Cone-driven ERGs are smaller, with components of shorter latency, compared with rod-mediated ERGs. Cone-driven ERGs can be distinguished by b-wave latencies around 30 to 35 ms, prominent a-waves, and "spikier" morphology. The rod ERG is rounder, with later and larger b-waves, around 50 to 60 ms, and the a-wave is less prominent, or may be nondetectable depending on stimulus intensity (Fig. 1-1).

The *a-wave* is the main corneal negative wave with a peak latency of 15 to 25 ms (depending on stimulus intensity and whether it is mainly being generated by cones or rods). In the dark, an influx of cations through channels kept open by cGMP depolarizes the rods, resulting in release of the neurotransmitter glutamate. Light stimulation causes closure of cation channels, resulting in diminution of the dark current, receptor hyperpolarization, and reduction of glutamate release. The a-wave is a reflection of the mass hyperpolarization of photoreceptors. The maximum amplitude of the photocurrent response is determined by the upper limit of dark, or circulating, current available. On illumination, the catalytically active form of rhodopsin, metarhodopsin II, binds to the membrane G-protein

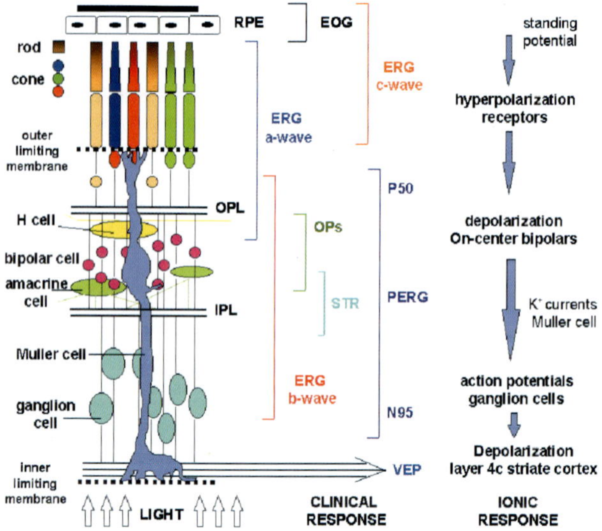

FIGURE 1-1. Schematic retina showing level of electroretinogram (ERG) component generators. Diagram represents ionic changes occurring in retinal thickness after light stimulation. The summation of these changes over time results in the ERG. The different parts of the ERG waveform are generated in different retinal levels.

(Gt) and initiates a signal-amplifying cascade of reactions.[163] Changes in the slope of the a-wave with intensity have been quantitatively related to the mechanisms involved in the G-protein-triggered phototransduction amplification cascade. Differences in amplification and maximal a-wave amplitude have been noted between retinitis pigmentosa (RP) and cone dystrophy.[28,29,91,171,178,197] Recent work has attempted to relate differences in the behavior of these parameters with RP genotypes.[222]

The *b-wave* is a corneal-positive component. Its latency is between 30 and 80 ms, depending on the relative contribution of cones and rods. b-wave activity is associated predominantly with depolarization of on-center bipolar cells. However, Sieving et al.[191] have recently demonstrated that the size and shape of the photopic ERG b-wave is limited by hyperpolarizing bipolars and represents the algebraic sum of both depolarizing and hyperpolarizing activity. The size of the b-wave changes systematically with stimulus intensity and can be approximated mathematically by the Naka–Rushton function, which is a derivation of the Michaelis–Menten equation and describes a saturating nonlinearity as follows:

$$\frac{V}{V_{max}} = \frac{Int}{Intensity + K}$$

where V = trough-to-peak amplitude of the b-wave
V_{max} = maximum value of trough-to-peak amplitude
Int = flash intensity in td-second
K = semisaturation value, i.e., when I = K V is $V_{max}/2$

Oscillatory potentials (OPs) are a series of high-frequency positive wavelets (four are usually discernible, but sometimes a late fifth wave is present also). OPs overlap with the rising phase of the b-wave. These wavelets are thought to reflect synaptic activity of inhibitory feedback pathways in association with retinal amacrine and ganglion cell activity. Early wavelets of OPs reflect rod function and "on" pathways, and later wavelets are linked with the cone system and "off" pathway activity.[225] OPs are most readily recorded under mesopic conditions. They represent both photopic and scotopic processes and the interaction between cone and rod pathways. They are sensitive to chemical agents that disrupt retinal inhibitory mechanisms (dopamine-, GABA-, and glycine-mediated) but are not selectively altered by excitatory amino acids.

The *c-wave* is a slow positive-going wave that is best recorded over several seconds using DC amplification. It shows variable presence among healthy controls, mainly as it represents the interaction of two retinal potentials with opposite polarity and similar time course. One is a slow positive retinal pigment epithelium (RPE) signal and the other a negative response caused by the presence of K^+ ions in subretinal space. The c-wave is difficult to record reliably and is little used clinically.

The *d-wave* is a positive wave that is closely associated with a reduction in light under photopic conditions. When very brief flashes are used, this component is not obviously discernible as it merges with the b-wave. It can only be isolated by separating on and off stimulation by 50 to 150ms.

Flicker ERGs elicited by stimuli rates greater than 20/s reflect cone photoreceptor activity. Rods are unable to respond to activation at these stimulation rates. There appears to also be an inner retinal contribution to the flicker response.[107] Stimulation rates of 8 to 10/s are used to elicit sinusoidal rod-mediated ERGs.

Scotopic Threshold Response (STR)

The STR is a slow negative response generated at the inner retina and peaking around 100 ms. It is elicited from a dark-adapted eye using very dim light at intensities lower than that which elicits the b-wave. Experimental evidence suggests that it is generated at the inner retina, most probably by amacrine cells.[193]

Pattern ERGs (PERGs)

PERGs are usually elicited for clinical purposes by using a reversing checkerboard, stimulating macular/paramacular retinal areas. The PERG has typically a biphasic configuration with a positivity at 50 ms (P50) and a negativity at 95 ms (N95). Clinical and experimental evidence indicates that the P50 reflects macula function and the N95 reflects ganglion cell function.[51,90] PERGs are small, of the order of 0.5 to 8 μV peak amplitude. They are best recorded with corneal electrodes that do not impede the eye's optics (e.g., DTL fiber, gold foil, HK silver wire electrodes). Interestingly, infraorbital skin electrodes pick up PERGs at about half the size of those detected by corneal electrodes, whereas, for flash stimulation, ERGs are about 80% to 90% smaller. ISCEV recommends a check size of 0.8°, presented in a field size of 16°.[12] Clear focus response, averaging up to 50 to 100 averages, and minimal blinking are needed to optimally record PERGs. This level of cooperation is more likely to be achieved in children aged 6 years and older.

ERG RECORDING METHODS

Electrodes

ERGs are recorded clinically from metal electrodes placed on, or very close, to the cornea. The electrode conductor may be mounted in a contact lens, or directly touch the eye's tear film (as with gold foil and DTL electrodes). There are warnings against multiuse contact lenses, and several guidelines are published regarding the risks of cross-contamination from electrodes used for clinical electrophysiology purposes. The greatest known risks are from AIDS, hepatitis B, and prions associated with Creutzfeld-Jakobs Disease (CJD) and human variant CJD. In clinical visual electrophysiology, disposable electrodes are strongly advocated. Single-use, contact lens JET electrodes and DTL fiber electrodes are favored for corneal ERG recordings and sticky pad electrodes for infraorbital recordings. Sterilizable silver/silver chloride EEG electrodes are commonly used to record VEPs.

Some centers routinely use contact lens electrodes to record flash ERGs from babies and young children. The recording is obtained while the child is unconscious, either under sedation or anesthetized as part of a fundus examination. Other centers find that reliable recordings can be obtained in most young children while the child is conscious but physically restrained. Very little has been published on the risks of corneal abrasion or serious damage associated with sedation or anesthesia for ERG recording in children. Indeed, there are medical practitioners and parents who feel the risks associated with induced unconsciousness are unacceptable when used to obtain the ERG only. Some departments use skin ERG recordings as "a last resort" when sedation is not an option for reasons of patient size or weight. Other departments (including the authors') find that, with signal averaging, reliable flash ERG recordings can be obtained from skin electrodes positioned immediately below the lower eyelids; this method allows the VEP to be recorded at the same session and has strong diagnostic advantages. The authors use DTL electrodes and ISCEV standard recordings for experimental purposes on cooperative older children and adults.

ERG amplitude is related to the type of recording electrode used. It is important for laboratories to standardize on one type. The authors compared six different forms of electrode in the same subjects. The Burian–Allen contact lens (with lid speculum) electrode gave the largest a-b amplitude for the mixed rod/cone ERG, which measured 470 μV on average. Relative to this, the amplitudes of the same component recorded from the other electrodes were as follows: Jet, 89%; C-glide, 77%; gold foil, 56%; DTL fiber 46%; and lower lid skin ERG, 12%.[53]

Physiological and physical factors also have important effects on the ERG. Physiological factors to consider include these:

1. Gender differences (females tend to produce larger and shorter latency responses compared with males).
2. Age.
3. Fundal pigmentation (light fundi are associated with larger b-wave amplitudes compared with darkly pigmented fundi).
4. Pupil size.
5. Refractive error.
6. Drugs (treatment and anesthesia).
7. Circadian rhythm.

Physical (stimulus) factors having important effects include these:

1. Intensity: illuminance rather than stimulus intensity, per se, should be used to study retinal responses. Illuminance depends on pupil size, which is small (around 3 mm diameter) in infants. In adults, however, it can vary between 5 mm and 9 mm after dilation. This variation of pupil area is significant, and it is important to note pupil size or, more pertinently, illuminance, especially if the pupils are unusually large or small.
2. Duration.
3. Interstimulus interval (ISI).
4. Color.

Technical Equipment

Amplification

ERGs and VEPs are relatively very small signals (5–10 thousandths of 1 volt). Differential amplification is needed to visualize responses. This technique involves recording the *voltage difference* between two points on the head (one "active," recorded over or very near where the response is generated, and the other relatively "inactive," little influenced by activity at the active site). The method is an effective way to remove background activity (called noise), common to both active and inactive sites. Differential amplifiers have filters to restrict the amplified range of high and low frequencies, which helps to distinguish response activity from electrical activity of other physiological and extraneous origins. DC amplifiers have no lower limit to their frequency response and can record both steady and fluctuating potentials. They are preferred for recording very slow potential changes (e.g., EOG fluctuations and the c-wave). AC amplifiers allow filtering of low-frequency activity, which can cause significant distortions in the recording of the ERG and VEP. Low-frequency interference mainly arises from eye movements and from ionic interactions at the electrode and body surface interface. Recent advances now permit digital DC amplification to be used, and with this technique corrections of slow potential changes can be made online while signal acquisition is taking place.

Averaging

Individual small evoked responses such as the PERG and VEP are often almost invariably difficult to discern, as they are intermixed with "noise" arising from physiological (usually muscle, heart, or spontaneous brain activity) and extraneous sources (power lines, hospital equipment, communication frequencies). The technique of signal averaging offers a powerful means to systematically add activity occurring immediately after each stimulus delivery; this has the effect of clarifying the signal and reducing background noise activity. The background noise reduces approximately in relation to the square root of the number averaged; for example, averaging 100 responses reduces background noise amplitude to one-tenth of the size of the response. Although children tend to produce larger VEPs than adults, they tend to be more restless (i.e., produce more eye movements and muscle activity), and a greater number of responses need to be averaged to achieve a good discrimination between the response and background activity.

THE ELECTRO-OCULOGRAM

Granit's process PI contributes to the c-wave of the ERG, and is also reflected in the standing potential of the electro-oculogram (EOG)[70] (see p. 91). Steady ionic currents flow between the pigment epithelium and the photoreceptors and generate the standing potential that is positive at the cornea relative to the posterior pole. ISCEV standards for the EOG, published in 1994 and reissued in 1998, are found on their Web site (www.ukl.uni-freiberg.de/aug/iscev)

The EOG is usually recorded using skin electrodes (nowadays, mainly EEG or sticky pad type) placed close to the inner and outer canthi of each eye. The potential difference between these electrodes is recorded, using DC or near-DC amplification, when the eye makes a saccade between two preset fixation points. This recording technique can also be used to depict and monitor nystagmus.

The amplitude of the EOG is closely linked with the size of the saccade and with the state of light adaptation of the eye. Patients are asked to alternate fixation between two lights placed centrally (commonly LEDS), with an angular separation at the eye between 20° and 30°, every 2 min or so. Eye movements are performed in the dark, when the EOG reaches a minimum amplitude, normally after 8 to 10 min (dark trough). Lighting conditions are then made strongly photopic and, after 8 to 10 min, the EOG usually increases to a maximum size (light peak), which is about twice the dark-trough size.[9]

Clinically, the ratio between the light peak against the dark trough is used as an index to gauge photoreceptor/pigment epithelium function. This is called the Arden index and, in many laboratories, values greater than 1.8 are considered normal.[9] In practice, children of approximately 6 years of age and older have the tolerance and discipline to reliably make saccades every 2 min, for a total of 30 min.

Fulton et al.[63] have described a technique for obtaining an EOG in younger children. A rotating chair (as used for eye movement studies) is utilized to elicit the vestibulo-ocular reflex (i.e., doll's head response). The child's fixation attention is held on a toy target while the chair rotates the child's body by a fixed amount (e.g., 30°). However, the technique is not widely applied because, in practice, it is difficult to reliably hold a child's attention for the long half-hour period required to gauge the light peak and dark trough.

THE VISUAL EVOKED POTENTIAL

Types of VEP: Transient, Steady State, Sweep, and Multifocal

The VEP is normally largest in the midline, around 3 to 5 cm above the inion. VEPs are elicited to stimulate a wide central area of the visual field, most commonly at stimulation rates less than 5/s; this ensures that all components of individual responses are clearly distinguished (the transient VEP). For clinical purposes, uniform light flashes and checkerboard pattern stimuli are usually used. Patterns either reverse (pattern reversal) or abruptly appear from a uniform background of the same overall stimulus luminance as the pattern and then disappear (pattern onset/offset). Recently, the technique of *multifocal VEP* has been introduced. The stimulation technique is similar to that used for multifocal ERG studies, but the VEP is usually recorded from a single midoccipital site following stimulation of small, well-localized areas of the visual field. Steady fixation during signal acquisition is vital, making its application to pediatrics very limited at this time.

When the stimulation frequency is increased so that the VEPs merge and appear to maintain a consistent sinusoidal waveform (noted at rates around 8–10/s or more), then responses are said to be "steady state." Steady-state techniques are used to elicit sweep VEPs where a predetermined range of different pattern sizes, or contrast levels, are presented sequentially. The changes in response amplitude and phase are analyzed using Fourier techniques, and the results are presented graphically (usually approximating a bell shape). Computations of the maximum and measures of regression relating to the rate of change of the rising and falling slopes are often used to summarize results.

Cortical Origins of the VEP

VEPs reflect surface activity of cortical gyri and, therefore, mainly reflect activity of areas of the visual field represented at the surface of gyri. Parts of the visual field represented within fissures are weakly recorded at the surface, at least by electrical means, and are best picked up using magnetic techniques. Experimental evidence indicates that the P100 component of the flash VEP arises from cortical activation by the retinogeniculate pathway. The arriving afferent volley causes depolarization in lamina 4c of the striate cortex (area V1).[68,184] Studies in the monkey indicate that pattern reversal stimulation activates the same cortical areas as diffuse flash stimulation but additionally activates supra- and infragranular layers of striate cortex. Other specialized visual areas are also activated, in particular, the V4 complex, which is also involved in generating later components of the flash VEP.[68] Topographic studies in adult humans suggest the pattern-onset VEP has spatially separate generator sources for its main three components, labeled CI, CII, and CIII.[98,99] The CII negativity, and probably CIII positivity, have an extrastriate origin whereas CI positivity arises from striate cortex. However, others have used dipole localization models and suggest that Cl originates in peristriate Brodmann area 18 and CII in a peripheral area adjoining.[162] In children, CI is the most prominent component and shows sensitivity to changes in contrast and luminance. CII shows sensitivity to the "contour" features of pattern (i.e., edges, corners), and inward, starting around 8 years of age and older. These maturational changes in the onset waveform can confound its application in the clinical context.

Flash VEPs

Bright-flash stimulation is used mainly when visual acuity is poor or when cooperation is limited. In patients with cataract, corneal opacity, severe retinal dystrophy, optic atrophy, or marked cortical defects, it is not possible to elicit pattern VEPs reliably. The flash VEP has a complex waveform and can show more variability across patients than pattern VEPs. This difference limits its clinical usefulness, as bright flashes must be markedly dimmed before significant changes in flash VEP are detected. This is the case also for changes in pupillary size.

Pattern Reversal VEPs

The *pattern reversal VEP (P.VEP)* is usually elicited by checks that alternate from black to white and vice versa. Some prefer to use vertical or horizontal gratings going through the same cycle. Horizontal gratings can be advantageous when nystagmus is present because stimulation is in the plane orthogonal to the eye movement. The P.VEP has a stereotype triphasic waveform, dominated by a major positive component at about 100 ms (P100), preceding (N80) and succeeding (N145) negative components.

Pattern-Onset VEPs

Pattern-onset VEPs are elicited by the brusque appearance of a pattern usually lasting between 100 and 300 ms. When onset durations are longer than about 80 to 100 ms, then VEPs both to the onset and offset are discernible; at shorter intervals, the VEPs merge and it is difficult to distinguish particular individual components. Interestingly, the waveform and response properties of the offset VEP are similar to those of the pattern reversal VEP (although component latencies are consistently about 10 ms later for offset VEPs).[188]

The pattern reversal VEP is used more widely in clinical assessment, as its waveform is maintained across the lifespan, and half-field abnormalities are more reliably detected with this stimulus mode. Pattern onset is valuable for assessing acuity in the older child, particularly if nystagmus is present. In older children, it is useful in identifying the abnormal pathway projection associated with albinism.[8] It is also more difficult to actively defocus the pattern with onset stimulation, and this stimulus mode is also valuable when assessing patients suspected of malingering or having hysterical visual loss. In their laboratory, the authors routinely perform both pattern reversal and onset/offset stimulation on patients with nystagmus and those who may be feigning visual loss, as the tests can be done rapidly, and complementary information is obtained in a recording session lasting approximately 35 to 40 min.

Color, Motion, Binocular, and Vernier VEPs

There are two main projecting systems from the retina: these parvocellular (P) and magnocellular (M) systems appear to maintain partial segregation in their projections to the many specialized cortical areas.[56] Although there is functional overlap between M and P systems, stimulus properties can be targeted so as to bias the contribution from one of these processing streams.[132,142,216] Isoluminant chromatic patterns, or high-contrast, high spatial frequency patterns, presented at low temporal rates preferentially stimulate the P system. The M system is more responsive to low-contrast, low spatial frequency stimuli presented at high temporal rates.[211] Stimuli at velocities less than 4°/s appear to preferentially elicit VEPs from cortical areas concerned with motion processing.[50,119,137,156]

The use of these specific stimuli has not yet significantly enhanced routine pediatric electrophysiological assessment.

However, experimental studies have reported interesting findings about normal visual development. Skoczenski and Norcia[195] have shown that vernier VEPs are strikingly immature, agreeing with what is found in psychophysical studies of vernier acuity. The slower normal maturation of the nasotemporal optokinetic nystagmus (OKN) (compared with temperonasal OKN) and the persistence of this asymmetry in infantile esotropia shows moderately good correlation with the degree of asymmetry in motion VEPs, eye alignment, fusion, and stereopsis.[20]

Paradoxical Lateralization of the Pattern Reversal VEP

It is well recognized that the posterior scalp distribution of the pattern reversal VEP is strongly asymmetrical if only one occipital hemisphere is activated; this occurs during half-field stimulation, or if a hemianopia is present. Half-field stimulation activates the contralateral striate visual area, represented at the occipital pole and medial surface on each side of the calcarine sulcus, near the pole (i.e., the right half-field activates the left hemisphere). The P.VEP P100 component is commonly largest over the midline and occipital scalp ipsilateral to the field (i.e., to right half-field). Stimulation P100 is largest over the right occiput, especially when moderate to large checks (>30′) are presented in a wide lateral half-field (>6° out from central fixation). Recording electrodes over the hemisphere ipsilateral to the stimulated field therefore are optimally placed to pick up the dipole-like activity generated by activation of the visual area of the contralateral hemisphere.[14] This has been called "paradoxical" lateralization, because the P.VEP P100 is mainly being recorded over the nonstimulated hemisphere.

It is very important to be aware of the changes in VEP distribution associated with hemianopia when clinically interpreting VEPs, particularly in pediatrics, when the abnormality may be unsuspected. The authors have described in several studies[97,125,166] how the detection of VEP asymmetry associated with hemianopia led to confirmation by imaging studies of unsuspected posterior cortical abnormalities in young infants. They disagree with others[37] who have asserted that VEP is not reliable in demonstrating hemianopia. When there is a P100 over one occiput and N100 over the other, the authors find that this is a strong and reliable indication of posterior hemisphere dysfunction (Fig. 1-2).[22,26–28]

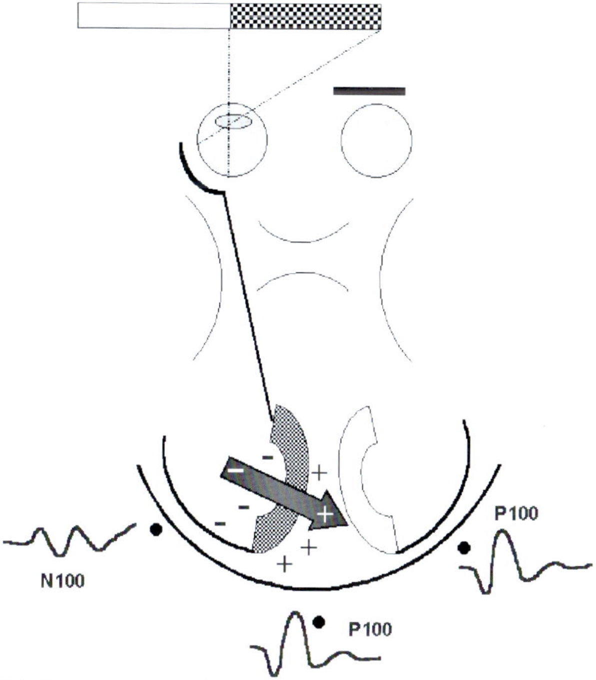

FIGURE 1-2. Diagram of paradoxical lateralization. The stimulation of the right half-field mostly activates the left hemisphere from the occipital pole along the calcarine fissure. If this hemisphere is regarded as a flat battery, the direction of the bioelectrical dipole (*arrow*) points to the opposite hemisphere. Thus, the electrode on the hemisphere ipsilateral to the field stimulated (contralateral to the activated hemisphere) is best placed to pick up the P100. This would be the occipital distribution if there were right hemisphere dysfunction and a homonymous left half-field defect. The distribution would be the same for each eye: an uncrossed asymmetry.

Macular and Paramacular P.VEP Components

As indicated previously, half-field stimulation in healthy controls and full-field stimulation in patients with hemianopia will produce asymmetrically distributed VEPs over the occiput, with the P100 component being largest on the side of the scalp ipsilateral to the stimulated or preserved half-field and an N100 component largest over the contralateral scalp. There is strong experimental and clinical evidence that activation of the macula area (up to about 6°) elicits P100 and its accompanying negative components at around 80 and 145 ms. However, activation of the paramacular areas of cortex (from about 6°–10° from central fixation) elicits a contralateral N100 (and its accompanying components, P75 and P145).[79] Patients with discrete central scotomas, such as those found with tobacco-alcohol amblyopia, will produce P.VEPs with an attenuated P100 but with relatively well-preserved N100 components best recorded over each side of the occipital midline.[78]

Recording VEPs in Children

VEPs are altered by the state of arousal and defocusing, more markedly so for P.VEPs elicited by smaller checks (<20′). Anesthesia and deeper levels of sedation can lead to all forms of VEP becoming broader, smaller, and later. However, Wright et al.[236–238] have described that P.VEPs obtained under chloral hydrate sedation can be useful in assessing interocular differences in amblyopia.

The authors much prefer to record from alert young children. Infants and toddlers sit on a parent's lap but are most likely to require encouragement to attentively fix on the stimulus target; this also helps to reduce myogenic activity associated with movement. The advice of parents is usually sought to help decide whether an older child should sit on a lap or sit independently. A large stimulus screen (about 10° to 15° out from central fixation) is important to ensure stimulation of both macular and paramacular cortical representations. It is useful to have the ability of switching from music videos or cartoons to pattern stimulation (but keeping the audio track constantly on). Toys making attention-grabbing noise and when dangled across the upper part of the stimulus field are also useful, as the cortical representation of the lower visual field is more represented mainly in occipital/parietal areas and predominantly contributes to full-field VEP recordings.

Closed-circuit television is valuable in helping to monitor fixation, and interrupted averaging, which acquires data only when fixation is adequate, greatly helps to obtain more reliable results. Repeated runs are necessary to confirm response consistency. The authors recommend using a series of different check sizes to assess consistency and subtle variations in response amplitude and latency. This methodology will also help give an indication of vision and refractive error (if P.VEPs become larger and of shorter latency when larger checks are used). Spectacles should be worn, but this is not always possible. Therefore, it is important to present an adequate range of check sizes that can withstand moderate refractive error. The authors use check sizes ranging from 400′ to 6.25′ presented in a 28° field, starting with a medium check size (50′), which is relatively robust to moderate refractive error and provides an indication of the general quality of P.VEPs likely to be recorded from that patient.[78] Marked changes in pupil size and eyelid droop will also deleteriously affect P.VEP amplitude and latency. Pattern-onset stimulation is the preferable stimulus mode when nystagmus is present or fixation is otherwise unstable. Slow stimulation rates (about 1/s), and longer acquisition times (about 500 ms) are more suitable when recording immature VEPs of infants less than about 8 weeks of age.

A transoccipital montage of at least three electrodes is essential for VEP detection of chiasmal or hemisphere anomalies. A monopolar recording derivation, in which a common reference is placed near the midfrontal location, is preferable for more optimal visualization of occipital VEP half-field asymmetries. Bipolar derivations, where separate references are placed at parietal/central location of each hemisphere (favored by some workers), can have the effect of reversing the apparent localization of the VEP.[78] Monocular stimulation should be part of the routine testing protocol, and pattern-onset stimulation used if latent nystagmus becomes evident. When cooperation is very limited, binocular and monocular ERG and VEP flash stimulation should be tried first, followed by attempts at pattern stimulation (onset and reversal). Many children are calmer by the end of this stage, and some may accept eye patching for monocular testing. If not, the session can be abandoned, having obtained useful details about retinal and postretinal function, and another appointment is given for 3 to 6 months later for another attempt at getting more detailed information using pattern stimulation.

STANDARDS AND GUIDELINES

Subcommittees of the International Society for Clinical Electrophysiology of Vision (ISCEV) have recommended standards for electroretinography, electro-oculography, and visual evoked potential recording. There are also guidelines for multifocal ERGs, and, as indicated earlier, guidelines for pediatric visual electrophysiology are in preparation. The International EEG Federation has endorsed the ISCEV standards (see also American EEG Society EP Guidelines, 1994).

ISCEV ERG Standards

These standards define a standard flash to be 1.5 to 3.0 photopic cd/m^2 intensity at the surface of the Ganzfeld stimulus bowl with a maximum duration of 5 ms. Use of a contact lens electrode with speculum is strongly advocated together with artificial pupillary dilation, a full-field Ganzfeld sphere, and at least 20 min of dark adaptation. The recording of five standard responses is recommended in the following order:

Dark-adapted responses:

1. A rod response from dark-adapted eyes, elicited after at least 20 min of dark adaptation by a dim white flash (2.5–3 log units dimmer than standard flash); the a-wave should be barely detectable and the b-wave should have a slow onset and be relatively large (200–400 μV).
2. Next, a maximal mixed rod/cone ERG recorded from a dark-adapted eye using the standard flash with well-defined a-wave, b-wave, and oscillatory potentials.
3. Finally, oscillatory potentials (OPs) are recorded to repetitive standard flashes, presented at 15-s intervals to the dark-adapted eye (the first few trials are discarded as OPs will become more conspicuous to later flashes). The slow activity of a- and b-waves is preferentially filtered (amplifier settings of 100–300 Hz), making OP high-frequency wave-lets more conspicuous. The number, size, and latency of OPs are noted.

Light-adapted responses:

1. The eye is then light adapted (rods saturate at levels above 30 cd/m^2) for at least 10 min as the patient stares into the internally illuminated Ganzfeld bowl. The cone-mediated ERG to the standard flash is then recorded.
2. Last, the cone-mediated ERG to the standard flash flickering at 30 Hz is acquired.

Recording from Young Children

ISCEV Approach

The ISCEV standards advocate that a contact lens, with lid speculum, also be used in young children. They indicate that for "unusually noncompliant" children (most often between 2 and 6 years), restraint may be necessary, or alternatively induced sedation or anesthesia (often linked with fundal examination) may be needed. It is acknowledged that heavy anesthesia can change the ERG. Light anesthesia is likely to have a small effect, compared with the variability expected in pediatric recordings. However, there is no discussion of the possibility of corneal abrasion and the rare, but potentially very serious, risk associated with general anesthesia or sedation. These issues are discussed from time to time on the ophthalmology Internet mail base (ped-ophth@ucsd.edu). The guidelines also acknowledge that the standard ISCEV protocol may need to be abbreviated and, when cooperation is poor, it may be possible to obtain only the ERG responses most pertinent to the diagnostic question (Fig. 1-3).

GOS Pediatric Protocol: Combined ERG/VEP Recording

Recording the ERG and VEP at the same session greatly enhances the diagnostic power of visual electrodiagnostic testing, particularly when assessing young children who appear to have poor vision. It is possible to rapidly and reliably gauge if the basis of the visual problem is retinal (involving predominantly cones, rods, or both), or whether it is postretina, primarily affecting the optic nerve, chiasm, or pathway beyond the chiasm (if multichannel recording and monocular stimulation are adopted). There is a degree of complementarity between the tests; thus, cone or macular abnormalities will be associated with poor VEPs also.

As mentioned previously, the authors do not routinely sedate or anesthetize young children, and still manage to achieve a low recording failure rate (about 2–3/1000 where no ERGs and VEPs could be recorded); this is accomplished by entertaining and encouraging children, and using the assistance of parents throughout the recording session. Skin ERG electrodes are positioned within 1 cm of the lower eyelid margin (this is comfortable for the child, and ERGs are relatively large). The authors

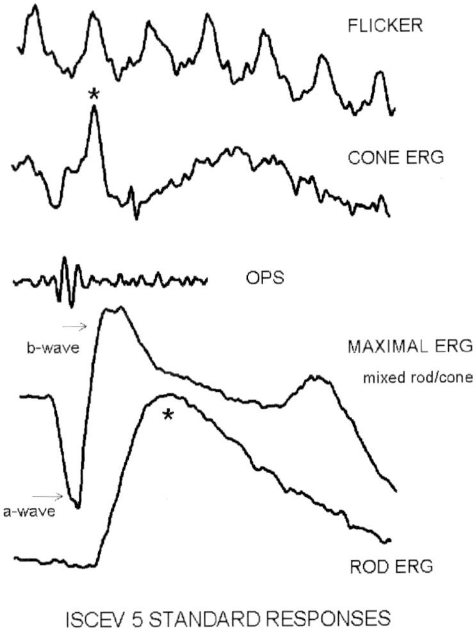

FIGURE 1-3. ISCEV responses. Diagram of the five ERGs recommended by the International Society for Clinical Electrophysiology of Vision (ISCEV), which ensure that rod and cone function are separated. The mixed rod/cone ERG shown is in response to a bright flash. As flash intensity increases in the dark-adapted eye, the a-wave grows and the b-wave becomes larger and early, until the opposite polarity responses start to interact and cancel one another. The morphology becomes more negative with a-wave = b-wave amplitude; this may occur from pale fundi, and it is always worthwhile varying flash intensity to observe the dynamic interaction of a- and b-waves. Compare also the waveform and b-wave latency change from rod ERG to cone ERG. Traces have been scaled individually for ease of illustration. *OPs*, oscillatory potentials.

use natural pupils so that cycloplegia does not affect pattern VEPs. Pupils are always inspected in case they are markedly constricted, as that will have an effect on both ERG and VEP recordings. The natural pupil mixed ERG a-b wave is, on average, 15% smaller when compared to those obtained under full dilation.[116]

A handheld Grass PS22 photic stimulator is held in front of the child's eyes at 25-cm distance. It is important to follow the head movements to ensure a degree of consistency in stimulation. Acquisition is halted if the child tightly closes their eyes or buries their head against the person who is holding them. The flash intensity 4 is normally used (3.7×10^5 cd m^2). Testing is carried out under fully darkened (scotopic) laboratory conditions. Spectrally matched stimuli are used to elicit similar amplitudes for rod- and cone-mediated ERGs using dim blue (450-nm) and red (670-nm) flashes, respectively. The flash stimuli are presented at a rate of 3/s, and 128 responses are averaged for each trial (Fig. 1-4); it takes 40 s to obtain an averaged response.

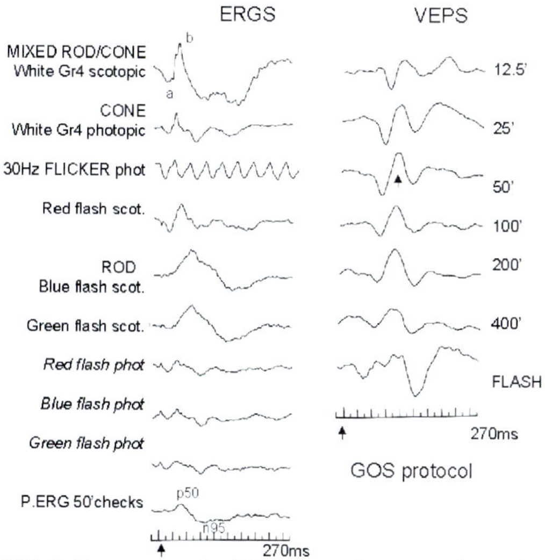

FIGURE 1-4. Responses to the (GOS) protocol. ERGs and visual evoked potentials (VEPs) are recorded in the same session. ERGs are recorded from skin electrodes placed beneath the eye to a range of flash intensities and colors. The mixed rod/cone responses show both a- and b-waves. First, record the mixed rod/cone ERG under scotopic (*scot.*) conditions and then use spectrally matched red, green, and blue flashes. Afterward, photopic (*phot*) conditions are introduced and cone-mediated ERGs are recorded. The colored filters under photopic conditions elicit poor responses, illustrating the predominant rod contribution to these stimuli and the P100 as labeled. As check size diminishes, the surrounding negative peaks, N80 and N145, become more prominent. Pattern reversal VEPs are recorded to a range of check sizes, and the midline channel is shown in this figure. The pattern electroretinogram (PERG) can be detected simultaneously and shows the p50 and n95 components. Flash VEP waveforms are more variable and complex.

RESPONSE MATURATION

Maturation of the ERG

The infant ERG is smaller and broader compared with that of the adult. By 6 months of age, the ERG is approximately within 10% of adult amplitude and latency values.[117] Maturation changes in the retina are due predominantly to changes in the structure of the rod outer segments and increased levels of rhodopsin.[62,21,158,230] The a- and b-waves precede the postnatal appearance of the first oscillatory activity, and earlier OPs emerge before later wavelets.[225]

Maturation of the VEP

Myelination progresses after birth, and this is partly reflected in the marked decrease of VEP latency during the first 6 months of life. It is advantageous to record at rates around 1/s, particularly in the first 6 to 8 weeks of life. Normally, there can be considerable interindividual variability in VEPs in the first few weeks after birth.[108] McCulloch et al.[141] have fit logistic curves to help laboratories that do not have young norms. As mentioned, the pattern-specific negativity of the CII pattern onset is poorly discerned, or even not detectable, in early childhood. The pattern-onset VEP waveform progressively becomes more complex and adult-like during later childhood (about 8–10 years of age).

Delayed Visual Maturation (DVM)

In DVM uncomplicated by other neurological or ophthalmologic disease, both the flash ERG and VEPs (to flash or pattern stimulation) are of normal size and latency, compared with age-matched controls.[123,181]

DIAGNOSTIC APPLICATIONS

The flash ERG probably plays its most vital role in conditions where ophthalmoscopy shows a normal, or questionably normal, fundus and optic disc appearance yet the child seems to have poor vision. In early childhood, this clinical picture frequently occurs in Leber's congenital amaurosis, congenital stationary night blindness (CSNB), cone monochromatism (congenital achromatopsia), progressive cone dystrophy, early stages of RP, and some toxic retinopathies.

Both Rod and Cone Function Are Markedly Abnormal

In Leber's congenital amaurosis (LCA), which accounts for at least 5% of all inherited retinal dystrophies, both rod and cone ERGs are most usually nondetectable, although occasionally they may be very severely attenuated and just barely detectable.[72] Concurrent recording of flash ERG and VEP is useful in assessing Leber's amaurosis, as the presence of flash VEP activity indicates cases who are likely to have some degree of rudimentary/navigational vision (as opposed to complete blindness). Lambert et al.[127] found attenuated, degraded flash VEPs in 19 of 43 LCA patients with vision limited to perception of light or hand movements. One patient (1/43) had P.VEPs to coarse checks (400′). If the successful gene transfer RPE65 mutation in the canine homologue holds for humans, then the demonstration of improved flash ERGs suggests that, in the future, visual electrophysiology will be useful in monitoring the functional success of young children treated by this means.[1]

Retinal Conditions in Which Rod Function Is Predominantly Abnormal

Rod dysfunction can occur in isolation as in retinitis pigmentosa (RP), or linked with a wide variety of conditions including hereditary and systemic disease, vitamin A or vitamin E deficiency, or disorders associated with high or prolonged drug therapy (e.g., chlorpromazine, thioridazine).

All these conditions, at least in the early stages of the disease process, share the picture of very attenuated, or nondetectable, mixed rod/cone and rod ERGs with partial preservation of cone ERG activity. In early RP, cone-mediated flicker ERGs can be delayed[19] and sometimes a negative ERG morphology is recorded.[41] Macular function tends to be preserved until later stages of the disease. In early and middle childhood, VEPs to flash and pattern stimulation are commonly of normal size and latency. However, as the retinal disease progresses centripetally, macular function is increasingly affected and the P.VEP is delayed and reduced in amplitude.[131] In addition, the P.ERG becomes much attenuated, or not detectable.[90]

The amplitude of the flash ERG can relate to the mutation site of the rhodopsin molecule (i.e., intradiscal, transmembrane, or cytoplasmic abnormality in dominant RP).[182] Compared with recessive and X-linked RP, autosomal dominant RP usually has a later onset and milder phenotype, and relatively mildly subnormal rod and cone ERGs are often recorded in these cases. Autosomal recessive and X-linked RP patients tend to have more deleteriously affected night vision. X-linked RP is phenotypically heterogeneous, and the two main genetic loci, RP2 and RP3, cannot be distinguished clinically.[60] RP3 is linked with mutations in the RPGR gene (retinitis pigmentosa GTPase regulator) and, on average, tends to show lower ERG amplitudes and smaller visual field areas than are seen in patients with RP2.[186] Flash ERG abnormalities in female carriers of X-linked RP appear to be correlated with the extent of fundal involvement, which manifests as the severity of tapetal sheen and peripheral pigment abnormalities increases.[74] AR RP is such a heterogeneous condition that prognosis is difficult.

The deeper understanding of the genetic basis of diseases has led to more complexity in the categorization and heterogeneity of phenotypes; this is demonstrated by the phenotypic variations associated with the ATP-binding cassette-transported gene, ABCR, ABCA4. Depending on mutation, this may present as an early macular dystrophy such as Stargardt's disease, an RP-like dystrophy, in the first decade or a cone/rod dystrophy with central chorioretinal atrophy in the second decade.[106,139,164] It is interesting that autosomal recessive RP has been mapped to the genetic interval encompassing the ABCR gene.[179]

Rod Dysfunction Associated with Systemic Disease, Syndromes, and Inborn Errors of Metabolism

Pigmentary retinopathy occurs also in association with a wide range of systemic diseases. *Gyrate atrophy* is an autosomal recessive defect of ornithine aminotransferase, causing chorioretinal disease that progressively affects rods more than cones, at least initially. The peripheral fundus has a characteristic hole-punched appearance. The mixed and rod-mediated flash ERGs are generally reduced and usually become extinguished by the second decade of life. The EOG also progressively diminishes as the disease process spreads toward the macula. The phenotype frequently occurs with reduced levels of ornithine but can also occur with normal levels.[104] A low-protein, low-arginine diet and/or supplementation with vitamin B_6 have had variable success in some patients.[18]

ABETALIPOPROTEINEMIA

In this autosomal recessive condition, the flash ERG can be of subnormal amplitude when the fundus appears normal on ophthalmoscopy. The EOG is abnormal when pigmentary retinopathy is observed. Injection or oral administration of both vitamins A and E are established treatments effectively reversing or stabilizing symptoms and exhibit abnormal flash ERG and EOG features.[54,180]

PEROXISOMAL DISEASE

Poggi-Travert et al.[168] have reviewed the clinical features distinguishing peroxisomal disease. At least 21 genetic disorders (mostly autosomal recessive) are linked with peroxisomal dysfunction. Nine of the 17 peroxisomal disorders with neurological involvement are associated with an accumulation of very long chain fatty acids. In *Zellweger's*, there is mostly severe neurological dysfunction and widespread photoreceptor and ganglion cell degeneration. The flash ERG and VEP are usually absent.[66,205] In autosomal recessive infantile Refsum's, the flash ERG is generally of subnormal size or nondetectable.[226] Berson[18] has reported that dietary restriction of phytanic acid and phytol can arrest the pigmentary retinopathy commonly observed in older children with this condition. Infantile adrenoleucodystrophy is an autosomal recessive condition in which there is marked demyelination within the brain. The flash ERGs and VEPs are usually not detectable beginning at an early age. However, in X-linked adrenoleucodystrophy, the flash ERG is normal, but VEP (to flash and pattern stimulation) is invariably delayed, probably in relation to the degree of visual pathway demyelination.[42,234]

BARDET–BIEDL SYNDROME

This heterogenous autosomal recessive condition, with at least six distinct loci and characterized by obesity, polydactyly, and renal malformations, is associated with a variable, progressive rod/cone dystrophy. Retinal pigmentary changes may not be detectable in early childhood, although some degree of night blindness may have already been noted by the parents or caregivers. Pattern VEPs tend to be smaller and later, compared with age-matched controls.[16,61,129] Recent research suggests that visual acuity is closely correlated with optic disc atrophy, and that the latter should be considered primary, rather than secondary, to retinal disease.[95]

Usher's Syndrome (US)

Usher's syndrome also has an autosomal recessive mode of transmission and is characterized by sensorineural hearing impairment associated with pigmentary retinopathy. Ten loci have been mapped so far. Clinically, three forms are recognized.[198] Type 1 Usher's syndrome is the most common and most severe. Patients present with severe to profound hearing impairment from birth, absent vestibular response, and progressive loss of night vision in the first decade. Type 1 accounts for 90% of all patients presenting with Usher's syndrome. The more common genotype is USH1B myosin VllA, which is detectable in 75% of type 1 and in 50% of all cases, taking into account all forms of Usher's syndrome. The type 2 form is clinically less severe, with relatively moderate sensorineural hearing loss (characterized by a steep sloping audiogram), normal vestibular responses, and pigmentary retinopathy. The type 3 form generally has a more variable clinical picture regarding onset of the progressive hearing loss, vestibular response abnormalities, and the degree of pigmentary retinopathy. The genetic heterogeneity of the disease obscures policy decisions regarding at what age hearing-impaired children should be screened for the progressive rod/cone dysfunction associated with Usher's.

Joubert Syndrome

Joubert et al.[102] first identified a condition in young children characterized by episodic tachypnea and apnea, oculomotor apraxia, developmental delay, ataxia, and absence of the cerebellar vermis clearly identified by imaging studies. Dekaban[46] described two siblings with the same clinical findings but indicated that retinal dystrophy was also a common feature. Visual electrophysiology studies commonly show a markedly attenuated or nondetectable mixed rod/cone ERG, but macular function is usually well preserved and reflected in normal, or near-normal, VEPs to both flash and pattern stimulation.[126] Longitudinal data that the authors have collected on six patients over an average 8-year period suggest there is some slow deterioration of pattern VEP over time.

Mucopolysaccharidosis and Neurolipidosis

In the majority of the different forms of mucopolysaccharidosis (MPS), there is infiltration at various levels of the visual pathway by one or more of the products of mucopolysaccharide such as heparan, dermatan, or keratan sulfate. Corneal deposition of heparan sulfate causes clouding in MPS I, II, and III. The authors have reviewed the mixed rod/cone ERGs and VEPs to flash and pattern stimulation in 21 patients with MPS: MPS I-H Hurler (9 patients), MPS I-HS Hurler Scheie (1 patient), MPS I-S Scheie (4 patients), II Hunters (X-linked) (3 patients), IV Morquio (2 patients), and VI Maroteaux–Lamy (2 patients). The mean age at the first recording was 6.2 years (range, 8 months to 18 years). Most of these young MPS patients had normal flash ERG and VEP results (43%); only in a minority of MPS children (10%) were there significantly attenuated mixed rod/cone flash ERGs. This finding contrasts with older cases reported in the literature, in which most of the patients in their second and third decades had subnormal or nondetectable flash ERGs. In 47% of patients, VEP degradation was present. In 28% of these patients, although flash VEPs were well preserved, pattern VEPs (especially those to small check sizes, <50′) were abnormally attenuated and degraded, suggesting that corneal clouding was significantly degrading vision. In the remaining 19% of patients, the flash ERG was normal, but VEPs to both flash and pattern stimulation were all generally markedly attenuated and degraded. This finding indicates marked postretinal involvement, most probably caused by compression of the optic nerve by infiltration of viscous mucopolysaccharide products and because of raised intracranial pressure. These findings did not correlate with specific groups. There is general agreement that pigmentary retinopathy does not occur in MPS IV and that ERG function is well preserved.

Neurolipidosis can also lead to accumulation of mucopolysaccharide products. Type IV, in particular, is linked with retinal degeneration and a generally abnormal ERG. In all forms of neurolipidosis, the VEP tends to be abnormally attenuated and degraded, especially in later stages of the disease.

Mitochondrial Disease

Different syndromes can have the same apparent genetic mutation, and different mutations can produce a similar syndrome. For example, in some forms of mitochondrial disease, the 4977-bp fragment is the "common deletion," which leads to three clinical manifestations: Pearson's syndrome, Kearne–Sayre syndrome (KSS), and chronic progressive external ophthalmoplegia (CPEO).[169] Pearson's syndrome is a potential precursor of KSS if patients survive the first year of hematological problems.[147] RPE degeneration has been associated with several of the more common mitochondrial DNA mutations. Atypical pigmentary retinopathy and subnormal ERGs have been reported in Kearne–Sayre syndrome and mitochondrial myopathy.[128,149] However, these fundal and flash ERG changes in KSS are more likely to be conspicuous in later childhood, around 8 to 12 years of age. In their clinic, the authors have observed an increased VEP latency and reduced amplitude pattern VEPs in KSS patients.

Flash ERGs are normal in Leigh's disease, but patients will manifest markedly attenuated VEPs in the first year of life when optic atrophy is also striking. Leber's hereditary optic atrophy (LHOA) has been shown to result from mutations in genes concerned with mediating oxidative phosphorylation. The clinical syndrome most frequently becomes manifest in the second decade of life. The flash ERG is generally normal, although the VEP becomes markedly attenuated and degraded.

Other conditions related to mitochondrial dysfunction include mitochondrial encephalomyopathy, lactic acidosis and stroke-like episodes (*MELAS*), myoclonic epilepsy with ragged red muscle fiber (*MERRF*), mitochondrial neurogastrointestinal encephalopathy (*MNGIE*), and the syndrome of neurogenic weakness, ataxia, and retinitis pigmentosa (*NARP*).

Retinal Conditions Predominantly Affecting Cones

Rod Monochromatism (Achromatopsia)

This rare, inherited condition is most commonly autosomally recessive. The rod-mediated ERG to dim white or blue flash is usually normal but, characteristically, the white flash cone-mediated ERG elicited under photopic conditions and those to red flash and 30/s flicker are all not detectable. The VEP is invariably significantly attenuated, degraded, and delayed. It is possible to electrophysiologically distinguish patients with X-linked blue cone monochromatism who have preservation of the normally sparse population of blue cones[55] from complete achromats (who have no functional cones of any type) by using blue flashes presented against a yellow-orange background. However, blue cone ERGs are normally very small, and contact lens ERG recording and good cooperation by patients (i.e., little or no background interference) is required to reliably discern the blue cone ERG. This condition is usually detected by psychophysical testing in older children and adults. The Berson color vision test has good specificity.[75,76] Young patients with achromatopsia usually have high-frequency nystagmus. Nystagmus undoubtedly contributes to degradation of the P.VEPs, particularly when using smaller checks (less than about 50′), depending on characteristics of the nystagmus and other factors. When nystagmus is present (be it congenital or latent), it is advantageous to use flash and pattern-onset stimulation and large checks (>100′) for pattern reversal stimulation.[124]

Alstrom's Disease

Alstrom's disease is an autosomal recessive multiple-system condition associated with a cone/rod dystrophy. In the first 6 months of life, cone function shows more severe abnormality compared with rod function.[218] By the age of 1 year, the cone ERG is not likely to be recordable. The rod-mediated ERG has a slower rate of deterioration and is commonly not recordable by 5 years of age. The earlier cone involvement helps to distinguish Alstrom's disease from other clinical conditions that also include pigmentary retinopathy, deafness, hypogonadism, obesity, chronic nephropathy syndrome, diabetes mellitus, and cardiomyopathy (i.e., Leber's amaurosis, Bardet–Biedl, Cohen's syndrome, Usher's syndrome).

Maculopathies

Best's disease is an autosomal dominant condition of unknown cause. It has a distinctive visual electrophysiological picture characterized by a normal ERG (for both photopic and scotopic activity) but a significantly reduced EOG. The Arden index is usually less than 1.5 in the early stages, when fundal abnormalities are conspicuous ("fried-egg" appearance) and acuity is reduced. In later stages, when the fundus has a "scrambled-egg" appearance, the PERG and P.VEP show mild amplitude abnormalities. Thus, the EOG is very valuable when testing for this condition. Usually, it is markedly subnormal from the onset (when ERG is wholly normal), and is valuable in identifying carriers in whom it is of subnormal size.

Stargardt's disease (STGD) is a macular dystrophy with an autosomal recessive mode of transmission. Bilateral visual loss usually occurs over a period of several months. *Fundus flavimaculatus* with macular involvement shows a more gradual visual loss in the second to third decade and maps to the same gene locus. These conditions display variable ERG abnormalities, loosely related to the severity of disease process and the fundal appearance. Some patients show additional marked involvement of cones, and others can show rod involvement.[133] In the early stages when acuity is mildly decreased, both the flash ERG and the EOG are likely to be normal. However, the PERG and P.VEP are likely to show mild abnormalities, as they more specifically test macular pathway function. Patients with retinal flecks (26/46) had a slightly greater incidence of flash ERG abnormalities, compared with patients without flecks (20/46).[206] Kretschmann et al.[110] have shown that, in Stargardt's disease, the multifocal ERG is more sensitive than the full-field flash ERG in demonstrating foveal dysfunction, at a stage before acuity or fundus signs are apparent. In advanced cases with poor acuity, the PERG is generally attenuated and P.VEP is usually attenuated and marginally delayed.[131] Mutations of the ABCR gene appear to be responsible for STGD/fundus flavimaculatus, autosomal recessive RP, and cone/rod dystrophy. Interestingly, an additional locus for Leber's amaurosis has been identified in a highly inbred family, mapping to chromosome 6, which is close to the loci for Stargardt's disease and Northern Carolina macular dystrophy.[72]

Inner Retinal Dysfunction and the "Negative" ERG

The normal bright-flash mixed rod/cone ERG has a b-wave that is 1.5- to 2-fold the size of the a-wave. When the b-wave amplitude is markedly attenuated or not detectable, the mixed ERG has a larger than average a-wave, as it is not partly reduced by the early phase of the electropositive b-wave activity. This a-wave-dominated ERG is described as a "negative" ERG and, when associated with X-L CSNB, some authors name it Schubert–Bornschein. The negative ERG morphology indicates preserved photoreceptor activity and dysfunction of the inner retina layers, usually affecting the bipolar and Müller cells (Fig. 1-5).

The negative ERG is associated with the following clinical conditions:

- X-linked CSNB[145]
- X-linked retinoschisis[25]
- Infantile and juvenile neuronal ceroid lipofuscinosis[227]
- Duchenne's muscular dystrophy[39]
- Early RP in a subset of RP patients[41]
- Bull's eye maculopathy[146]
- Cone dystrophies[105]

Negative ERGs also occur in association with birdshot retinopathy, CRVO, and melanoma-associated retinopathy (MAR IgG circulating antibodies[130]). Lachapelle et al.[121] reported a family in which 4 of 11 children had cone dystrophy and a negative photopic ERG, mainly ascribed to absence of OP4. In CSNB,

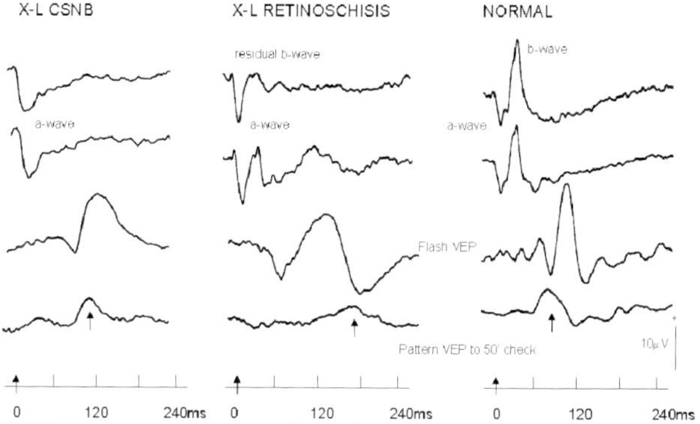

FIGURE 1-5. Negative ERGs: *first column*, from a 5-year-old patient with X-L congenital stationary night-blindness (CSNB); *second column*, from a 5-year-old with X-L retinoschisis; *third column*, normal morphology trace. It is noticeable that the CSNB patient does not appear to have any b-wave activity whereas there is some attenuated activity in the retinoschisis patient. The very poor pattern reversal VEP indicates macula pathway involvement in the patient with retinoschisis and suggests poor vision. In CSNB, the pattern reversal VEP (P.VEP) is better preserved but marginally delayed.

OP2 and OP3 are selectively abolished. Recently, Fitzgerald et al.[57] described three generations of a family all of whom had nystagmus, moderate myopia, and visual developmental delay. They all produced negative ERGs but, interestingly, compared to Duchenne's muscular dystrophy patients, there was no clinical evidence of night blindness or fundal abnormalities.

Congenital Stationary Night Blindness (CSNB)

Patients with dominant CSNB (also called Nougaret type) have near-normal cone-mediated ERGs, but rod-mediated ERGs are not usually detectable. In autosomal recessive CSNB (Riggs type) without myopia and fundus albipunctatus, both rod and cone pigment take a long time to regenerate after bleaching by light. The flash ERG and EOG attain normal amplitudes only after very long periods of dark adaptation, sometimes as long as 3h, compared with 20min for normal rod function. This feature is distinct from that encountered in autosomal recessive *Oguchi's disease*, where the rod-mediated flash ERG is of normal size and configuration for the first couple of flashes or so but then attenuates markedly. The cone ERG is normal.[143]

In X-linked CSNB, there is a functional deficiency affecting the ON-rod pathway. X-L CSNB is commonly associated with myopia greater than 4 diopters. The P.VEP tends to be of normal, or marginally increased latency; however, it is often smaller than average,[124] which may be partly due to the nystagmus that is frequently present in these patients, although subtle abnormalities affecting the cone system have also been reported for this condition.

Miyake et al.[145] have subdivided X-linked CSNB into two types: complete CSNB and incomplete CSNB. Patients with incomplete CSNB show a small positive rod ERG to dim flash, negative bright-flash mixed rod/cone ERG, delayed but intact rod-mediated oscillatory potentials (OPs), nondetectable photopic OPs, and attenuated cone and flicker ERGs. Indeed, cone function appears to be more deleteriously affected than in complete CSNB.[144,219] OPs 2 and 3 are commonly not detectable in patients with complete CSNB.[121] Complete CSNB is characterized by near-normal cone ERGs, but negative bright-flash ERGs and very attenuated negative rod ERGs have been recorded.[122]

These CSNB subtypes have a different genetic basis. Incomplete CSNB has been linked with mutations affecting specific calcium channel alpha-1 subunit (CACNA1F) in a retina.[24,151] Complete CSNB is related to mutations involving nyctalopin and is postulated to disrupt development of retinal bipolar connections.[17] Incomplete CSNB and Aland Island eye disease lie within the same gene interval, Xp11.23–p11.22, and there is a suggestion that the two conditions are allelic.[89]

X-Linked Retinoschisis

X-linked juvenile retinoschisis is a vitreoretinal disorder in which there is vitreous degeneration and a separation within the retinal nerve fiber layer. Both central and peripheral fundal areas are affected. Radial (cartwheel-like) folds consisting of perifoveal microcysts with radiate plications of overlying internal limiting membrane are commonly seen around the fovea. The cysts tend to coalesce with time, followed by pigmentation and atrophy. Mechanical separation of the inner layer affects retinal function and leads to selective attenuation of the b-wave. X-linked retinoschisis patients usually show a negative ERG to a bright flash and attenuated rod- and cone-mediated ERGs. Interocular ERG and VEP are not uncommon. P.VEPs are frequently delayed, depending on the fovea involvement. Bradshaw et al.[25] reported considerable heterogeneity of ERG response without clinical, age, or genetic correlates in 19 patients. They suggest retinal function is relatively stable throughout life, and found abnormal a-waves suggesting some receptor involvement as well. Sieving et al.[192] have cautioned that it is possible to have a normal flash ERG in the presence of known X-L juvenile retinoschisis mutation, XLRS1 Arg213Trp. They report a grandfather and grandson, each showing characteristic fundoscopic macular changes, but a negative ERG was recorded from the grandfather. The grandson produced normal ERGs. Retinoschisis with both clinical and electrophysiological features can occur in females.

Duchenne's Muscular Dystrophy

The majority (65%–100%) of patients with Duchenne's muscular dystrophy and Becker muscular dystrophy (the milder form of Duchenne's) can produce a negative ERG for bright flash stimulation delivered under scotopic condition and markedly attenuated or nondetectable rod-mediated ERGs.[39] Interestingly, there is no effect on dark adaptation, suggesting the defect relates to truncation or absence of retinal glia dystrophin affecting ERG generation but not the direct neural pathway.[100] The presence of increased macular pigmentation and normal photopic ERGs distinguished in patients with Duchenne's muscular dystrophy mutations separates them from other X-linked retinal disorders with negative-shaped ERGs (e.g., iCSNB).[58,194] The authors have not found any ERG abnormalities in patients with merosin-positive or -negative congenital muscular dystrophy.

Neuronal Ceroid Lipofuscinosis (NCL or Batten's Disease)

All four childhood-onset forms of Batten's disease are inherited by autosomal recessive transmission and are associated with retinal degeneration, severe visual failure, and nondetectable flash ERG at advanced stages. However, in early stages of both infantile and juvenile Batten's disease, patients can have negative ERGs before the ERG becomes finally extinguished.[227] In both conditions, the flash VEP is commonly not detectable. In late infantile Batten's Disease, the "flash VEP" is reported to be markedly enlarged, from 12 to 20 times larger than normal.[83] However, this response may not be true occipital VEP, as each flash elicits what appears to be "epileptic-like" activity with different morphology and distribution to a normal VEP (analogous to the very large myoclonic response following somatosensory stimulation).[116] In the early stages, the cone b-waves are severely attenuated and markedly increased in b-wave latency. The rod responses are mildly abnormal, but more preserved than in infantile NCL or juvenile NCL. In Kuf's disease, the adult form of Batten's disease, the flash ERG and VEP are normal.[227]

Vitreoretinal Disorders

X-linked retinoschisis is characteristically associated with a negative ERG and has been discussed previously.

Goldmann Favre Syndrome

This syndrome is an autosomal recessive condition that may present in the second and third decade. The flash ERGs are markedly attenuated, the EOG is subnormal, and flash VEPs are attenuated and degraded. It has been suggested that the rare "enhanced S-cone sensitivity" (ESCS) syndrome may fall within the spectrum of Goldmann Favre syndrome, as the retinal appearance is similar with yellowish retinal pigment epithelial lesions in the region of the retinal vascular arcades.[138] ESCS is characterized by night blindness and cystoid maculopathy, and both scotopic and photopic ERGs are of similar morphology characterized by a large slow response.[138] ESCS is thought to be caused by a mutation of the nuclear receptor gene NR2E3 that drives pluripotent cells into S-cones.[77]

Wagner's Vitreoretinal Degeneration and Erosive Vitreoretinopathy

These diseases are both allelic autosomal dominant conditions manifesting as atrophy of the RPE, with choroidal and lenticular changes that distinguish them from Stickler's syndrome. Patients have poor night vision and attenuated ERGs.

Stickler's Syndrome

This syndrome is a dominantly inherited disorder of collagen connective tissue causing an abnormal vitreous, myopia, variable orofacial abnormality, deafness, and arthropathy. Almost two-thirds of the families affected by Stickler's syndrome have mutations in type 2 procollagen (COL2A1).[199] COL2A1 is present in the vitreous. The flash ERG changes appear to be directly proportional to the extent of retinal detachment and myopic fundal changes.

DIAGNOSTIC APPLICATIONS OF PERG

The combination of flash ERG and P.VEP can indicate if the macular pathway is compromised. The PERG can further help to distinguish macular retinal dysfunction from postretinal macula pathway dysfunction. PERGs are most frequently used to investigate possible early maculopathies (e.g., Stargardt's). The P50 component is expected to be attenuated in these circumstances. Attenuation of the P50 component is also reported in diabetes, central serous retinopathy, and age-related maculopathy, whereas the N95 reflects more proximal retina and is abnormal in optic nerve dysfunction[51,90] (e.g., optic neuritis, optic nerve compression, and optic atrophy associated with Leber's optic neuropathy) linked with 11778 mutations and with dominant optic atrophy linked with OPA1 locus 3q abnormalities. These abnormalities can be present before clinical signs are evident.[90] Usually, the ratio N95/P50 amplitude is greater than 1.

DIAGNOSTIC APPLICATIONS OF EOG

A main indication for an EOG in young children is to investigate the possibility of Best's disease maculopathy. Here the ERG is likely to be normal, but the EOG will be conspicuously abnormal. This picture contrasts with established Stargardt's disease, RP, and myopic choroidal degeneration, in which both the EOG and ERG are abnormal. If there is severe RPE photoreceptor dysfunction, then the EOG can be too small to record eye movements. Recently, Arden and Wolf[10] have described how alcohol directly affects the RPE to elicit the same voltage changes as produced by light. In patients with RP, both light rise and alcohol rise are diminished, suggesting that secondary abnormalities of RPE function have occurred in these RP patients.

DIAGNOSTIC APPLICATIONS OF VEP

It is worth briefly stressing again that there are overwhelming advantages, particularly in pediatric practice, to record both the ERG and VEP together in diseases that affect the retina or ocular structures anterior to the retina. By these means, it is possible to gauge deleterious involvement of macular and extramacular areas and to obtain an indication of the quality of macular pathway function, including acuity levels. The pattern VEP indicates the functioning of the postretinal macula pathway and optic nerve. Thus, the presence of a pattern VEP with an attenuated ERG indicates relative preservation of the macula region.

Ocular Opacities

Bright flashes usually penetrate all but the densest ocular opacities, and flash VEPs and ERGs are particularly valuable when ocular opacities prevent adequate ophthalmoscopic visualization of the perimacular fundus.[223,228]

Corneal Opacity

Mucopolysaccharidoses and homocystinuria are associated with corneal opacification. The flash ERG can help in gauging the degree of retinal dysfunction, often before retinal pigmentary changes are apparent, and the VEP (particularly those to pattern stimulation) can provide an estimate of the degree of optic nerve dysfunction and visual acuity.

Congenital Hereditary Endothelial Dystrophy (CHED)

CHED 1 is autosomal dominant inherited, and corneal opacification tends to occur between 1 and 2 years of age. CHED 2 is more common and is an autosomal recessive condition. Corneal clouding is noted usually at birth, but progression is very slow. Treatment for both conditions is penetrating keratoplasty, which has better success rates when recipients are older. Schaumberg et al.[183] reviewed graft success and commented that it was difficult deciding when to intervene because acuity measurement in these children is difficult. In the authors' experience, pattern VEPs provide a good means of monitoring visual function (Fig. 1-6).

Lens Opacity

Flash ERGs are usually normal, even in the presence of dense cataracts that lead to rudimentary perception-of-light acuity level, provided, of course, that the retina is functionally normal. Indeed, it is possible to record larger-than-normal flash ERGs, as the cataract may increase the degree of light scattering to the very peripheral retinal areas (also called *Ganzfeld* effect).[64] However, the cataract is likely to reduce the intensity of light reaching the macular area, and the VEP, to both pattern and standard flash stimulation, will be markedly attenuated or, most probably, not recordable. Galloway[64] recommends that exceptionally bright flashes be used on these patients before commenting on macular pathway function. When lens opacities are less severe and acuity is at moderate levels, then pattern VEP is likely to be present but is reduced in amplitude and moderately increased in latency, particularly to small check stimulation.[113] When cataracts are small and of low density, using a small stimulus field and small check sizes ($<20'$) may increase the sensitivity pattern VEPs in detecting its degrading visual effects.

Vitreous Opacity

The size and latency of the flash ERG and VEP can be a useful indicator of the likely visual outcome in intraocular hemorrhage associated, for example, with advanced diabetic eye disease or a

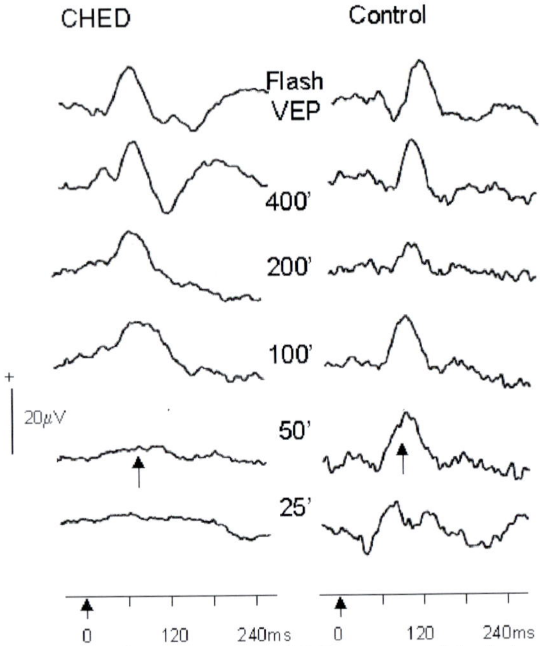

FIGURE 1-6. Midline pattern reversal VEPs to a range of check sizes presented binocularly to a 3-year-old with congenital hereditary endothelial dystrophy (CHED) compared to P.VEPs from an age-matched control, shown in the next column. As check size decreases to 100′, the P.VEP morphology becomes degraded by the corneal opacity, and the P100 is attenuated, indeed barely detectable, to checks smaller than this. This method provides an objective measure of vision that can be monitored in a child at an otherwise difficult age to obtain reliable behavioral measures. This illustration, however, is typical of the VEP acuity assessment in any condition.

traumatic ocular injury.[94] However, flash ERGs and VEPs may not be detectable in the acute stage, but can reemerge as the hemorrhage clears and allows more light to reach the retina.[45,135]

Maculopathy

Both the PERG and P.VEP reflect macular function well and, ideally, both should be recorded when a maculopathy is suspected. It is best to record the PERG with corneal noncontact lens electrodes but, if this is not practicable, then infraorbital skin electrodes may be useful. If the PERG is not detectable, then it can be inferred more confidently from the P.VEP that the dysfunction is affecting the macular pathway beyond the retina. The N105 P.VEP component has been shown to arise from stimulation of paramacular areas of the visual field (between 10° and 15° eccentricity) and becomes prominent in macula dysfunction, especially if accompanied by central scotoma at lateral occipital locations, about 5 cm from the midline.[79,114,236] In experimental studies, central scotoma shows the P.VEP P100 component to be distributed over the side of the scalp ipsilateral to the stimulus field (called paradoxical lateralization). Latency increases are usually only mild, often less than 10 ms.[114] As an example, in central serous retinopathy the P100 latency has been reported to show an average increase of 7 ms.[165] The flash VEP is less sensitive than the P.VEP in showing abnormalities related to maculopathy.

In autosomal recessive incomplete color defect (dyschromatopsia) and in some forms of X-linked dyschromatopsia, there is deficiency affecting one of the cone types only, most frequently either green or red type. The P.VEP is commonly of good size and normal latency when black and white check stimulation is used.[174] Detection of a VEP abnormality in patients with isolated red or green defects relies on using appropriate and accurately balanced isoluminant stimuli.[174,175]

Optic Nerve Disorders

It is worth stressing, again, that monocular stimulation and transoccipital multichannel VEP recording will help indicate whether a disease process is affecting the optic nerve, chiasm, or pathway beyond the chiasm. Half-field testing will improve sensitivity in detecting VEP abnormalities associated with homonymous or bitemporal defects.[26,78] However, this form of testing demands sustained fixation and is most commonly performed satisfactorily by older children (usually 6 years of age or older).

Optic Neuritis

In optic nerve demyelination related to optic neuritis and in multiple sclerosis with visual involvement, the P.VEP is almost invariably markedly delayed (of the order of 20–40 ms) when testing is done following the acute stage. Once acuity has recovered, P.VEP levels rise to moderate to good levels. The P.VEP tends to have a well-preserved waveform and is of moderate to good amplitude. During the acute stage when acuity is poor, the P.VEP is likely not to be detectable, or is very attenuated and delayed.[80]

In a follow-up study of 39 cases of childhood optic neuritis (average follow-up period, 8.8 years), it was found that only 20% had developed multiple sclerosis.[115] In another study of 20 children who had had optic neuritis, with a mean age of onset of 9.4 years, it was found that 45% had significantly delayed VEPs at follow-up and that, on average, this was 9.3 years after the onset of the attack.[81] In 64% of the eyes that showed significant delays, P.VEP latencies were increased by 15 to 35 ms, compared with 10 to 20 ms in optic nerve compression that is described next. This finding contrasts with optic neuritis in adulthood, where 90% of cases maintain significant delays in P.VEPs.[78]

Optic Nerve Hypoplasia (ONH)

Both flash and pattern VEPs are markedly attenuated, or not detectable, in cases of severe ONH. In moderate hypoplasia, the VEP (both to flash and large checks, >100′) is variably attenuated, probably related to the degree of hypoplasia,[117] and latency may be moderately increased.[7] ONH can occur in albinism and is also frequently associated with de Morsier's septooptic dysplasia, a syndrome linked with other midline brain abnormalities, particularly pituitary and hypothalamic dysfunction, and achiasmia. The flash VEP is valuable for indicating achiasmia in young children, a condition that may miss detection on routine CT or MRI scanning.[212]

Optic Nerve Compression

The P.VEP is usually degraded, attenuated, and mildly delayed (of the order of 10–20 ms) in optic atrophy caused by compressive, ischemic, or degenerative conditions. P.VEPs show a greater change compared with flash VEPs and often involve amplitude, latency, morphology, and occipital distribution.[78] The authors have monitored a rare situation where the amplitude of P.VEPs (and PERGs) progressively reduced and became nondetectable concurrent with a gaze-evoked amaurosis when the patient (who had neurofibromatosis type 2) held his eyes in leftgaze. The transient blindness was caused by a mass at the apex of the left orbit compressing the optic nerve.[196]

Infantile osteopetrosis is an autosomal recessive disease caused by inadequate bone shaping by osteoclasts, which leads to excessive deposition of bone throughout the body. Patients are of short stature and characteristically have a pronounced forehead. The visual and auditory systems are adversely affected by the narrowing of the cranial foramina.[67] The condition has a characteristic "bone-within-bone" radiologic appearance. The flash ERG has been reported to be attenuated;[93,103] however, in a series by the authors, the majority of young children (13/15 patients) had normal mixed rod/cone flash ERGs.[213] An abnormal flash ERG is likely to indicate associated neurological disease and would contraindicate a bone marrow transplant (BMT). However, it is worth noting that one of the cases had a pigmentary retinopathy and macular chorioretinal degeneration and did not show signs of central nervous system (CNS) degeneration 2 years after a BMT. The flash and P.VEP are abnormal in most cases of infantile osteopetrosis. In this same series, most patients had delayed (on average, 14 ms above laboratory norms) and attenuated flash VEPs. This finding can provide an early sign of anterior optic pathway compromise, often before detection by neuroimaging or fundoscopy.[213]

For *craniofacial dysostosis*, flash and P.VEPs can similarly provide an early indication of visual pathway dysfunction in syndromic and nonsyndromic craniosynostoses. Visual compromise is mainly ascribed to elevated intracranial pressure and physical distortion of the optic pathway. The authors have recently reviewed 130 craniofacial patients, most of whom have autosomal dominant syndromic conditions (e.g., Crouzon's, Apert's, Pffeifer's, and Saethre chotzen syndromes). These syndromes have been associated with mutations in fibroblast growth factor receptor genes.[173,232] In the authors' series, Crouzon's syndrome patients tended to have fewer ocular complications, compared with the other syndromes. Breathing difficulties, especially obstructive sleep apnea due to midfacial anomalies, may also contribute to the papilledema and optic neuropathy observed in these patients;[172] this may explain why some cases show progressive deterioration in P.VEPs despite surgery to expand the vault. The authors have also observed recovery of small check P.VEPs after surgery and found that P.VEPs are a sensitive monitor of visual function in these instances. VEP changes can be conspicuous before optic pallor is frankly present and can indicate functional changes when the appearance in chronically swollen discs is difficult to judge. Electrodiagnostic assessment has become an important part of the multidisciplinary protocol for assessing and managing such patients in the authors' hospital.

Optic nerve glioma usually leads to a broadening, attenuation, and mild delay of the P.VEP from the affected eye. The transoccipital distribution of monocular P.VEPs can indicate any chiasmal involvement, caused by either backward spread of the disease process or primary involvement of the chiasm. Groswasser et al.[73] found that the P.VEP P100 from the affected eye was, on average, delayed by about 20 ms and attenuated by 5 to 12 μV, compared with the fellow unaffected eye. P.VEPs were much more sensitive than flash VEPs in showing eye differences and transoccipital asymmetries. In 20% of patients, occipital P.VEP asymmetry was mirror imaged when comparing eyes (called crossed asymmetry) and strongly indicative of compromised optic fibers subserving the temporal visual field of each eye. Interestingly, remission can occur occasionally in this condition, and visual function can improve spontaneously. Jabbari et al.[96] stressed P.VEPs were useful in identifying patients with neurofibromatosis who also have optic nerve glioma. Primary involvement of the chiasm usually leads to marked attenuation and degradation of P.VEPs.

Hereditary Optic Atrophy and Cerebellar Ataxias

P.VEPs are commonly attenuated, degraded, and sometimes mildly delayed, in all forms of hereditary optic atrophy, although there may be differences between conditions in the tendency to which VEP components are affected.

Leber's Optic Neuropathy

In Leber's optic neuropathy, there is bilateral subacute optic neuropathy linked with mutations in the mitochondrial genome in one of three nucleotide positions: 3460, 11778, or 14484. The illness is commonly similar to that in multiple sclerosis (MS) in females with 11778 mutation. P.VEPs are invariably markedly attenuated at the initial stage when visual acuity is poor, and although there may be some visual improvement subsequently, P.VEPs remain attenuated and degraded compared with controls.[32,49,78]

Dominant Optic Atrophy

Many patients with dominant optic atrophy show "W," or bifid morphology, in both their P.VEPs and flash VEPs.[51,165] For P.VEPs, at least, this "W" waveform can be demonstrated by scotomatous changes in which the macular P100 is attenuated and there is predominance of paramacular VEP components.[79] However, other patients may have more widespread central vision involvement in which P.VEPs are generally markedly attenuated and mildly delayed (Fig. 1-7).

In some cerebellar ataxias, there may be pigmentary retinopathy, not necessarily linked with optic atrophy. In Friedreich's ataxia, mild axonal degeneration of the optic nerve

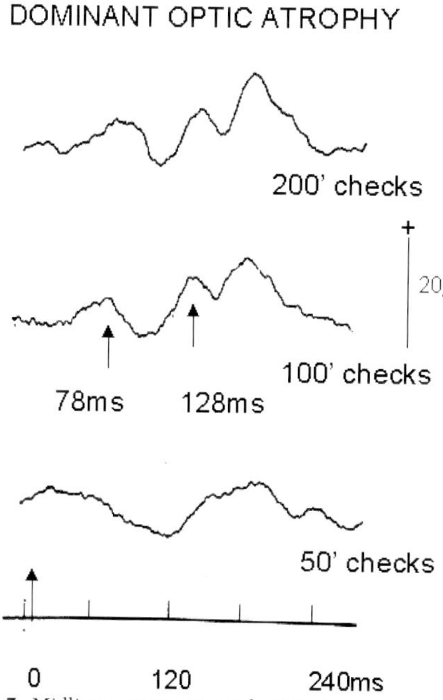

FIGURE 1-7. Midline pattern reversal VEPs to a range of check sizes elicited in a boy with dominant optic atrophy. The P100 is replaced by early and later positivities (*arrows*), most likely because of an attenuation of macula contribution. Compare these to the control subject in Figure 1-5.

occurs and P.VEPs are moderately attenuated and marginally delayed.[33] Vitamin E therapy for a Friedreich-like ataxia associated with RP has been shown to be effective in the short term.[71] Reports of P.VEPs changes in olivopontocerebellar atrophy (OPCA) are somewhat variable. Some authors describe delayed and attenuated P.VEPs in about 20% to 50% of patients;[159,204] however, others find P.VEPs to be normal.[38]

Drug Toxicity

Vigabatrin

Vigabatrin is used to control infantile spasms and appears to achieve this antiepileptic effect by inhibiting action of gamma-aminobutyric acid transaminase (GABA). However, it also produces a nonreversible loss of peripheral vision (in 1%–29% of adult patients) that is often binasal.[52,231] Visual electrophysiology results are somewhat variable. There are reports of reduced EOG and oscillatory potentials,[11,84] sometimes associated with cone system dysfunction[109] and rod dysfunction.[11] The current guidelines from the Vigabatrin Pediatric Working Party[224] advise testing the cone system, and Harding et al.,[85] endorsed by the American editorial board of *Neurology*, suggest that photopic cone-mediated flicker ERG is an effective screening protocol. Visual field testing is the most sensitive measure, but multifocal ERG and VEP testing also appear to be useful in detecting visual side effects of Vigabatrin.

Other Antiepileptic Medication

Other antiepileptic medicines have also been linked with visual field defects, including valproic acid, lamotrigine, gabapentine, diazepam, phenotoin, and carbamazepine.[207,235] Carbamazepine and phenytoin reduce b-wave amplitude and OPs.[15] Some of these drugs are often taken in combination, complicating the interpretation of studies on side effects.

Indomethacin

This medicine is used as a prophylactic to reduce the incidence of severe intraventricular hemorrhage in very low birth weight infants (less than 1500 g) and as an antipyretic in newborns and infants. Prolonged use can cause changes in scotopic a- and b-waves.[78]

Chloroquinine

The side effects of chloroquine include bull's eye maculopathy. The dysfunction is confined to the macula, and flash ERG findings are usually normal. However, P.VEPs often show abnormalities relating to the central scotoma, the macula P100 being replaced by paramacular PNP complex.[157]

Vincristine and Vinblastin

These two medicines can lead to rod and cone b-wave attenuation[177] and cause an abnormal VEP when there is optic neuropathy.

Deferoxamine

Deferoxamine can produce subtle changes in b-wave sensitivity when stimulus intensity is altered.[152] It has been suggested that it is the iron accumulation in the retina, rather than deferoxamine per se, which underlies the rod dysfunction often found in older thalassemic patients.[101]

Ethambutol

Ethambutol can induce an optic neuropathy, and the P.VEP is of reduced amplitude and mildly increased latency. However, there is often good visual and electrophysiological recovery when treatment dosage is reduced or ceased.[87,241]

Vitamin Deficiency

Vitamin B_{12} Deficiency

Vitamin B_{12} deficiency can lead to patchy demyelination of the visual pathway and spinal cord, particularly affecting the visual papillomacular bundle and the spinal posterior columns.[2] Abnormally attenuated P.VEPs are found in patients with pernicious anemia, subacute combined degeneration, and tobacco-alcohol amblyopia. In all these conditions, partial improvement of vision and P.VEPs can occur following treatment with vitamin B_{12}.[78]

Vitamin E Deficiency

Vitamin E is a fat-soluble vitamin. Deficiency is associated with spinocerebellar degeneration, neuromuscular weakness, ophthalmoplegia, and pigmentary retinopathy. In cystic fibrosis and abetalipoproteinemia, there is fat malabsorption in the gut that leads to vitamin E deficiency. Flash ERG and VEP abnormalities (attenuation and increases in latency of both flash and pattern responses) have been reported in humans.[120,180]

Chiasmal Abnormalities

Chiasmal anomalies are optimally detected by VEP studies when patterned left- and right half-field testing is carried out on each eye.[27,78] P.VEP half-field testing is difficult to perform in young children because sustained fixation is not dependable. However, it is possible to reliably detect an occipital asymmetry on monocular full-field testing that reverses in distribution when the other eye is tested. As mentioned previously, this change in occipital distribution is called *crossed asymmetry* and is an important VEP indicator of a chiasmal defect.[78] This form of VEP asymmetry is of greatest significance when there is activity of opposite polarity on either side of the occipital midline. The authors find that VEPs are particularly valuable in pediatrics when demonstrating chiasmal and posterior hemisphere abnormalities. However, these authors disagree with others who assert that P.VEPs are not useful in detecting hemisphere abnormalities.[37] Binocular VEP testing is not helpful in identifying chiasmal abnormalities, as there will be cancellation of activity recorded at lateral electrodes due to an algebraic summation (Fig. 1-8).

Crossed asymmetry anomalies can be of two opposite occipital distributions:

1. A negativity contralateral to the stimulated eye (as occurs in albinism)
2. An ipsilateral negativity (as occurs in chiasmal compression and achiasmia)

Chiasmal Glioma

As indicated previously, optic nerve glioma can spread toward the chiasm and affect visual fibers from the fellow eye. Gliomas intrinsically located within the chiasm usually have a seriously deleterious effect on the VEPs from both eyes.[73,120]

Craniopharyngioma

Craniopharyngioma commonly leads to visual pathway compression at the chiasm. The authors have reviewed 75 children

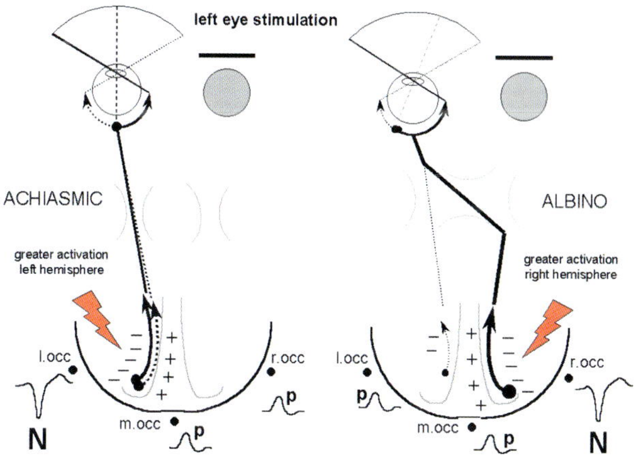

FIGURE 1-8. Schematic representation of crossed asymmetry, which characterizes chiasmal anomalies. The asymmetrical distribution over the occiput reverses if the other eye is stimulated. In achiasmia (*left*), the asymmetry is due to disproportionate activation of the ipsilateral hemisphere to the stimulated eye; in albinism (*right*), too many fibers cross at the chiasm and innervate the contralateral hemisphere.

treated for craniopharyngioma and, in 87% of the patients, there were preoperative ophthalmic signs such as optic atrophy, papilledema, or strabismus.[111] In 44% of these patients, both flash and pattern VEPs were very attenuated and degraded or not detectable at all. In 20% of patients, there was a P.VEP crossed asymmetry, with poor temporal field responses from each eye. Also, 10% had an *uncrossed asymmetry* (same occipital distribution when stimulating each eye), indicating postchiasmal compression affecting one hemisphere only. In 2%, the VEPs from one eye only were markedly degraded and attenuated, indicating optic nerve compression, and P.VEPs were within normal limits in 24%. There was good agreement between the type of field loss indicated by P.VEPs and Goldmann visual field studies, except for a small minority of patients who had peripheral field loss confined to the upper quadrants. In these patients, the P.VEPs were deemed normal. Others have similarly emphasized the value of P.VEPs in detecting and monitoring chiasmal compression caused by craniopharyngioma or pituitary tumors.[27,59,78,90]

ACHIASMIA

In achiasmia, the chiasm fails to develop normally and the majority of fibers from one eye project to the ipsilateral hemisphere. Apkarian et al.[6] and Dell'Osso[47] described two patients with isolated achiasmia who showed a crossed asymmetry for the first positive component (CI) of the pattern-onset VEP. The authors have detected chiasmic hypoplasia in more than seven young children using the flash VEP. Most had nystagmus, which was either seesaw or pendular. The achiasmal abnormality was often overlooked in MRI studies and, in most of the authors' cases, was detected only after a rereview of images following VEP reporting (Fig. 1-9).[212]

ALBINISM

The crossed asymmetry VEP distribution in albinism is opposite to that of chiasmal compression or achiasmia. In infancy,

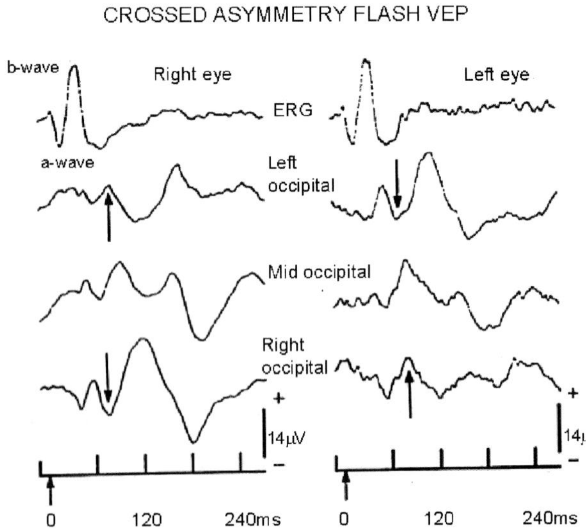

FIGURE 1-9. Achiasmia traces of crossed asymmetry from a patient with chiasmal hypoplasia show how the responses (*arrows*) invert when the eyes are compared (i.e., crossed asymmetry). The negative and positive peaks occur typically in the 70–120 ms time period after the flash stimulation.

the "albino" crossed asymmetry is best shown by using flash stimulation. In older children and adult albinos, the VEP abnormality is most conspicuous when using pattern-onset stimulation.[5,44] Almost all albinos have nystagmus and foveal hypoplasia, and it is best to use large check sizes for eliciting P.VEPs. A small minority of albinos (8%–10%) may have near-normal acuity and no nystagmus; however, they all show an albino-like crossed asymmetry for pattern-onset and pattern reversal stimulation.[118] The authors have recently used half-field stimulation to estimate the proportion of fibers crossing at the chiasm using the VEP. It was found that this proportion can vary widely between patients and does not correlate well with the presence or absence of nystagmus or vision. Soong et al.[202] compared five methods of gauging transoccipital asymmetry and commented on the interindividual variability in the methods; asymmetry was not detected by some techniques and was picked up by others. However, no patient with a confirmed molecular diagnosis of albinism gave symmetrical responses for all five paradigms. The variability, in part, can be related to optic nerve hypoplasia that can be marked in albinism. Optic nerve hypoplasia can be associated with very attenuated VEPs from which it is difficult to make judgment about distribution.

There is some debate whether iCSNB is allellic with Aland Island eye disease. Tremblay et al.[217] have described an albino-like crossed asymmetry in iCSNB, using a bipolar interhemispheric electrode montage. The albino P-gene effects can also manifest as crossed asymmetry in Prader–Willi (PWS) and Angelman's syndrome (AS).[43,214] These syndromes are associated with the loss of imprinted gene expression from chromosome 15q11–q13; a loss from the paternal chromosome gives PWS and from the maternal chromosome, AS. The OCA2 gene can be involved in the common deletion site of these syndromes, and patients manifesting albinism are thought to have a deleterious mutation on their second P-gene allele as well.

Postchiasmal Dysfunction

Generalized

In hypoxic, infective, ischemic, hydrocephalus, and most neurodegenerative conditions affecting the visual cortex, flash and P.VEPs are usually attenuated and degraded, although they tend to have normal, or near-normal, latencies. There are case reports of individuals who appear cortically blind yet have normal flash VEPs.[23,34] Other studies assessing a large number of young children with acute-onset cortical blindness report preserved F.VEPs, predicting a good recovery of vision regardless of etiology.[209] There is agreement that patients with persistent and abnormally attenuated degraded F.VEPs were likely to remain behaviorally blind.[174,176,210]

In spite of these findings, one must always be mindful of the underlying condition. For example, a patient later diagnosed as having maple syrup urine disease presented to the authors with cortical visual impairment and absent flash VEPs. She responded to treatment with oral thiamine, with vision recovering and the white matter changes resolving on MRI. These findings were mirrored by the recovery of P.VEPs.[13] Conversely, the authors have also recorded normal VEPs from an infant with apparent delayed visual maturation; however, when behavioral vision had not improved by 5 months of age, MRI studies were performed and showed lissencephaly. VEPs indicate that visual information reaches the visual cortex, but cannot yet provide information about the child's ability to integrate and interpret this visual information.

Perinatal Hypoxia

Perinatal hypoxia often causes cerebral palsy with damage to visual cortical areas.[170] The F.VEP during the acute stage can give an indication of the degree of visual function and eventual outcome.[209] In milder cases of cerebral palsy, P.VEPs are attenuated and recordable to the larger (>100′) check sizes only. The authors found that some severe cases of cerebral palsy with rudimentary vision have a flash VEP with a consistent, but unusual, morphology and distribution. There is an early pronounced positivity at 80 ms, with maximal amplitude 3 to 5 cm lateral to the midocciput. Shepherd et al.[189] have described a delayed N3 and absent positive P2 at term age as correlating with adverse outcomes in premature infants.

Hydrocephalus

A common electrodiagnostic picture associated with hydrocephalus is normal flash ERG and attenuated, degraded, and delayed flash and pattern VEPs. Often, this picture is evident before optic atrophy is seen on fundoscopy. VEP latency shows a close relationship with intracranial pressure (ICP) and parallels improvements after shunting and deterioration with shunt blockage.[3]

Neurodegenerative Conditions

In *Neuronal ceroid lipofuscinosis* (*Batten's disease*), in the late infantile form, the flash VEP is reported to be unusually large, but this appears to be an epileptic activity with a different distribution to a normal VEP.

Tay-Sachs disease (GM2 type 1) is an autosomal recessive condition with defective hexosaminidase A causing GM2 ganglioside to build up in neurous. The mixed rod/cone flash ERG is usually normal throughout the course of the disease, but the F.VEP is poorly defined during early stages and not detectable in the later stages. *Leucodystrophies* are characterized by de- or dysmyelination. In AR *metachromatic* leucodystrophy and X-linked adrenoleucodystrophy, the flash ERG is normal but the VEP findings are somewhat variable. In some patients they are normal, but in others they are poorly formed and delayed, or even absent.

Pelizaus–Merzbacher disease is X-linked and associated with poor central myelination. Patients have markedly delayed VEPs.[5,65]

Unilateral Occipital Hemisphere Dysfunction

This situation produces certain hallmark VEP features that warrant emphasizing. In young children, P.VEPs usually show a conspicuous occipital asymmetry when there is dysfunction of one hemisphere associated with hemianopia. The authors have described asymmetrical changes for both flash and P.VEP stimulation in patients with space-occupying vascular lesions and damage due to amniocentesis where clinical signs are not obvious. VEPs provided initial evidence, which subsequently led to obtaining MRI or CT studies.[97,125,166] The uncrossed VEP asymmetry does not vary and is the same for monocular or binocular stimulation. As mentioned previously, the P100 of the P.VEP and the main positivity of the flash VEP (also around 100ms) occur over the midline and over the dysfunctional hemisphere (paradoxical lateralization). A negativity with peak latency of about 100ms is usually recorded over the opposite hemisphere.

COMBINED ERG/VEP IN INFANTS WITH NYSTAGMUS

Nystagmus in infancy is likely to be a sign of poor vision resulting from retinal, optic nerve, or chiasmal abnormalities or arising from neurological disease involving the brainstem or cerebellum. The majority of patients (up to 79% in one study) with congenital nystagmus have retinal or optic nerve disease.[40,134] Nystagmus is rarely seen in postchiasmal disorders even though vision is very poor. Combined ERG/VEP recording helps greatly in establishing a diagnosis. Patients with Leber's amaurosis, achromatopsia, or X-linked CSNB will produce abnormal flash ERGs with characteristic features; whereas patients with albinism (not always easily recognized clinically), osteopetrosis, optic nerve hypoplasia, glioma, and craniopharyngioma have normal ERGs but abnormal monocular VEPs, indicating optic nerve and chiasmal postretinal visual pathway dysfunction. In infancy, all these conditions may present with a normal or near-normal fundus, and nystagmus is the only conspicuous clinical sign.[124]

If both flash ERGs and VEPs are normal, then the nystagmus is likely to be idiopathic or associated with brainstem or cerebellar disease. Eye movement studies are useful in characterizing the nystagmus waveform and, combined with electrophysiological recording, can help in deciding which cases require neuroimaging.[88]

THE VEP IN ACUITY TESTING AND AMBLYOPIA

Objective estimates of visual acuity can be inferred by noting the smallest pattern size to consistently elicit a P.VEP when refractive error is corrected (it is important to test after correction of any refractive errors).[137,140] This method is particularly useful in preverbal children or older children with expressive or motor communication difficulties. Pattern-reversal, pattern onset VEPs, and flashed patterns have all been used to give a quantitative assessment of vision.[7,48,137,140,160,161,200]

Amblyopia

Behavioral measures of detection, resolution, and recognition acuity measure different abilities. A strabismic amblyope may give a higher resolution acuity than recognition acuity secondary to spatial distortion. VEP acuity is also a different measure, and it would be unrealistic to expect a direct relationship between objective and behavioral acuity measures. Nevertheless, P.VEP findings do provide a good benchmark and are especially useful in highlighting interocular differences associated with amblyopia. In particular, these findings include clinically unrecognized indications of iatrogenic effects of patching on the unaffected eye. The authors have noted irreversible and significant VEP amplitude loss in the fellow (patched) eye of a 3-month-old patient with unilateral congenital cataract (followed up until 7 years of age).[113] Conversely, patching 50% of waking hours was stopped in a 3-month-old with a lid hemangioma because the P.VEP from the fellow eye showed degradation and attenuation. The P.VEP amplitude and definition showed clear improvement in a recording done 3 months later.

Unilateral congenital cataracts are a particular challenge for amblyopia occlusive therapy. Although the lensectomized eye shows significant improvements in acuity, overall, the authors find that the fellow (patched) eye shows smaller transient P.VEPs and reduced LogMAR acuity compared with untreated unilateral cataract patients and healthy controls.[215]

Transient P.VEP amplitudes demonstrate an inverted "U-shaped" spatial tuning curve. The peak of the tuning curve is broadly associated with the size of the stimulus field that, for clinical work, is greater than 10°. For these field sizes, patterns with element sizes of 10° to 20° arc give the largest P.VEPs from 5 to 6 years onward.[229] In amblyopia, the P.VEP is slightly increased in latency and relatively attenuated as check size diminishes, losing the inverted U-shaped tuning curve. If the amblyopia is very profound, such that large checks and flash VEPs are affected, it is not possible to distinguish amblyopia from other causes of postretinal dysfunction.

Wright et al. have reported on the use of chloral hydrate sedation for obtaining pattern visual evoked potential in children with amblyopia. Eye-to-eye comparison of P1 amplitudes provided an indication of the presence of amblyopia and gross quantification of the amblyopia. Chloral hydrate P.VEPs can be used in infants whose diagnosis of amblyopia is equivocal, and appropriate management is dependent on knowledge of visual function. Decisions regarding surgery for partial cataracts and corneal opacities that split the visual axis may be aided by information obtained by the chloral hydrate pattern visual evoked potential.[236–238]

Amblyopia affects the broad spectrum of visual subsystems that constitute vision, including contrast and color, motion, and vernier discriminations. P.VEP studies show that the pursuit of high-contrast acuity does not ensure optimum performance at lower contrasts. Rather than relying on just one measure to monitor amblyopia therapy (e.g., high-contrast recognition acuity), it is likely that a battery of specific stimuli may provide an enhanced profile of amblyopia against which the results of occlusion can be better monitored.

Sweep VEPs

P.VEP amplitudes tend to fall off linearly with spatial frequency near the limit of acuity.[30,31] The extrapolation of the high spatial frequency limb of the spatial tuning function to zero amplitude (or the noise level) produces an intercept that correlates with subjective visual resolution; this has been the basis of the sweep VEP techniques. Transient pattern VEP recording can take 20 to 40 s to obtain an average for one spatial frequency. When the stimulation rate is speeded up, steady-state VEPs are recorded. Sweep techniques can progressively and rapidly test (usually in 8–16 s) a range of spatial frequencies (checks or gratings) to determine a VEP threshold.[174,220] Each spatial frequency is presented for a discrete interval (usually for 5–10 s), and the change in pattern size can be continuous or sampled.[185] It is found that the "optimal" temporal frequency giving the largest VEPs increases with maturation;[148] it is around 8 reversals/s in adults and about 4 reversal/s in young infants less than 3 months of age. There is some degree of intersubject and age-related variability in the spatial tuning function of the sweep VEP. It may monotonically decrease with increasing spatial frequency or may have two or three maximal peaks. A double peak is not uncommon in older infants and adults.[208,221] Pattern onset/offset stimulation gives larger amplitude responses than P.VEPs to equivalent pattern sizes and also has a simpler tuning function. However, the phase change with spatial frequency (which is a useful indicator of signal reliability with pattern reversal stimulation) is not present for onset/offset stimulation. VEP contrast sensitivity threshold to a reversing sinusoidal grating over a range of spatial frequencies can also give an acuity estimate.[4,153,203] There is good correlation between subjective perceptual judgments and P.VEP amplitude estimates of contrast threshold (Fig. 1-10).[4,30]

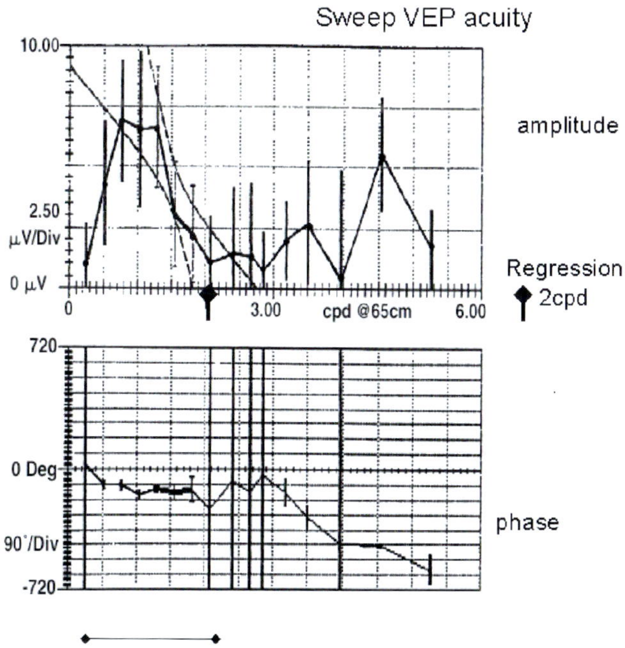

FIGURE 1-10. Example of a monocular sweep acuity VEP from a 3-month-old baby. A range of rapidly reversing, 16/s sine wave gratings steadily decreased in size every second. Amplitude is plotted versus spatial frequency, and regression analysis estimates the intersection or acuity threshold. Confidence limits on the regression are shown by the *curved lines*. The area of quiet phase highlighted distinguishes the response from background noise. *cpd*, cycles per degree.

VEP Acuity Development

Transient P.VEP estimates of acuity indicate that adult levels are reached between 6 to 10 months.[48,137,200] Sweep VEP estimates indicate acuities of about 4.5 cycles per degree (cpd; a cycle is made up of one black and one white bar) in the first month of life, increasing to the adult level of 20 cpd by 8 months of age.[4,154,155] During the first year of life, sweep VEP acuity is higher and has a slower developmental course compared with transient VEPs. Sweep VEP estimates exceed behavioral forced-choice preferential looking (FCPL) acuity in the first year of life, but they become similar after this.[4,82,201,215]

The differences between electrophysiological and behavioral acuity assessments may be accounted for by stimulus differences (i.e., central field for VEPs versus smaller peripheral field for FCPL) or by static stimulus versus changing stimulus involving motion for pattern reversal VEPs. There is good agreement between interocular acuity estimates between the two methods. Children with good optotype acuity tend to have higher sweep acuity at lower temporal frequency, and those with poor optotype acuity tend to have better sweep acuity at higher temporal rates.[69] This difference reflects the contrast sensitivity function: lower spatial frequencies are more visible when they move whereas high spatial frequencies are best seen when static or slow moving.

Hysterical (or Functional) Visual Loss

Hysterical visual loss is associated with normal flash and pattern VEP findings. It is particularly important to carefully monitor fixation performance (e.g., with closed-circuit TV) and also not to use too small a check size ($<15'$), because voluntary changes in accommodation by patients may lead to apparently significant VEP changes affecting both amplitude and latency. Larger check sizes are more resistant to such maneuvers by patients.[78]

Suppression and the Pattern Visual Evoked Potential

Visual potential can be useful in investigating the mechanisms of suppression associated with amblyopia and strabismus.[239,240] Central suppression associated with monofixation syndrome and anisometropic amblyopia has been shown to reduce and, essentially, extinguish the P1 of the P.VEP. These results imply that suppression inhibits neuronal activity at the level of the visual cortex.[239] P.VEP evidence of suppression has also been identified in childhood-onset strabismus with suppression and adults with acquired strabismus where diplopia was ignored. Wright et al. demonstrated that patients with childhood-onset and adult-onset "ignored" diplopia similarly showed essentially no response when the nonpreferred eye was stimulated during binocular viewing. The study suggests that adults with acquired strabismus who ignore the diplopic image actually have suppression of cortical visual activity.[240]

FUTURE OF VISUAL ELECTROPHYSIOLOGY

Objective measures of function are invaluable to pediatric examination. Visual electrophysiology is objective and will be used in the future for assessing the success of retinal gene therapies and visual pathway rescue. Improvements in pediatric visual electrophysiology practice will lie with techniques that minimize patient contact; for example, using smart electrodes and amplifiers that require no skin preparation for good signal-to-noise ratios. Eventually, there may be remote detection of bioelectric activity. Visual stimulation will be developed to mimic normal visual space, yet allow the systematic manipulation of individual visual parameters and independent stimulation of each eye. The functional significance and specificity of treatment will be enhanced with topographic montages that directly and immediately relate to an individual's brain image or retinal image. Finally, the integration of these data with measures of higher cortical function will become a very active area of study. It will help to understand how our ability to interpret the processed afferent visual information is assembled.

References

1. Acland G, Aguirre G, Ray J, et al. Gene therapy restores vision in a canine model of childhood blindness. Nat Genet 2001;28(1):92–95.
2. Agamanolis D, Chester E, Victor M, et al. Neuropathology of experimental vitamin B_{12} deficiency in monkeys. Neurology 1976;26: 905–914.
3. Alani S. Pattern-reversal visual evoked potentials in patients with hydrocephalus. J Neurosurg 1985;62(2):234–237.
4. Allen D, Tyler C, Norcia A. Development of grating acuity and contrast sensitivity in the central and peripheral visual field of the human infant. Vision Res 1996;36(13):1945–1953.
5. Apkarian P. Electrodiagnosis in paediatric ophthalmogenetics. Int J Psychophysiol 1994;16(2–3):229–243.
6. Apkarian P, Bour L, Bart P. A unique achiasmatic anomaly detected in non-albinos with misrouted retinal fugal projections. Eur J Neurosci 1994;6:501–507.
7. Apkarian P, Spekreijse H. The use of the electroretinogram and visual evoked potentials in ophthalmogenetics. In: Desmedt JE (ed) Visual evoked potentials. Amsterdam: Elsevier, 1990:169–223.

8. Apkarian P, Reits D, Spekreijse H. Component specificity in albino VEP asymmetry: maturation of the visual pathway anomaly. Exp Brain Res 1984;53:285–294.
9. Arden G, Kelsey J. Changes produced by light in the standing potential of the human eye. J Physiol 1962;61:189–204.
10. Arden G, Wolf J, Singbarti F, et al. Effect of alcohol and light on the retinal pigment epithelium of normal subjects and patients with retinal dystrophies. Br J Ophthalmol 2000;84(8):881–883.
11. Arndt C, Derambure P, Defoort-Dhellemmes S, et al. Outer retinal dysfunction in patients treated with vigabatrin. Neurology 1999; 52(6):1201–1205.
12. Bach M, Hyalina M, Holder G, et al. Standard for pattern electroretinography. Doc Ophthalmol 2000;101:11–18.
13. Backhouse O, Leitch R, Thompson D, et al. A case of reversible blindness in maple syrup urine disease [letter]. Br J Ophthalmol 1999;83(2):250–251.
14. Barrett G, Blumhardt L, Halliday A, et al. A paradox in the lateralization of the visual evoked response. Nature (Lond) 1976;261: 253–255.
15. Bayer A, Zrenner E, Ried S, et al. Effect of anticonvulsant drugs on retinal function. Pyschophysical and electrophysiological findings in patients with epilepsy. Investig Ophthalmol Vis Sci 1990;31:427.
16. Beales P, Elcioglu N, Woolf A, et al. New criteria for improved diagnosis of Bardet-Biedl syndrome: results of a population survey. J Med Genet 1999;36(6):437–446.
17. Bech-Hansen NT, Naylor M, Maybaum T, et al. Mutations in NYX, encoding the leucine-rich proteoglycan nyctalopin, cause X-linked complete congenital stationary night blindness. Nat Genet 2000; 26(3):319–323.
18. Berson E. Nutrition and retinal generations. Int Ophthalmol Clin 2000;40(4):93–111.
19. Berson E. Electrical phenomena in the retina. In: Hart WH (ed) Adler's physiology of the eye: clinical application. St. Louis: Mosby Yearbook, 1992:641–707.
20. Birch E, Fawcett S, Stager D. Co-development of VEP motion response and binocular vision in normal infants and infantile esotropes. Investig Ophthalmol Vis Sci 2000;41:1719–1723.
21. Birch E, Birch D, Uauy R. Retinal and cortical function of very low birthweight infants at 36 and 57 weeks post conception. Clin Vis Res 1990;5:363–373.
22. Blumhardt L, Barratt G, Kriss A, et al. The pattern-evoked potential in lesions of the posterior visual pathways. Ann NY Acad Sci 1982;388:264–289.
23. Bodis-Wollner I. Recovery from cerebral blindness: evoked potential and psychophysical measurements. Electroencephalogr Clin Neurophysiol 1977;42(2):178–184.
24. Boycott K, Maybaum T, Naylor M, et al. A summary of 20 CACNA1F mutations identified in 36 families with incomplete

X-linked congenital stationary night blindness, and characterization of splice variants. Hum Genet 2001;108(2):91–97.

25. Bradshaw K, George N, Moore A, et al. Mutations of the XLRS1 gene causing abnormalities of photoreceptor as well as inner retinal responses of the ERG. Doc Ophthalmol 1999;98:153–173.
26. Brecelj J, Stirn-Kranjc B, Skrbec M. Visual electrophysiology in children with tumors affecting the visual pathways. Doc Ophthalmol 2000;101:125–154.
27. Brecelj J. Electrodiagnosis of chiasmal compressive lesions. Int J Psychophysiol 1994;16:263–272.
28. Breton M, Schueller A, Lamb T, et al. Analysis of ERG a-wave amplification and kinetics in terms of the G-protein cascade of phototransduction. Investig Ophthalmol Vis Sci 1994;35(1):295–309.
29. Breton M, Quinn G, Schueller A. Development of electroretinogram and rod phototransduction response in human infants. Investig Ophthalmol Vis Sci 1995;36(8):1588–1602.
30. Campbell F, Gubisch R. Optical quality of the human eye. J Physiol 1966;186(3):558–578.
31. Campbell F, Maffei L. Electrophysiological evidence for the existence of orientation and size detectors in the human visual system. J Physiol 1970;207(3):635–652.
32. Carroll W, Mastaglia F. Leber's optic neuropathy: a clinical and visual evoked potential study of affected and asymptomatic members of a six-generation family. Brain 1979;1102:559–580.
33. Carroll W, Kriss A, Baraitser M, et al. The incidence and nature of visual pathway involvement in Friedreich's ataxia: a clinical and visual evoked potential study of 22 patients. Brain 1980;103: 413–434.
34. Celesia G, Archer C, Kurroiwa Y, et al. Visual function of the extrageniculate-calcarine system in man. Arch Neurol 1980;37:704–706.
35. Celesia G, Brigell M. Recommended standards for pattern electroretinograms and visual evoked potentials. The International Federation of Clinical Neurophysiology. Electroencephalogr Clin Neurophysiol Suppl 1999;52:53–67.
36. Celesia G, Brigell M, Peachey N. Recommended standards for electroretinograms. The International Federation of Clinical Neurophysiology. Electroencephalogr Clin Neurophysiol Suppl 1999;52: 45–52.
37. Celesia G, Meredith J, Pluff K. Perimetry, visual evoked potentials spectrum in homonymous hemianopsia. Electroencephalogr Clin Neurophysiol 1983;56:16–30.
38. Chokroverty S, Duvoisin R, Sachdeo R, et al. Neurophysiologic study of olivopontocerebellar atrophy with or without glutamate dehydrogenase deficiency. Neurology 1985;35:652–659.
39. Cibis G, Fitzgerald K, Harris D, et al. The effects of dystrophin gene mutations on the ERG in mice and humans. Investig Ophthalmol Vis Sci 1993;34(13):3646–3652.

40. Cibis G, Fitzgerald K. Abnormal electroretinogram associated with developmental brain anomalies. Trans Am Ophthalmol Soc 1995;93: 147–158; discussion 158–161.
41. Cicedyian A, Jacobsen S. Negative electroretinograms in retinitis pigmentosa. Investiag Ophthalmol Vis Sci 1993;34:3253–3263.
42. Cohen S, Brown F, Martyn L, et al. Ocular histopathologic and biochemical studies of the cerebrohepatorenal syndrome (Zellweger's syndrome) and its relationship to neonatal adrenoleucodystrophy. Am J Ophthalmol 1983;96:488–501.
43. Creel D, Bendel C, Wiesner G, et al. Abnormalities of the central visual pathways in Prader-Willi syndrome associated with hypopigmentation. N Engl J Med 1986;314(25):1606–1609.
44. Creel D, Spekreijse H, Reits D. Evoked potentials in albinos: efficacy of pattern stimulation in detecting misrouted optic fibres. Electroencephalogr Clin Neurophysiol 1981;52:595–603.
45. Crews S, Thompson C, Harding G. The ERG and VEP in patients with severe eye injury. Doc Ophthalmol 1978;15:203–209.
46. Dekaban A. Hereditary syndrome of congenital blindness (Leber), polycystic kidneys and maldevelopment of the brain. Am J Ophthalmol 1969;689:1029–1036.
47. Dell'Osso L. Seesaw nystagmus in dogs and humans: an international, across discipline, serendipitous collaboration. Neurology 1996;47:1372–1374.
48. De Vries Khoe L, Spekreijse H. Maturation of luminance and pattern EPs in man. Doc Ophthalmol 1982;31:461–475.
49. Dorfman L, Nikoskelianen E, Rosenthal A, et al. Visual evoked potentials in Leber's optic neuropathy. Ann Neurol 1977;1:565–568.
50. Drasdo N, Edwards L, Thompson D. Models of the visual cortex based on visual evoked potentials. In: Gulyas B, Ottoson D, Roland P (eds) Functional organization of the human visual cortex. Wenner Gren international series, vol 61. Oxford: Pergamon Press, 1993: 255–270.
51. Drasdo N, Thompson D, Arden G. A comparison of pattern ERG amplitudes and nuclear layer thickness in different zones of the retina. Clin Vis Sci 1990;5:415–420.
52. Eke T, Talbot J, Lawden M. Severe persistent visual field constriction associated with vigabatrin [see comments]. Br Med J 1997; 314(7075):180–181.
53. Esakowitz L, Kriss A, Shawkat F. A comparison of flash electroretinograms recorded from Burian Allen, JET, C-Glide, gold foil, DTL, and skin electrodes. Eye 1993;7:169–171.
54. Fagan E, Taylor M. Longitudinal multimodal evoked potential studies in abetalipoproteinaemia. Can J Neurol Sci 1987;14:617–621.
55. Farley M, Heckenlively J. Blue cone monochromatism. In: Heckenlively J, Arden G (eds) Principles and practice of clinical electrophysiology of vision. St. Loius: Mosby, 1991:753–755.
56. Fellman D, Van Essen D. Distributed hierarchical processing in the primate visual cortex. Cereb Cortex 1991;1:1–47.

57. Fitzgerald K, Hashimoto T, Hug T, et al. Autosomal dominant inheritance of a negative electroretinogram in three generations. Am J Ophthalmol 2001;131(4):495–502.
58. Fitzgerald K, Cibis G, Giambrone S, et al. Retinal signal transmission in Duchenne muscular dystrophy: evidence for dysfunction in the photoreceptor depolarising bipolar cell pathway. J Clin Investig 1994;93:2425–2430.
59. Flanagan J, Harding G. Multichannel visual evoked potentials in early compressive lesions of the optic chiasm. Doc Ophthalmol 1987;69:271–282.
60. Flaxel C, Jay M, Thiselton D, et al. Difference between RP2 and RP3 phenotypes in X linked retinitis pigmentosa. Br J Ophthalmol 1999;83(10):1144–1148.
61. Fulton A, Hansen R, Glynn R. Natural course of visual functions in the Bardet-Biedl syndrome. Arch Ophthalmol 1993;111(11):1500–1506.
62. Fulton A, Hansen R. Electroretinography: application to clinical studies of infants. J Pediatr Ophthalmol Strabismus 1985;22(6): 251–255.
63. Fulton A, Hartmann E, Hansen R. Electrophysiological testing techniques for children. Doc Ophthalmol 1989;71:341–354.
64. Galloway N. Electrophysiological testing of eyes with opaque media. Eye 1988;2:615–624.
65. Garbern J, Cambi F, Shy M, et al. The molecular pathogenesis of Pelizaeus-Merzbacher disease. Arch Neurol 1999;56(10):1210–1214.
66. Garner A, Fielder A, Primavesi R, et al. Tapetoretinal degeneration in the cerebro-hepato-renal (Zellweger) syndrome. Br J Ophthalmol 1982;66:422–431.
67. Gerritsen E, Vossen J, van Loo, et al. Autosomal recessive osteopetrosis: variability of findings at diagnosis and during the natural course. Pediatrics 1994;93:247–253.
68. Givre S, Schroeder C, Arezzo J. Contribution of extra striate area V4 to the surface recorded flash VEP in the awake macaque. Vision Res 1994;34:415–428.
69. Gottlob I, Fendick M, Guo S, et al. Visual acuity measurements by swept spatial frequency visual-evoked-cortical potentials (VECPs): clinical application in children with various visual disorders. J Pediatr Ophthalmol Strabismus 1990;27(1):40–47.
70. Granit R. Sensory mechanisms of the retina. London: Oxford University Press, 1947.
71. Grant C, Berson E. Treatable forms of retinitis pigmentosa associated with systemic neurological disorders. Int Ophthalmol Clin 2001;41(1):103–110.
72. Grieshaber M, Boltshauser E, Niemeyer G. Leber's congenital amaurosis. Clinical heterogeneity and electroretinography in 27 patients. In: Hollyfield X, et al. (eds) Retinal degenerative diseases and experimental therapy. New York: Kluwer, 1999:95–104.

73. Groswasser Z, Kriss A, Halliday AM, et al. Pattern and flash evoked potentials in the assessment and management of optic nerve gliomas. J Neurol Neurosurg Psychiatry 1985;48:1125–1134.
74. Grover S, Fishman G, Anderson R, et al. A longitudinal study of visual function in carriers of X-linked recessive retinitis pigmentosa. Ophthalmology 2000;107(2):386–396.
75. Haegerstrom-Portnoy G, Schneck M, Verdon W, et al. Clinical vision characteristics of the congenital achromatopsias. II. Color vision. Optom Vis Sci 1996;73(7):457–465.
76. Haegerstrom-Portnoy G, Schneck M, Verdon W, et al. Clinical vision characteristics of the congenital achromatopsias. I. Visual acuity, refractive error, and binocular status. Optom Vis Sci 1996;73(7):446–456.
77. Haider N, Jacobsen S, Cideciyan A, et al. Mutation of a nuclear receptor gene, NR2E3, causes enhanced cone syndrome, a disorder of retinal cell fate. Nat Genet 2000;24:127–131.
78. Halliday A. Evoked potentials in clinical testing, 2nd edn. Edinburgh: Churchill Livingstone, 1993.
79. Halliday A, Barrett G, Blumhardt L, et al. The macular and paramacular components of the pattern evoked response. In: Lehmann D, Calloway E (eds) Human evoked potentials: applications and problems. New York: Plenum Press, 1979:135–151.
80. Halliday A, McDonald W, Mushin J. Delayed pattern evoked responses in optic neuritis in relation to visual acuity. Trans Ophthalmol Soc UK 1973;93:315–324.
81. Halliday A, Kriss A, Cuendent F, et al. Childhood optic neuritis: a study of flash and pattern evoked potentials. In: Gallai V (ed) Maturation of the CNS and evoked potentials. Amsterdam: Elsevier, 1986:41–50.
82. Hamer R, Norcia A, Tyler C, et al. The development of monocular and binocular VEP acuity. Vision Res 1989;29(4):397–408.
83. Harden A, Pampiglione G. Neurophysiological studies (EEG/ERG/VEP/SEP) in 88 children with so-called neuronal ceroid lipofuscinosis. In: Armstrong D, Koppang N, Rider JA (eds) Ceroid lipofuscinosis (Batten's disease). Amsterdam: Elsevier, 1982:61–70.
84. Harding G, Wild J, Robertson K, et al. Separating the retinal electrophysiologic effects of vigabatrin: treatment versus field loss [see comments]. Neurology 2000;55(3):347–352.
85. Harding G, Wild J, Robertson K, et al. Electro-oculography, electroretinography, visual evoked potentials, and multifocal electroretinography in patients with vigabatrin-attributed visual field constriction. Epilepsia 2000;41(11):1420–1431.
86. Harding G, Crews S. The VER in hereditary optic atrophy of the dominant type. In: Mauguiere F, Courjon F (eds) The clinical applications of evoked potentials in neurology. New York: Raven Press, 1982:21–30.
87. Harding G, Williams D, Innes J. The visual evoked potentials and psychophysics during ethambutol therapy. In: Nodar RH, Barber

C (eds) Evoked potentials, vol II. Boston: Butterworth, 1984:339–344.

88. Harris C. Nystagmus and eye movement disorders. In: Taylor D (ed) Pediatric ophthalmology. Oxford: Blackwell, 1997:869–896.
89. Hawksworth N, Headland S, Good P, et al. Aland Island eye disease: clinical and electrophysiological studies of a Welsh family. Br J Ophthalmol 1995;79(5):424–430.
90. Holder G. Pattern electroretinography (PERG) and an integrated approach to visual pathway diagnosis. In: Fishman GA, Birch D, Holder GE, Brigell M (eds) Electrophysiological testing in disorders of retinal optic nerve, and visual pathway. 2001.
91. Hood D, Birch D. Abnormalities of the retinal cone system in retinitis pigmentosa. Vision Res 1996;36(11):1699–1709.
92. Hood D, Birch D. Assessing abnormal rod photoreceptor activity with the a-wave of the electroretinogram: applications and methods. Doc Ophthalmol 1996–97;92(4):253–267.
93. Hoyt C, Billson F. Visual loss in osteopetrosis. Am J Dis Child 1979;133:955–958.
94. Hutton W, Fuller D. Factors influencing final visual results in severely injured eyes. Am J Ophthalmol 1984;97:715–722.
95. Iannoccone A, De-Propris G, Roncati S, et al. The ocular phenotype of the Bardet-Biedl syndrome. Comparison to non-syndromic retinitis pigmentosa. Ophthalmic Genet 1997;18:13–26.
96. Jabbari B, Maitland C, Morris L, et al. The value of visual evoked potential as a screening test in neurofibromatosis. Arch Neurol 1985;42:1072–1074.
97. Jacobs M, Shawkat F, Harris C, et al. Eye movement and electrophysiological findings in an infant with hemispheric pathology. Dev Med Child Neurol 1993;35(5):431–435.
98. Jeffreys D, Axford J. Source localisations of pattern-specific components of human visual evoked potentials I. Component of striate cortical origin. Exp Brain Res 1972;6:1–21.
99. Jeffreys D, Axford J. Source localisations of pattern-specific components of human visual evoked potentials. II. Component of extrastriate cortical origin. Exp Brain Res 1972;6:22–40.
100. Jensen H, Warburg M, Sjo O, et al. Duchenne muscular dystrophy: negative electroretinograms and normal dark adaptation. Reappraisal of assignment of X-linked incomplete congenital stationary night blindness. J Med Genet 1995;32(5):348–351.
101. Jiang C, Hansen R, Gee B, et al. Rod and rod mediated function in patients with beta-thalassemia major. Doc Ophthamol 1998–99;96(4):333–345.
102. Joubert M, Eisenring J, Robb J, et al. Familial agenesis of the cerebellar vermis: a syndrome of episodic hyperapnea, abnormal eye movements, ataxia, and retardation. 1969 [classical article]. J Child Neurol 1999;14(9):554–564.
103. Keith C. Retinal atrophy in osteopetrosis. Arch Ophthalmol 1968;79:234–241.

104. Kellner U, Weleber R, Kennaway N, et al. Gyrate atrophy-like phenotype with normal plasma ornithine. Retina 1997;17(5):403–413.
105. Kellner U, Foerster M. Cone dystrophies with negative photopic electroretinogram. Br J Ophthalmol 1993;77(7):404–409.
106. Klevering B, van-Driel M, van de Pol D, et al. Phenotypic variations in a family with retinal dystrophy as result of different mutations in the ABCR gene. Br J Ophthalmol 1999;83(8):914–918.
107. Kondo M, Sieving P. Primate photopic sine-wave flicker ERG: vector modeling and component origins using glutamate analogs. Investig Ophthalmol Vis Sci 2001;42(1):305–312.
108. Kraemer M, Abrahamsson M, Sjostrum A. The neonatal development of the light flash visual evoked potential. Doc Ophthalmol 1999;99:21–39.
109. Krauss G, Johnson M, Miller N. Vigabatrin-associated retinal cone system dysfunction: electroretinogram and ophthalmologic findings [see comments]. Neurology 1998;51(6):1778–1779; discussion 1779–1781.
110. Kretschmann U, Seeliger M, Ruether K, et al. Multifocal electroretinography in patients with Stargardt's macular dystrophy. Br J Ophthalmol 1998;82(3):267–275.
111. Kriss A, Thompson D, Lavy T, et al. Pattern VEPs and craniopharyngiomas in children. Investig Ophthalmol Vis Sci 1996;37: 1075.
112. Kriss A, Russell-Eggitt I, Harris C, et al. Aspects of albinism. Ophthalmol Paediatr Genet 1992;13:89–100.
113. Kriss A, Thompson D, Lloyd I, et al. Pattern VEP findings in young children treated for unilateral congenital cataract. In: Cottlier E (ed) Congenital cataracts. Austin: Landes, 1994:79–88.
114. Kriss A, Carroll W, Blumhardt L, et al. Pattern and flash evoked potential changes in toxic (nutritional) optic neuropathy. In: Courjon J, Maugiere F, Revol M (eds) Clinical applications of evoked potentials in neurology. Advances in neurology, vol 32. New York: Raven Press, 1982:11–19.
115. Kriss A, Francis D, Cluendet F, et al. Recovery from optic neuritis in childhood. J Neurol Neurosurg Psychiatry 1988;51:1253–1258.
116. Kriss A, Thompson D. Visual electrophysiology. In: Taylor D (ed) Pediatric ophthalmology. Oxford: Blackwell, 1997:93–121.
117. Kriss A, Russell-Eggitt I. Electrophysiological assessment of visual pathway function in infants. Eye 1992;6:145–153.
118. Kriss A, Russell-Eggitt I, Harris C, et al. Aspects of albinism. Ophthalmol Paediatr Genet 1992;13:89–100.
119. Kubova Z, Kuba M. Clinical application of motion onset potentials. Doc Ophthalmol 1992;81:209–218.
120. Kupersmith M, Siegel I, Carr R, et al. Visual evoked potentials in chiasmal gliomas in four adults. Arch Neurol 1981;38:362–366.
121. Lachapelle P, Rousseau S, McKerral M, et al. Evidence supportive of a functional discrimination between photopic oscillatory potentials

as revealed with cone and rod mediated retinopathies. Doc Ophthalmol 1998;95(1):35–54.

122. Lachapelle P, Little J, Polomeno R. The photopic electroretinogram in congenital stationary night blindness with myopia. Investig Ophthalmol Vis Sci 1983;24:442–450.
123. Lambert R, Kriss A, Taylor D. Delayed visual maturation; a longitudinal clinical and electrophysiological assessment. Ophthalmology 1989;96:534–529.
124. Lambert S, Taylor D, Kriss A. The infant with nystagmus, normal appearing fundi but an abnormal ERG. Surv Ophthalmol 1989;34:176–186.
125. Lambert S, Kriss A, Taylor D. Detection of isolated occipital lobe anomalies during early childhood. Dev Med Child Neurol 1990;32(5):451–455.
126. Lambert S, Kriss A, Taylor D. Joubert syndrome. Arch Ophthalmol 1989;107:709–713.
127. Lambert S, Taylor D, Kriss A, et al. Follow-up and diagnostic reappraisal of 75 patients with Leber's congenital amaurosis. Am J Ophthalmol 1989;107:624–631.
128. Lang G, Maumenee I. Retinal dystrophies associated with storage diseases. In: Newsome DA (ed) Retinal dystrophies and degenerations. New York: Raven Press, 1988:319–340.
129. Lavy T, Harris C, Shawkat F, et al. Electrophysiological and eye movement abnormalities in children with the Bardet-Biedl syndrome. J Pediatr Ophthalmol Strabismus 1995;32(6):364–367.
130. Lei B, Bush R, Milam A, et al. Human melanoma-associated retinopathy (MAR) antibodies alter the retinal ON-response of the monkey ERG in vivo. Investig Ophthalmol Vis Sci 2000;41(1):262–266.
131. Lennerstrand G. Delayed visual evoked cortical potentials in retinal disease. Acta Ophthalmol (Copenh) 1982;60:497–504.
132. Livingstone M, Hubel D. Segregation of form, colour, movement and depth: anatomy, physiology and perception. Science 1988;240:740–750.
133. Lois N, Holder G, Bunce C, et al. Phenotypic subtypes of Stargardt's macular dystrophy-fundus flavimaculatus. Arch Ophthalmol 2001;119(3):359–369.
134. Lorenz B, Gampe E. Analyse von 180 Patienten mit sensorischem Defektnystagmus (SDN) und kongenitalem idiopathischen Nystagmus (CIN). [Analysis of 180 patients with sensory defect nystagmus (SDN) and congenital idiopathic nystagmus (CIN).] Klin Monatsbl Augenheilkd 2001;218(1):3–12.
135. Mandelbaum S, Cleary P, Ruan S, et al. Bright flash electroretinography and vitreous haemorrhage. Arch Ophthalmol 1980;98:1823–1828.
136. Marg E, Freeman D, Peltzman P, et al. Visual acuity development in human infants: evoked potential measurements. Investig Ophthalmol Vis Sci 1976;15:150–153.

137. Markwardt F, Gopfert E, Muller R. Influence of velocity, temporal frequency and initial phase position of gratings on the motion VEP. Biomed Biochim Acta 1988;47:753–760.
138. Marmor M, Jacobsen S, Foerster M, et al. Diagnostic findings of a new syndrome with night blindness, maculopathy, and enhanced s cone sensitivity. Am J Ophthalmol 1990;110:124–134.
139. Maugeri A, Klevering B, Rohrschneider K, et al. Mutations in the ABCA4 (ABCR) gene are the major cause of autosomal recessive cone-rod dystrophy. Am J Hum Genet 2000;67(4):960–966.
140. McCulloch D, Skarf B. Pattern reversal visual evoked potentials following early treatment of unilateral, congenital cataract [see comments]. Arch Ophthalmol 1994;112(4):510–518.
141. McCulloch D, Orbach H, Skarf B. Maturation of the pattern reversal VEP in human infants: a theoretical framework. Vision Res 1999;39:3673–3680.
142. Merigan W. P and M pathway specialisation in the macaque. In: Valberg A, Lee B (eds) From pigments to perception: advances in understanding visual processes. NATO ASI series no. 203. New York: Plenum Press, 1991;117–125.
143. Miyake Y, Horiguchi M, Suzuki S, et al. Electrophysiological findings in patients with Oguchi's disease. Jpn J Ophthalmol 1996;40(4): 511–519.
144. Miyake Y, Horiguchi M, Terasaki H, et al. Scotopic threshold response in complete and incomplete types of congenital stationary night blindness. Investig Ophthalmol Vis Sci 1994;35:3770–3775.
145. Miyake Y, Yagasaki K, Horiguchi M, et al. Congenital stationary night blindness with a negative electroretinogram: a new classification. Arch Ophthalmol 1986;104:1013–1020.
146. Miyake Y, Shiroyama N, Horiguchi M, et al. Bull's eye maculopathy and negative electroretinograms. Retina 1989;9:210–215.
147. Mohri I, Taniike M, Fujimura H, et al. A case of Kearns-Sayre syndrome showing a constant proportion of deleted mitochondrial DNA in blood cells during 6 years of follow-up. J Neurol Sci 1998;158(1): 106–109.
148. Moskowitz A, Sokol S. Spatial and temporal interaction of pattern-evoked cortical potentials in human infants. Vision Res 1980;20(8): 699–707.
149. Mullie M, Harding A, Petty R, et al. The retinal manifestations of mitochondrial myopathy: a study of 22 cases. Arch Ophthalmol 1985;103:1825–1830.
150. Multifocal electroretinography: special issue. The multifocal technique: topographic ERG and VEP responses. Doc Ophthalmol 2001; 100:49–251.
151. Nakamura M, Ito S, Terasaki H, et al. Novel CACNA1F mutations in Japanese patients with incomplete congenital stationary night blindness. Investig Ophthalmol Vis Sci 2001;42(7):1610–1616.
152. Niemeyer G. Pharmacological effects in retinal electrophysiology. In: Heckenlively JR, Arden GB (eds) Principles and practice of

clinical electrophysiology of vision. St. Louis: Mosby, 1991:151–162.

153. Norcia A, Tyler C, Hamer R, et al. Measurement of spatial contrast sensitivity with the swept contrast VEP. Vision Res 1989;29(5):627–637.
154. Norcia A, Tyler C. Infant VEP acuity measurements: analysis of individual differences and measurement error. Electroencephalogr Clin Neurophysiol 1985;61(5):359–369.
155. Norcia A, Tyler C. Spatial frequency sweep VEP: visual acuity during the first year of life. Vision Res 1985;25(10):1399–1408.
156. Norcia A, Garcia H, Humphrey R, et al. Anomalous motion VEPs in infants and infantile esotropia. Investig Ophthalmol Vis Sci 1991;32:436–439.
157. Novack G. Ocular toxicology. Curr Opin Ophthalmol 1997;8(6):88–92.
158. Nusinowitz S, Birch D, Birch E. Rod photoresponses in 6-week and 4-month-old human infants. Vision Res 1998;38(5):627–635.
159. Nuwer M, Perlman S, Packwood J, et al. Evoked potential abnormalities in the various inherited ataxia. Ann Neurol 1983;13:20–27.
160. Orel-Bixler D, Norcia A. Differential growth for steady state pattern reversal and transient onset offset VEPs. Clin Vis Sci 1987;2:1–10.
161. Orel-Bixler D, Haegerstrom-Portnoy G, Hall A. Visual assessment of the multiply handicapped patient. Optom Vis Sci 1989;66(8):530–536.
162. Ossenblock P, Spekreijse H. The extra-striate generators of the EP to checkerboard onset. A source localisation approach. Electroencephalogr Clin Neurophysiol 1991;80:181–193.
163. Palczewski K. Is vertebrate phototransduction solved? New insights into the molecular mechanism of phototransduction. Investig Ophthalmol Vis Sci 1994;35(10):3577–3581.
164. Papaioannou M, Ocaka L, Bessant D, et al. An analysis of ABCR mutations in British patients with recessive retinal dystrophies. Investig Ophthalmol Vis Sci 2000;41(1):16–19.
165. Papakostopoulos D, Hart C, Cooper R, et al. Combined electrophysiological assessment of the visual system in central serous retinopathy. Electroencephalogr Clin Neurophysiol 1984;59(1):77–80.
166. Patel C, Taylor D, Russell-Eggitt I, et al. Congenital third nerve palsy associated with mid-trimester amniocentesis. Br J Ophthalmol 1993;77:530–533.
167. Pepperberg D, Birch D, Hood D. Photoresponses of human rods derived from paired flash ERGs. Vis Neurosci 1997;14:73–82.
168. Poggi-Travert F, Fournier B, Poll B, et al. Clinical approach to inherited peroxisomal disorders. J Inherit Metab Dis 1995;18(suppl 1):1–18.
169. Porteous W, James A, Sheard P, et al. Bioenergetic consequences of accumulating the common 4977-bp mitochondrial DNA deletion. Eur J Biochem 1998;257(1):192–201.

170. Pryds O, Greisen G. Preservation of single flash visual evoked potentials at very low cerebral oxygen delivery in preterm infants. Pediatr Neurol 1990;6:151–158.
171. Pugh E, Lamb T. Phototransduction in vertebrate rods and cones: molecular mechanisms of amplification, recovery and light adaptation. In: Stavenga DG, de Grip WJ, Pugh EN Jr (eds) Handbook of biological physics, vol 3. Amsterdam: Elsevier, 2000:183–254.
172. Purvin V, Kawasaki A, Yee R. Papilledema and obstructive sleep apnea syndrome. Arch Ophthalmol 2000;118:1626–1630.
173. Reardon W, Winter R. The molecular pathology of syndromic craniosynostosis. Mol Med Today 1995:432–437.
174. Regan D. Human brain electrophysiology. Amsterdam: Elsevier, 1989.
175. Regan D, Spekreijse H. Evoked potential indicators of colour blindness. Vision Res 1974;14:89–95.
176. Regan D, Regal D, Tibbles J. Evoked potentials during recovery from blindness recorded serially from an infant and his normally sighted twin. Electroencephalogr Clin Neurophysiol 1982;54:465–468.
177. Ripps H, Mahaffy L, Siegel I, et al. Vincristine-induced changes in the retina of isolated arterially perfused cat eye. Exp Eye Res 1989;48:771–790.
178. Robson J, Frishman L. Dissecting the dark-adapted electroretinogram. Doc Ophthalmol 1998–99;95(3–4):187–215.
179. Rozet J, Gerber S, Ghazi I, et al. Mutations of the retinal specific ATP binding transporter gene (ABCR) in a single family segregating both autosomal recessive retinitis pigmentosa RP19 and Stargardt's disease: evidence of clinical heterogeneity at this locus. J Med Genet 1999;36(6):447–451.
180. Runge P, Muler D, McAllister J, et al. Oral vitamin E can prevent the retinopathy of abetalipoproteinaemia. Br J Ophthalmol 1986;70: 166–173.
181. Russell-Eggitt I, Harris M, Kriss A. Delayed visual maturation: an update. Dev Med Child Neurol 1998;40:130–136.
182. Sandberg M, Wiegel-DiFranco C, Drya T, et al. Clinical expression correlates with location of rhodopsin mutation in dominant retinitis pigmentosa. Investig Ophthalmol Vision Sci 1995;36:1934–1942.
183. Schaumberg D, Moyes A, Gomes J, et al. Corneal transplantation in young children with congenital hereditary endothelial dystrophy. Multicenter Pediatric Keratoplasty Study. Am J Ophthalmol 1999; 127(4):373–378.
184. Schroeder C, Tenke C, Givre S, et al. Striate cortical contribution to the surface recorded pattern reversal VEP in the alert monkey. Vision Res 1991;3197(80):1143–1157 [also published erratum Vision Res 191;31(11):1].
185. Seiple W, Holopigian K. An examination of VEP response phase. Electroencephalogr Clin Neurophysiol 1989;73(6):520–531.
186. Sharon D, Bruns G, Mcgee T, et al. X-linked retinitis pigmentosa: mutation spectrum of the RPGR and RP2 genes and correlation with visual function. Investig Ophthalmol Vis Sci 2000;41:2712–2721.

187. Sharpe L, Stockman A. Rod pathways: the importance of seeing nothing. Trends Neurosci 1999;22:497–504.
188. Shawkat F, Kriss A. A study of the effects of contrast change on pattern VEPs, and the transition between onset, reversal and offset modes of stimulation. Doc Ophthalmol 2000;101(1):73–89.
189. Shepherd A, Saunders K, McCulloch D, et al. Prognostic value of flash visual evoked potentials in preterm infants. Dev Med Child Neurol 1999;41:9–155.
190. Sieving P. Photopic ON- and OFF-pathway abnormalities in retinal dystrophies. AOS thesis. Trans Am Ophthalmol Soc 1993;LXXXXl: 701–773.
191. Sieving P, Murayama K, Naarendorp F. Push-pull model of the primate photopic electroretinogram: a role for hyperpolarizing neurons in shaping the b-wave. Vis Neurosci 1994;11:519–532.
192. Sieving P, Bingham E, Kemp J, et al. Juvenile X-linked retinoschisis from XLRS1 Arg213Trp mutation with preservation of the electroretinogram scotopic b-wave. Am J Ophthalmol 1999;128(2): 179–184.
193. Sieving P, Frishman L, Steinberg R. Scotopic threshold response of proximal retina in cat. J Neurophysiol 1986;5694:1049–1061.
194. Sigesmund D, Weleber R, Pillers D, et al. Characterization of the ocular phenotype of Duchenne and Becker muscular dystrophy. Ophthalmology 1994;101(5):856–865.
195. Skoczenski A, Norcia A. Development of VEP vernier acuity and grating acuity in human infants. Investig Ophthalmol Vis Sci 1999;40:2411–2417.
196. Smith L, Kriss A, Gregson R, et al. Gaze evoked amaurosis in neurofibromatosis type ll. Br J Ophthalmol 1998;82:584–585.
197. Smith N, Lamb T. The a-wave of the human electroretinogram recorded with a minimally invasive technique. Vision Res 1997; 37(21):2943–2952.
198. Smith R, Berlin C, Hejtmancik J, et al. Clinical diagnosis of the Usher syndromes. Am J Med Genet 1994;50:32–38.
199. Snead M, Payne S, Barton D, et al. Stickler syndrome: correlation between vitreoretinal phenotypes and linkage to COL 2A1. Eye 1994;8:609–614.
200. Sokol S. Measurements of infant visual acuity from pattern-reversal evoked potentials. Vision Res 1978;18(1):33–39.
201. Sokol S, Moskowitz A. Comparison of pattern VEPs and preferential-looking behavior in 3-month-old infants. Investig Ophthalmol Vis Sci 1985;26(3):359–365.
202. Soong F, Levin A, Westall C. Comparison of techniques for detecting visually evoked potential asymmetry in albinism. J Am Assoc Pediatr Ophthalmol Sci 2000;4:302–310.
203. Spileers W, Maes H, Van Hulle M, et al. Contrast modulated steady state evoked potentials (CMSS VEPS) measuring static and dynamic contrast sensitivity. Clin Vis Res 1992;7:93–106.

204. Sridharan R. Visual evoked potentials in spinocerebellar degenerations. Clin Neurol Neurosurg 1983;85:235–243.
205. Stanesu Segal B, Evrard P. Zellweger syndrome, retinal involvement. Metab Pediatr Syst Ophthalmol 1989;9:96–99.
206. Stavrou P, Good P, Misson G, et al. Electrophysiological findings in Stargardt's-fundus flavimaculatus disease. Eye 1998;12(pt 6):953–958.
207. Stefan H, Bernatik J, Knorr J. Gesichtsfeldstorungen bei Antiepileptikabehandlung. [Visual field defects due to antiepileptic drugs.] Nervenarzt 1999;70(6):552–555.
208. Strasburger H, Remky A, Murray I, et al. Objective measurement of contrast sensitivity and visual acuity with the steady-state visual evoked potential. Ger J Ophthalmol 1996;5(1):42–52.
209. Taylor M, McCulloch D. Visual evoked potentials in infants and children. J Clin Neurophysiol 1992;9:357–372.
210. Taylor M, McCulloch D. The prognostic value of VEPs in young children with acute onset cortical blindness. Pediatr Neurol 1991;7:86–90.
211. Thompson D, Drasdo N. Temporal patterns and the topography of the visual evoked potential. In: Non-invasive assessment of the visual system, vol 1. Tech digest series. Ophthalmology Society of America, 1992;1:150–153.
212. Thompson D, Kriss A, Chong K, et al. Visual evoked potential evidence of chiasmal hypoplasia. Ophthalmology 1999;106:2354–2361.
213. Thompson D, Kriss A, Taylor D, et al. Early VEP and ERG evidence of visual dysfunction in autosomal recessive osteopetrosis. Neuropediatrics 1998;29:137–144.
214. Thompson D, Kriss A, Cottrell S, et al. Visual evoked potential evidence of albino-like chiasmal misrouting in a patient with Angelman syndrome with no ocular features of albinism. Dev Med Child Neurol 1999;41(9):633–638.
215. Thompson D, Lloyd I, Dowler J, et al. The development of spatial resolution measured by swept VEP and forced choice preferential looking techniques. Investig Ophthamol Vis Sci 1993;34:1354.
216. Tolhurst D. Separate channels for the analysis of the shape and movement of a moving visual stimulus. J Physiol 1973;231:385–402.
217. Tremblay F, De Becker I, Cheung C, et al. Visual evoked potentials with crossed asymmetry in incomplete congenital stationary night blindness. Investig Ophthalmol Vis Sci 1996;37:1783–1792.
218. Tremblay F, LaRoche R, Shea S, et al. Longitudinal study of the early electroretinographic changes in Alstrom's syndrome. Am J Ophthalmol 1993;115(5):657–665.
219. Tremblay F, Laroche R, De-Becker I. The electroretinographic diagnosis of the incomplete form of congenital stationary night blindness. Vision Res 1995;35(16):2383–2393.
220. Tyler C, Apkarian P, Levi D, et al. Rapid assessment of visual function: an electronic sweep technique for the pattern visual evoked potential. Investig Ophthalmol Vis Sci 1979;18(7):703–713.

221. Tyler C, Apkarian P, Nakayama K. Multiple spatial-frequency tuning of electrical responses from human visual cortex. Exp Brain Res 1978;33(3–4):535–550.
222. Tzekov R, Locke K, Hood D, et al. Cone and rod phototransduction parameters in retinitis pigmentosa patients. Investig Ophthalmol Vis Sci 2001;42:420.
223. van-Lith G, Hekkert-Wiebenga W. Cataract, pattern stimulation and visually evoked potentials. Doc Ophthalmol 1983;28;55(1–2):107–112.
224. Vigabatrin Paediatric Advisory Group Guideline for prescribing vigabatrin in children has been revised. Br Med J 2000;320:1404.
225. Wachtmeister L. Oscillatory potentials in the retina: what do they reveal. Prog Retina Eye Res 1998;17(4):485–521.
226. Weleber R, Kennaway N. Infantile Refsum's disease. In: Gold DH, Weingeist TA (eds) The eye in systemic disease. Philadelphia: Lippincott, 1990:409–411.
227. Weleber R. The dystrophic retina in multisystem disorders: the electroretinogram in neuronal ceroid lipofuscinoses. Eye 1998;12(pt 3b): 580–590.
228. Wendel R, Mannis M, Keltner J. Role of electrophysiologic testing in the preoperative evaluation of corneal transplant patients. Ann Ophthalmol 1984;16(8):788–793.
229. Wenzel D, Brandl U. Maturation of pattern evoked potentials elicited by checkerboard reversal. Dev Ophthalmol 1984;9:87–93.
230. Westall C, Paton C, Levin A. Time courses for maturation of electroretinogram responses from infancy to adulthood. Doc Ophthalmol 1999;96:355–379.
231. Wild J, Martinez C, Reinshagen G, et al. Characteristics of a unique visual field defect attributed to vigabatrin. Epilepsia 1999;40(12): 1784–1794.
232. Wilkie A. Craniosynostosis: genes and mechanisms. Hum Mol Genet 1997;6:1647–1656.
233. Willison H, Muller D, Matthews S, et al. A study of the relationship between neurological function and serum vitamin E concentrations in patients with cystic fibrosis. J Neurol Neurosurg Psychiatry 1985;48:1097–1102.
234. Wilson W. Peroxisomal disorders. In: Gold DH, Weingeist TA (eds) The eye in systemic disease. Philadelphia: Lippincott, 1990:402–406.
235. Wohlrab G, Boltshauser E, Schmitt B, et al. Visual field constriction is not limited to children treated with vigabatrin. Neuropediatrics 1999;30(3):130–132.
236. Wright K, Eriksen K, Shors T. Recording pattern evoked potentials under chloral hydrate sedation. Arch Ophthalmol 1986;104:718–721.
237. Wright K, Eriksen K, Shors T. Detection of amblyopia with P-VEP during chloral hydrate sedation. J Pediatr Ophthalmol Strabismus 1987;24(4):170–175.

238. Wright K, Fox B, Shors T, Eriksen K. The use of the PVEP with multiple large check stimuli for quantitating amblyopia in children. Binoc Vis Q 1990;5(1):19–26.
239. Wright K, Ary J, Shors T, Eriksen K. J Pediatr Ophthalmol Strabismus 1986;23(5):252–257.
240. Wright K, Fox B, Eriksen K. PVEP evidence of true suppression in adult onset strabismus. J Pediatr Ophthalmol Strabismus 1990;27(4): 196–201.
241. Yiannikas C, Walsh J, McCleod J. Visual evoked potentials in the detection of sub-clinical optic toxic effects secondary to ethambutol. Arch Neurol 1983;40:645–648.

2

The Pediatric Low-Vision Patient

Anne Frances Walonker

The American Academy of Pediatrics states that 75% of learning during the early years is processed through vision; because vision is a learning sense, children with visual impairment may not learn to perform many tasks as quickly as those with normal vision. Children with subnormal vision often look and act like any other child in the classroom and on the playground making it difficult to distinguish them from normally sighted children. Children with low vision may wear thick glasses or even dark glasses, but they will run and jump as fearlessly as their playmates.

Never having known any other vision, these children are often unaware that their vision is less than that of other children, and the majority adapt quite well to their environment. Only a few children with low vision need special schools or a protected environment. The majority of these low-vision children function much better in a standard school system with the help of a resource teacher for some part of the school week. As much as is possible, these children need to be mainstreamed. They need to be expected to perform the same tasks and to assume the same responsibilities as normally sighted children of the same age.

INCIDENCE

According to the Centers for Disease Control (CDC), nearly 1 in 1000 children in the United States has some degree of low vision or is legally blind.[1] Not being able to see can alter how a child understands and functions in the world. Impaired vision can affect a child's emotional, neurological, and physical development by potentially limiting the range of experiences and the kinds of information to which a child is exposed.

CLINICAL FEATURES

Decreased vision in a child can be caused by many different processes, each one requiring a different method of treatment: either medical, surgical, or optical. If normal vision cannot be restored, then the use of both optical and nonoptical aids to enhance the remaining vision is necessary.

Whatever the cause of the decreased vision, early intervention is of the utmost importance for the child to adapt to the environment and to continue the learning processes without interruption. The clinical features that could alert a parent to signs of a visual problem in their child include, but are not limited to, nystagmus, strabismus, random eye movements, leukocoria, and corneal opacity.

CLINICAL ASSESSMENT

Clinical assessment of a child with a suspected visual impairment always consists of a very detailed clinical evaluation by a pediatric ophthalmologist, with ancillary testing such as electrophysiology and ultrasonography when appropriate.

The measurement of visual function should be done with targets appropriately sized for both the age of the child and the level of vision suspected, moving the child closer to the testing targets both for near and for distance. The visual requirements for each child should also be assessed because the various therapeutic modalities are age and task appropriate.

The importance of early diagnosis of the child's visual disability cannot be overstated. The earlier the disability is diagnosed, the earlier treatment intervention can begin. Early treatment may produce a better outcome by allowing a stepwise approach to planning the use of aids, both visual and nonvisual, for the short and long term. For those children with an inherited process, early diagnosis makes it possible to provide expedient and appropriate counseling for the families involved. Innumerable low-vision aids of various types are available for enhancing both distance and near vision. The type of device that is appropriate will change as the child becomes older and their visual requirements change and increase. The low-vision devices that are useful for children bear no relationship to those used by most adults.

Because reading is the child's access to learning, a visual aid that makes this task possible is one of the most important devices for these children. The phakic school-age child has an enormous range of accommodation. These children find that reading can be a simple matter of bringing the print close enough to their faces to magnify the image. A fixed-stand low-power magnifier (Fig. 2-1) to enhance these images is probably the most useful low-vision aid for these young children. When the magnifier is placed directly on the page, its fixed focus keeps the

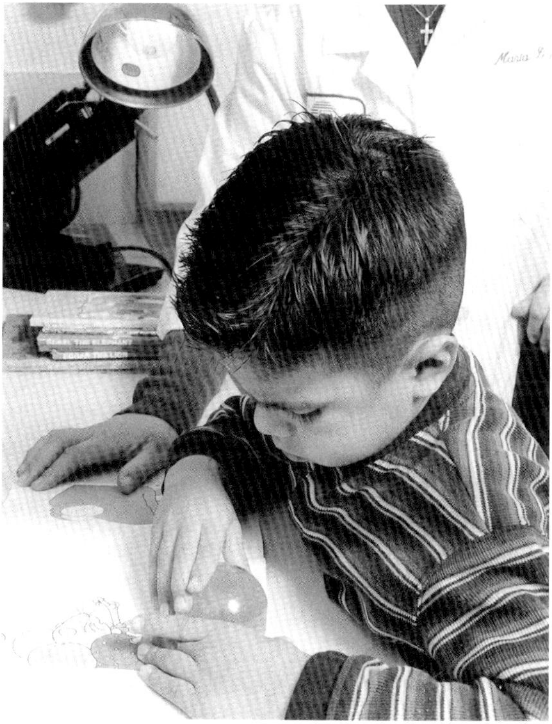

FIGURE 2-1. Low-power stand magnifier.

print clear at all times and lets the child run the device along the page. Even very young children learn to manipulate these devices, and they have been found more useful than many of the more technically sophisticated and costly aids available today.

The aphakic child has different needs. However, glasses or contact lenses with reading additions and the same fixed-focus stand magnifiers can be of great help to these children. The other aid that is exciting to young children with decreased vision is a monocular telescope (Fig. 2-2). It takes a little longer to master this device, but, once the child learns to use it, it opens up a whole new world. The small size of these telescopes makes

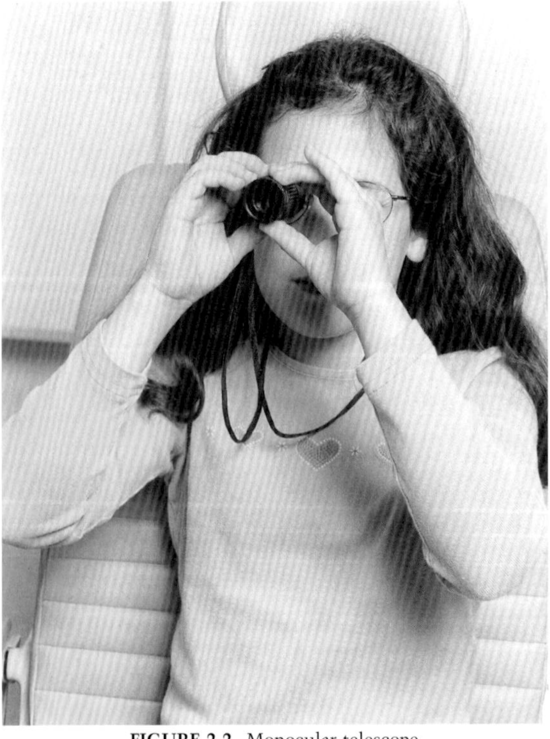

FIGURE 2-2. Monocular telescope.

them highly portable. A child can use this device anywhere and can share it with normally sighted friends, thus erasing the stigma associated with the use of a low-vision aid.

The social and academic success of a child with a visual disability depends largely on the expectations of the family and the understanding of the teachers and the school administrators; the focus should not be on the limitations that the visual disability creates but on the heights that these children can achieve. Teachers, classroom aides, and playground supervisors should be encouraged to treat these children no differently than they treat the others in the class. However, staff need to remain aware of the children's special needs and address these needs appropriately. Where these children are seated in the classroom, the distance between them and the blackboard, the size of the letters on the board, the color of the chalk used, and the angle of the glare from the windows are all as important as any optical or nonoptical visual aid being used.

Furnishing the family and the teachers with a detailed report of the size of print that the child can see for both near and distance work is most helpful. When there are problems with contrast on homework assignments (some copies are so poor that enlarging the print makes them impossible to read), a different type of copy for these children is important. For some children, a closed-circuit television (Fig. 2-3) facilitates reading when increased magnification is required, as the magnifying glass of increased power decreases the field of view. These devices are expensive, but an older child will find them very useful. Most schools with resource centers make them available, as do public libraries.

With increased awareness of and attention to those things that make schoolwork easier to handle, most children will adapt well to their less-than-normal vision, which will do more for their self-confidence than any expensive magnifier or complicated reading machine can possibly do. However, as the child becomes older and reading demands increase, these more sophisticated instruments will become appropriate and should be added to the armamentarium. Newer instruments include closed-circuit television cameras that can be used with computers and portable handheld devices that scan curved surfaces and have large-print readouts on the handles. There are many headborne devices, used for both distance and near reading, that are appropriate for adults who need them to maintain a career. These newer devices are not really necessary in the elementary

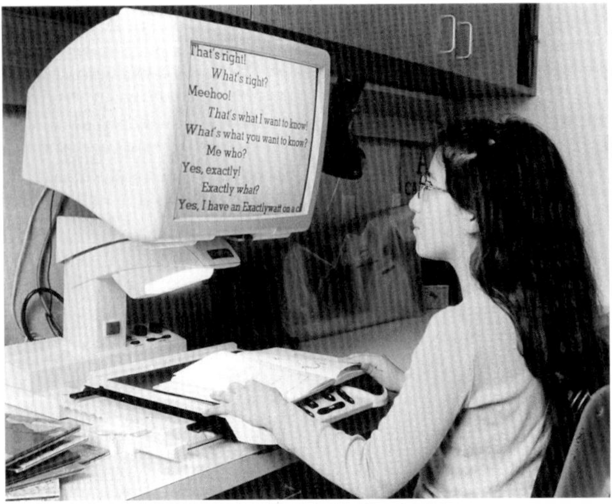
That's right!
What's right?
Meehoo!
That's what I want to know!
What's what you want to know?
Me who?
Yes, exactly!
Exactly what?

FIGURE 2-3. Closed-circuit television.

and high school classroom, but they may be more useful to college students who sit in large classrooms and who may find it necessary to copy notes from distant blackboards or screens.

There are some points to remember when evaluating a child for visual aids:

- Amblyopia can occur in the presence of another visual abnormality and should be treated vigorously. The better the vision, the less magnifying power needed.
- It is acceptable for moderate to high myopes to remove their glasses for near work.
- The accommodative range will decrease as these children get older, and a change in vision does not necessarily mean a worsening of a previously stable condition.
- There is no limit to the amount of reading aid that can be prescribed so long as this aid improves near vision.
- Only those visual aids that are needed for the currently performed tasks should be prescribed. For the young child, this will probably mean a stand magnifier for near tasks and a telescope for distance tasks.

RESOURCES

Bibliography from Pediatric Ophthalmology Consumer Resources

Madelyn Hall
Good Samaritan Hospital and Medical Center
1040 N.W. 22nd Avenue
Portland, OR 97219

"Vision and Vision Impairment" (a bibliography of books for children)
Pediatric Projects Incorporated
P.O. Box 1880
Santa Monica, CA 90406

"Selected readings for parents of preschool handicapped children"
National Library Service for the Blind and Physically Handicapped
Library of Congress
1291 Taylor Street NW
Washington DC 20542
1-800-424-8567

Additional Resources

National Association for the Visually Handicapped (NAVH)
305 East 24th Street
New York, NY 10010

American Foundation for the Blind
Customer Service Division
15 West 16th Street
New York, NY 10010

Reference

1. Centers for Disease Control. NECH Publ no 99-0444. National Center for Environmental Health, Centers for Disease Control. Washington, DC: 1999.

3

Breaking the News: The Role of the Physician

Nancy Chernus-Mansfield

Janet and Marc thought their life was as close to perfection as any family's life could be. Married for 8 years, they had one daughter, Missy, age 5, and Brian, age 3 months, their long-awaited son. At Brian's 3-month routine well-baby checkup, the pediatrician remarked that Brian might have strabismus because his eyes appeared to turn in and weren't "working together," as Janet later described it. The pediatrician was very reassuring, however, and told Marc and Janet that he would like the baby to be examined by a pediatric ophthalmologist "just to be on the safe side." Marc had recently started a new and more responsible job so it was decided that Janet would take Brian for the eye examination herself, to minimize the amount of time Marc was away from the office.

Thursday, July 14, began like many others for Janet. She got Missy off to kindergarten, kissed Marc goodbye, and packed up for the day's outing, an eye doctor's appointment. Preparing a 3-month-old to meet a new doctor was a challenge for Janet. She wanted Brian not only to look his best but to be his most alert and charming self.

When Janet arrived for the appointment, everything seemed easy enough. She filled out the routine medical information and was brought into the examining room. The doctor came in, introduced himself, and asked Janet some questions about Brian's development and about the pregnancy. As Brian was being examined, Janet began to feel twinges of anxiety. Brian was screaming. For the doctor to get a good look at his eyes, he explained to Janet that he would have to put a speculum in Brian's eyes to keep them open and in position. Unprepared for the papoose board they placed him on, or for the torturous-looking instrument the doctor used, Janet was becoming extremely upset. Finally the examination was complete, or so Janet thought. The doctor said he couldn't give a diagnosis, however, without some additional tests. Janet didn't understand. Why would crossed eyes require additional tests? The doctor would not comment. He told Janet he wanted more information and would arrange for her to go across the street to a facility that could do the tests. Quickly, Janet called her neighbor to make arrangements for Missy to be picked up from kindergarten. Although she was feeling upset by the morning's examination, Janet thought it best not to call and alarm Marc because she thought the doctor was probably just being thorough.

Janet took Brian across the street to the laboratory where they did electrophysiological tests. Fortunately, Brian had fallen asleep and the flashing lights and electrodes did not seem to bother him. The person who did the tests did not give Janet any information. He told her to return to her physician's office.

When Janet entered the doctor's office this time, she was feeling very apprehensive. She was ushered into the doctor's office, instead of an examining room. After about 15 long minutes, the doctor appeared. He sat down behind his desk, took out Brian's chart, and began to speak. From what Janet can remember, he said something like this: "The test confirmed what I have suspected. Your baby has a condition known as Leber's congenital amaurosis. This condition affects the optic nerves and, from my experience, I believe he is totally blind. There is no treatment. I am sorry. I wish you and your family the best of luck."

Janet can't remember what happened after that. She has no memory of her drive home, of picking up Missy, or of calling Marc. What she does remember is feeling that her life, Brian's life, Marc's life, and Missy's life were over. Nothing would ever be the same again.

Thursdays were busy days for Jack Smith, M.D. He had private patients in the morning and clinic patients all afternoon. At 38, he had achieved his dream of becoming a successful pediatric ophthalmologist. He had always had an interest in ophthalmology but, after his pediatric rotation, he decided that pediatric ophthalmology was a truly exciting field. Jack felt lucky that his wife of 12 years was always supportive of him and that all three of his children, Jack Jr., 10, Jennifer, 8, and Jason, 6, seemed happy and were proud of their dad. He enjoyed the challenge of his work in his private office as well as his research and teaching at the medical school. He had developed a particular interest in treating strabismus and had become the leading specialist in his area.

After arriving at his office, Jack surveyed his schedule and buzzed Karen, his "right arm," to send in the first patient. As he entered the examining room he saw Janet, an attractive thirtyish woman, gazing lovingly at her infant. Jack suspected that the baby had strabismus. The call from the pediatrician was brief, and indicated nothing out of the ordinary. Jack introduced himself and began the examination. Almost immediately he could feel a knot beginning in his stomach as he noted the presence of a nystagmus. By the time the baby was papoosed and the speculum was in place, he was really concerned. He thought, "Maybe it won't be as bad as I think it is; wait for the ERG." He would feel his discomfort build as he told Janet he wanted some additional tests. "No need to alarm her at this point," he thought. So he sent Janet across the street and proceeded to see the many other children waiting for their examinations.

At 11:45 A.M., the call came from the electrophysiology lab. Jack's suspicions were confirmed: Leber's—a totally blind baby. In 45 minutes he would be face-to-face with Janet. This was the only part of his practice he dreaded—giving bad news. What should he tell her? He wished he knew. "Does anyone?" he wondered. "I will just give her the facts. There's no way to sugarcoat this," he thought. Nothing had prepared him to break people's hearts.

Jack doesn't remember the details of Janet's reaction. He knew, of course, that she was extremely upset. Primarily, though, he felt overwhelming helplessness. None of his hard-won expertise could fix this baby; no patching, no surgery, no nothing. All Jack could do was hope that this family had the strength to cope with the diagnosis. The thought came, "If it was one of my kids, what would I do?" He dismissed that thought quickly. It was too painful. "I'm getting morbid; probably most of the kids do great, and their parents can handle their problems." At least Jack wanted to think so. He loved being a pediatric ophthalmologist because he could really help kids. It was so satisfying to see a child who had amblyopia, for example, and to know that with patching the child's vision would be assured. He didn't really know that much about what happened to the few blind children he had encountered. They seemed okay, but, Jack thought, to be fully honest, they were the patients with whom he spent the least time. There was, after all, nothing he could do for them.

Yet that day he couldn't shake the feeling of discomfort as he continued to see patients. His mind kept returning to Janet and the pain on her face. What would life be like for her and for her family? Janet seemed shocked when she heard the diagnosis, but she was very quiet. She hadn't said very much or even asked any questions other than, "Are you sure there is nothing that can be done?" He had said "No." Maybe, he thought in retrospect, just saying "no" was too brusque. He hated to admit there was nothing more he could do and that he was unable to offer further hope. Maybe he should have said more. Is there something else he could have done for her? He just didn't know.

PARENTAL REACTIONS TO THE DIAGNOSIS OF BLINDNESS

The impact of blindness on all family members is tremendous. Before the birth of any baby, we all have dreams and expectations about what the future holds. Expecting a child is a special time for most parents. Mothers and fathers love their baby long before it is born. They love the baby because they project onto their child all their dreams, fantasies, and expectations. For many parents, their hopes are realized when a healthy child is born. But for a moment try to imagine all these expectations and dreams destroyed by hearing the doctor say, "Your baby is blind." Parents are devastated. They experience a blow that is totally shattering. As Pearl Buck said when learning her daughter was mentally retarded, "All the joy of my life was gone."

Author Renee Nastoff, the parent of a child with a disability, eloquently described her pain when she wrote, "I fight the unseen enemy. I have reason for revenge but nothing against which to vent my outrage. My child is held hostage by a cruel twist of fate. Only a parent can comprehend the frustration of fighting an attacker that can't possibly be hurt. It is in the air all around me every moment of my life, overshadowing all decisions about my child, crushing and destroying the simple parental right to dream—about Little League, college, marriage, grandchildren. I can feel the enemy now, its fingers tightening at my throat, forcing what I thought were controlled tears. Sometimes it loosens its painful clasp, but never does it desert its hold on my life. I can't kill this stranger, and I can't break away. Yet it tries to force the very spirit of life from me. It will remain with me forever."

A parent experiences one of life's most devastating losses when a child is born with a disability. What the parent has lost is the anticipated perfect child—that very-much-loved-and-dreamed-of child to whom they have already become attached. Surprisingly, the degree of the baby's impairment is not always the crucial factor in determining the parent's reactions. The most important determinant is the parent's dreams for that child. Loss is the hardest thing that we, as human beings, experience. It is not an uncommon event that affects only certain people, nor is loss merely defined as death of a loved one. It actually touches each of us many times and in many ways in our lifetime. Loss shatters the dreams that are the most basic to a person's existence. Major losses with which we are all familiar include divorce, death, or illness. However, less profound losses can include the loss of physical attractiveness, career recognition, money, etc. The significance of the loss varies for each person and depends on how meaningful that particular loss is to the individual's identity. Loss is a common human experience cutting across all socioeconomic lines. The loss of the expected perfect baby is a major trauma in a family's life. The kinds of feelings that parents have in response to their child's visual impairment may be confusing to them. Feelings of shock, helplessness, fear, denial, depression, sadness, anger, guilt, disappointment, and uncertainty are natural and occur with intensity. Many parents have called this time a "mourning period" because the feeling of sadness is so acute. As one mother said: "I felt like my perfect baby had died and I had a different baby—a blind one." Another parent said, "I was so confused. What I expected to be the happiest time of my life turned out to be the saddest."

Grieving is a normal and spontaneous reaction to loss, but in our culture this normal reaction is often regarded as abnormal. Society may view people who are grieving appropriately as though they are behaving inappropriately. Grieving is the process that enables human beings to deal with loss. Yet parents report that the expression of their grief often cuts them off from the very support they need. As one father said, "I haven't cried since I was 12, but now whenever anyone asks about my son, I start to cry. I know that I make people uncomfortable and they often try to avoid me." This father's expression of his feelings is a healthy response that will eventually enable him to cope with his grief. It is part of the process of detaching from the child he wished for and forming an attachment to his actual child.

Another important and universal reaction parents express is an overwhelming need to understand the reason for their child's impairment. Parents say:

"The question 'why' is always in the back of my mind. Am I to blame?"

"When I was pregnant, I moved the furniture."

"There were various medications I was taking for my asthma. I often wonder, 'Was the medicine the cause of my baby's handicap?' "

"When I was pregnant with John, I couldn't quit work. We had no insurance, and I sometimes think maybe I could have taken it easier and should not have worried about the money. When I'm alone I start blaming myself."

It is natural for parents to look for reasons to explain their child's blindness. When a painful event occurs, it is human nature to feel that perhaps we could bear the pain better if we would understand why it happened, if we could make sense of something so senseless. When people feel lost, they want a road map, and answers seem to provide the needed map. For some people, medical explanations are helpful; for others, religious beliefs provide comfort; but for the vast majority of parents, there are no satisfying answers that relieve the pain or diminish the feeling that "life is not fair." Most of us have a deep sense of justice and fairness, and it is terribly hard to think that something this tragic can happen without a reason. Some fortunate families who are religious believe that, although they don't understand why, God has a purpose and this helps them cope with their child's disability. Many parents never find a reasonable explanation. People find it hard to think that a catastrophic disability happens randomly or that the world could be so chaotic that who or what a person is, or does, is of no consequence. Most of us grow up believing that justice prevails, that bad things happen to bad people and good things happen to good people. Reconciling this view with one's own life is very difficult for all of us. A physician once said, in helping a family deal with this issue: "Often people think that, because they took drugs in high school or had a teenage abortion, they may be responsible for the child's disability. I reassure my patients that all of us can find fault with ourselves in reviewing our lives. However, I tell parents that their previous behaviors have nothing to do with their child's disability. It is simply a random event, and they were unlucky. I find that my patients are very relieved when I reassure them about these issues."

Most parents do begin to cope quickly and in tandem with grieving. Although parents love their disabled child and make the necessary adjustments, their lives are never the same. The pain comes and goes forever.

BREAKING THE NEWS: THE ROLE OF THE PHYSICIAN

Physicians are often unaware the their role has a direct effect on the family's adaptation process. The way the physician presents the diagnosis to the family is crucial. For the rest of their lives, parents will remember not just what they were told, but the way in which it was communicated by the physician.

The following ingredients are necessary in a successful doctor–patient or doctor–parent interaction: consideration, truth, clarity, awareness, compassion, trust, accessibility, and professional kindness.

Consideration

Always sit down when talking to a family. Sit down in a private place, with no spectators. Do not appear rushed, even though you may have a waiting room full of patients. Look directly at the parents, make eye contact, and do not write or dictate into a recorder as you are talking. Try not to be interrupted when giving bad news; the family needs your undivided attention. During the diagnostic process, don't think out loud. This causes unnecessary anxiety. Don't talk with other medical personnel in front of the family; this can be accomplished before or after you have finished explaining the diagnosis. Above all, treat people as you would like to be treated in a like situation.

Truth

It is understandably difficult for the physician to give bad news. It is best to be direct, but not blunt. As one physician said, "There are many ways to say the same thing: truth doesn't mean brutality. Your face can stop a clock—when I'm with you, time stands still." Although both statements convey the same cognitive information, the emotional impact is significantly different.

Clarity

Give information using plain language. When parents are anxious, it interferes with understanding. Often physicians use medical jargon to protect themselves in this time of stress. Physicians must give the information clearly and directly. Sometimes in their discomfort, doctors unconsciously resort to excessive discussion or speculation about the disease or use too much intellectual discourse. This is not helpful to the family.

Awareness

Be aware of how the family is feeling. Acknowledge your own feelings as well. Recognize how you feel as a doctor giving a diagnosis for which there is no cure. Remember that the family is frightened and in more pain than you are and think about how the news is affecting them. Often physicians talk about disease or body parts to depersonalize the information and to depersonalize the enormity of the task of giving a difficult diagnosis.

Compassion

Allow yourself to feel compassion for your patient, for their parents, and for yourself. Compassion will not distort the professional relationship. Rather, your concern and discomfort about the diagnosis can be helpful to a family. Even if you are ill at ease or uncomfortable, the human connection your feelings can create may help the family to cope. Your expression, body language, and tone of voice are important. Your words will be etched forever in the memory of the family.

Trust

Parents must trust you not only as a physician who is medically competent, but as someone that they can count on to help them in this critical period. They must trust you to be honest at all times. Parents must also be able to trust that you recognize their pain and sorrow and will not abandon them.

Accessibility

Because of the emotional impact of the diagnosis, parents need to be able to talk with you more than once. Often it is helpful to leave the room for a period of time after the initial diagnosis has been delivered. Anxiety often blocks the ability to absorb information, and the family may need to have the diagnosis explained more than once. This response is normal and has nothing to do with their intelligence. Allow them some private time and then return 10 to 15 minutes later to review the information. Let the family know that you are available if they would like to schedule another appointment to talk about the diagnosis again or to answer any questions.

Professional Kindness

Professional kindness is the key to giving bad news. It encompasses all the ingredients previously discussed. It enables physicians to communicate with their patients in a helpful and meaningful way. It helps parents to come to terms with the diagnosis. Professional kindness is a tool, a means of helping people in a kind and humane way. Professional kindness lets parents know you care and are concerned about their welfare and the welfare of their child. Professional kindness will not tax the personal resources of a physician. Rather, it provides a concrete set of behaviors that can be relied upon even in the most serious situation.

SUMMARY

- Professional kindness works. Parents, and physicians themselves benefit.
- Treating families with professional kindness affects those families for the rest of their lives. Families who experience the lack of kindness are negatively affected forever, whereas those who experienced their doctor's concern feel cared about, which strengthens their ability to cope.
- Points to remember:
  a. Sit down.
  b. Make eye contact.
  c. Say you are sorry to have to give bad news.
  d. Give the diagnosis in a private setting.
  e. Explain the diagnosis simply and clearly.
  f. Do not take calls or allow interruptions while telling the news.
  g. Allow the parents to cry or to express shock, grief, anger, or any other emotion they feel.
  h. If you are too busy to spend sufficient time, arrange for another appointment so that parents can have adequate time to ask questions.

i. Do not try to ameliorate grief by saying such things as "It could be worse."
j. Try to give appropriate referrals. It helps both the family and the physician to be able to do something.
k. If possible, do not request payment from a family in shock. A staff member can contact the family at a later date.
l. Teach your staff about all these points. Insist on professional kindness in your office.

Acknowledgment. I thank Marilyn Horn, L.C.S.W., for all her hard work with the original subject matter.

APPENDIX

Parents need referrals. Contacting resources is something concrete parents can do for their child, and for many individuals, taking action also relieves anxiety. Resources are different in each state. We have prepared a list that gives you a place to start. Parents can use this list to find out what other resources may exist in their community.

Cancer

American Cancer Society
46 First St. NE
Atlanta, GA 30308
800/ACS-2345
404/320-3333

Candlelighters Childhood Cancer Foundation
1312 18th St. NW, Suite 300
Washington, DC 20036
800/366-2223
202/659-5136
(See also Visual Impairments for Retinoblastoma resources)

Cerebral Palsy

Canadian Cerebral Palsy Association
800 Wellington St., Suite 612
Ottawa, Ontario
Canada K1R 6K7
800/267-6572 (in Canada)
613/235-2144

United Cerebral Palsy Association
7 Penn Plaza, Suite 804
New York, NY 10001
800/USA-1UCP
212/268-6655

CHARGE Syndrome

CHARGE Accounts
c/o Quota Club
2004 Parkade Blvd.
Columbia, MO 65202
314/442-7604

Chronic Illness

N.O.R.D.
National Organization for Rare Disorders
P.O. Box 8923
New Fairfield, CT 06812
http://www.rarediseases.org

Magic Foundation
(Optic Nerve Hypoplasia)
1327 N. Harlem Ave.
Oak Park, IL 60302
709/383-0808
http://www.magicfoundation.org

Parents of Chronically Ill Children
1527 Maryland St.
Springfield, IL 62702
217/522-6810

Deaf/Blind

John Tracy Clinic
806 West Adams Blvd
Los Angeles, CA 90007
800/522-4582

Hydrocephalus

Hydrocephalus Association
2040 Polk St., Box 342
San Francisco, CA 94109
415/776-4713

Hydrocephalus Support Group
c/o Kathy McGowan
6059 Mission Rd., #106
San Diego, CA 92108
619/282-1070

National Hydrocephalus Foundation
22427 S. River Rd.
Joliet, IL 60436
815/467-6548

Lawrence Moon Bardet Biedl Syndrome

Lawrence Moon Bardet Biedl Syndrome Network
18 Strawberry Hill
Windsor, CT 06095
203/688-7880

Marfan Syndrome

National Marfan Foundation
382 Main St.
Port Washington, NY 10050
516/883-8712

Mental Retardation

Association for Retarded Citizens of the U.S.
500 E. Border St., Suite 300
Arlington, TX 76010
817/261-6003

Neurofibromatosis

National Neurofibromatosis Foundation
141 Fifth Ave., Suite 7-S
New York, NY 10010
800/323-7938
212/460-8980

Visual Impairments

American Foundation for the Blind
15 West 16th St.
New York, NY 10011
800/AF-BLIND (232-5463)
212/620-2043

American Printing House for the Blind
1839 Frankfort Ave.
P.O. Box 6085
Louisville, KY 40206-0085
502/895-2405

Association for Macular Diseases
210 East 64th St.
New York, NY 10021
212/655-3007

The Institute for Families of Blind Children
P.O. Box 54700
Mailstop #111
Los Angeles, CA 90054-0700
323/669-4649

National Association for the Visually Impaired
P.O. Box 317
Watertown, MA 02272-0317
800/562-6265
Fax: 617/972-7444
(Some areas have a state organization as well; NAPVI can direct the parent)

National Organization for Albinism and Hypopigmentation (NOAH)
155 Locust St., Suite 1816
Philadelphia, PA 19102
800/473-2310
215/545-2322

Parents and Cataract Kids (PACK)
c/o Geraldine Miller
P.O. Box 73
Southeastern, PA 19399
215/352-0719

Retinoblastoma International
4650 Sunset Blvd., M.S. 88
Los Angeles, CA 90027
323/669-2299
www.retinoblastoma.net

New England Retinoblastoma Support Group
603 Fourth Range Road
Pembroke, NH 03275

General Resources

The Family Resource Coalition
230 N. Michigan Avenue
Suite 1625, Dept. W
Chicago, IL 60601
(Identification of parent support groups all over the country)

Reaching Out: A Directory of National Organizations Related to Maternal and Child Health
38th and R Streets, NW
Washington, DC 20057
202/625-8400

Team of Advocates for Special Kids
100 W. Cerritos Ave.
Anaheim, CA 92805
714/533-8275

Other National Toll-Free Numbers:

American Council of the Blind 800/424-8666
Better Hearing Institute 800/424-8576
Epilepsy Information Line 800/332-1000
Cystic Fibrosis Foundation 800/344-4823
Downs Syndrome 800/221-4602
Easter Seal Society 800/221-6827
Health Information Clearinghouse 800/336-4797
Spina Bifida 800/621-3141
Fragile X Foundation 800/835-2246
American Kidney Fund 800/835-8018
National Information Center for Orphan Drugs and Rare Disease 800/336-4797
Sickle Cell Association 800/421-8453
Retinitis Pigmentosa (RP) Association International 800/344-4877
Local School Districts or State Departments of Special Education

Search on the Internet for most current information.

4

Heritable Disorders of RPE, Bruch's Membrane, and the Choriocapillaris

Arlene V. Drack

This chapter covers disorders characterized by ophthalmoscopically visible changes in structures deep to the neurosensory retina. A prominent component of many of these conditions is the accumulation of yellowish material within and beneath the retinal pigment epithelium (RPE) associated with a progressive loss of macular RPE cells. A number of toxic and inflammatory conditions can also cause dots and spots at the level of the RPE, but these conditions can usually be distinguished by history from those in this chapter and are considered elsewhere in this volume (Chapter 11). Choroideremia, gyrate atrophy, and some forms of congenital stationary night blindness are also associated with ophthalmoscopically visible abnormalities in structures beneath the photoreceptors. However, these diseases share some psychophysical, electrophysiological, and symptomatic features with the photoreceptor degenerations and are discussed in Chapter 5. Last, myopia (Chapter 12) can be associated with several abnormalities at the level of the RPE that can be ophthalmoscopically similar to the entities discussed in this chapter.

The disorders discussed here are a source of distress for many ophthalmologists for a variety of reasons. Some of the conditions can cause legal blindness at a relatively young age while others usually have a very benign clinical course. Despite the descriptive nature of many of their names (e.g., butterfly dystrophy), it is often quite difficult to distinguish between them in individual patients using ophthalmoscopy alone. Several different terms have been used to describe each disorder in the literature, and there seem to be more different classification schemes than diseases themselves.

These difficulties notwithstanding, some of these entities are common enough that they are encountered from time to time in most general and pediatric ophthalmology practices and, so long as the ophthalmologist can provide a discussion of prognosis and risk of recurrence to the affected patient and their family, then the exact name attached to the condition is of little importance.

The main goal of this chapter is to provide the general or pediatric ophthalmologist with a practical approach to patients with these disorders that will allow most cases to be correctly diagnosed with a minimum of laboratory investigation and which allow the most serious errors in diagnosis and genetic counseling to be avoided. A secondary goal is to give the reader an appreciation of the history and genetic complexity of these diseases and their potential importance to our understanding of normal and pathological macular physiology.

HISTORICAL ORIGIN OF AN OPHTHALMOSCOPICALLY BASED NOMENCLATURE

Some of the diseases discussed in this chapter were recognized shortly after the introduction of the direct ophthalmoscope and were initially thought to be inflammatory. The familial nature of these conditions was clarified in the first decades of the twentieth century. Despite the variable expressivity of many of these disorders, the near-total reliance on the ophthalmoscope for diagnosis resulted in the evolution of a descriptive nomenclature that persists to the present day.

A tacit assumption in any system that classifies diseases on the basis of their ophthalmoscopic appearance is that lesions that look alike are similar in other ways; that is, for such a system to be clinically useful, a lesion's appearance should have some relationship to its clinical behavior. This notion is often extended to include an expectation that similar-appearing diseases have similar pathophysiological mechanisms and even similar responses to therapy.

Unfortunately, such assumptions are frequently not valid and can cloud one's thinking; this is especially true for the dystrophies discussed in this chapter as well as the heritable photoreceptor degenerations discussed in the next.

INEQUALITY BETWEEN OPHTHALMOSCOPIC APPEARANCE AND BIOCHEMICAL ABNORMALITY

The mechanical analogy depicted in Figure 4-1 is useful for understanding why ophthalmoscopically similar diseases can behave very differently. At the level of ophthalmoscopy, the retina is a "black box" whose individual molecular components cannot be visualized. Only the end result of the function or dysfunction of the parts can be seen, depicted in Figure 4-1 as a pair of clock hands that move as a result of the movement of the other parts. Note that an electrical generator is also connected at one point in the power train such that additional diagnostic information can be obtained by sampling the output of the generator.

In this system, loss of gears "a," "b," "c," "d," "e," or "f" would result in an identical result: lack of movement of the

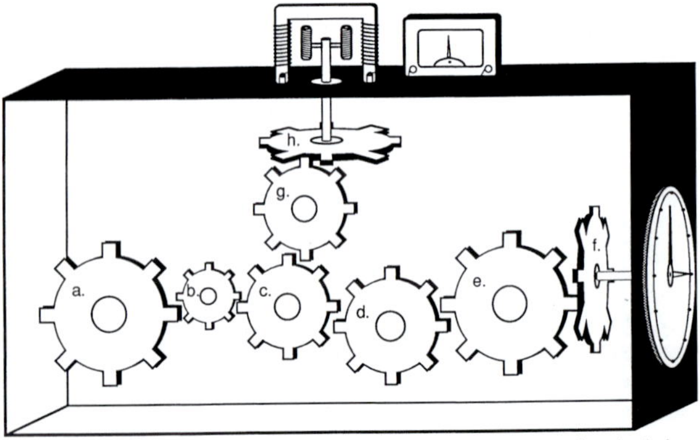

FIGURE 4-1. Mechanical analogy of inherited eye disease. The clock face on the right-hand side of the machine represents the function of the retina (or retinal pigment epithelium) as visualized by ophthalmoscopy. The meter at the top of the machine represents a detectable voltage produced by the generator connected to gear *h*. The various gears inside the machine correspond to specific components, all of which must be normal if the clock hands and the electric generator are to function normally.

hands. Measurement of the voltage produced by the generator could distinguish between lesions proximal and distal to gear "c" but not between lesions in each group. An enlargement of gear "a" would make the hands move faster, and a reduction in size would make the hands move more slowly. Thus, lesions affecting the same part can look different to the observer while lesions affecting different parts can look the same. A nomenclature based upon clock movement would not correctly group the disorders according to the components actually affected.

In human beings, the situation is further complicated by the diploid nature of the genetic material. That is, there are potentially two different blueprints (genes) for each component—one inherited from each parent. Consider the situation in which each parent carries one inactive gene for "gear a." Both parents are phenotypically normal because their normal gene for "gear a" is capable of directing the manufacture of a sufficient quantity of that gear that all their machines still work normally. In contrast, if one of their children inherits both defective genes, the child is not able to make "gear a" at all and none of his machines work, which is the situation for disorders with a recessive inheritance pattern.

If a parent has a gene for an enlarged "gear a," some of the machines in that parent will have rapidly moving clocks that might be detectable clinically. Any child who inherits the gene for the enlarged gear would have a similar phenotype, the situation for dominantly inherited conditions. Note that this example illustrates that different defects in the same gene can cause phenotypes with different inheritance patterns.

Suppose a fraction of the population have genes that result in clock hands that are more fragile than the rest and that this fragility causes no problems so long as the rate of clock movement is normal. If a child with fragile clock hands inherits a large "gear a" from a parent, the outcome might be more severe than if his sibling with strong clock hands inherited it. Thus, the presence of other genes (the genetic background) can alter the effect of a disease-causing gene.

The ideal nomenclature for referring to defects in the machine depicted in Figure 4-1 would precisely describe each defect; for example, "gear 'a' missing" or "gear 'a' has 32 teeth with 50% fragile clock hands." Molecular biology is making such a component-based nomenclature a reality for ophthalmic diseases. As discussed more fully in the next chapter (Chapter 5), some retinal diseases can now be diagnosed by identifying the precise genetic defect to the level of a single nucleotide, allowing patients with identical defects to be grouped for study even if they are seen by different investigators in different centers. Thus, within the past few years we have been able to ascertain whether such similar disorders as Stickler syndrome and Wagner syndrome are really the same genetic and biochemical disorder.

The advent of molecular biology holds great promise not only for the diagnosis and classification of heritable diseases but also for understanding the pathophysiology well enough to design effective therapy. To return to the mechanical analogy, one would be hard pressed to design an effective therapy knowing only that the clock hands did not move. Even worse, if the patient population consisted of patients with all possible gear abnormalities, one might statistically overlook the beneficial effect of replacing "gear a" in patients lacking that part because this treatment would have no benefit in the phenotypically identical patients with defects in other components.

After extolling the virtues of molecular biology, it is important to add that this new technology in no way lessens the importance of skillful clinical ophthalmology. On the contrary, for a molecular biologist to find a disease-causing gene, clinicians must first identify families affected with the disease and correctly diagnose various family members. Moreover, as different mutations are identified in patients with inherited diseases, it will be the correlation of a clinical phenotype with each mutation that will give molecular diagnosis real prognostic power. Last, even though the clinician may be aided by the availability of molecular diagnosis, he or she still must interpret the meaning of such tests for patients and their families.

GENERAL APPROACH TO PATIENTS WITH BILATERAL LESIONS OF THE POSTERIOR POLE

Table 4-1 gives a differential diagnosis of flecks, drusen, vitelliform lesions, atrophy, and pigment disruption affecting the posterior pole. There are several general questions that apply to patients who have such lesions which should be addressed before the individual disease entities are considered.

When a lesion of the posterior pole is discovered either incidentally or because the patient has visual complaints, a few bits

TABLE 4-1. Differential Diagnosis of Flecks, Drusen, Vitelliform Lesions, Atrophy, and Pigment Disruption in the Posterior Pole.

1. Stargardt's disease
2. Best's vitelliform dystrophy
3. The pattern dystrophies
4. Drusen
5. North Carolina macular dystrophy
6. Sorsby's macular dystrophy
7. Fenestrated sheen macular dystrophy
8. Crystalline macular dystrophy
9. Congenital stationary night blindness (see Chapter 5)
10. Inflammatory lesions of the retina and retinal pigment epithelium (see Chapter 11)
11. Toxic retinopathies (see Chapter 11)
12. Myopia (see Chapter 12)
13. Systemic diseases (see Chapter 13)
14. Cone dystrophies (see Chapter 5)

of historical data coupled with some features of the clinical examination can rule out a large number of entities from the differential diagnosis. First, are the lesions bilaterally symmetrical? Most heritable dystrophies affecting the posterior pole are quite symmetrical. Of course, one eye may have already progressed to a more atrophic stage than the other eye and thus the lesions might appear ophthalmoscopically different, but it is unusual for one macula to be totally normal while the other macula has an easily observable lesion. Unilateral lesions should lead one to seriously consider other diagnoses such as choroidal hemangiomas or nevi or the sequelae of trauma or inflammation. The next information to gather is a family history. One should ask whether any relatives have poor vision even with glasses, whether anyone has been unable to obtain or keep a driver's license, or if any have been diagnosed with "macular degeneration." The latter diagnosis is often given to patients with familial disorders of the posterior pole who manage to reach their fifth decade before coming to ophthalmologic attention. If any relatives have accompanied the patient to the clinic, it is wise to try to examine them as well. It is not uncommon to discover macular lesions similar to those in the patient in an asymptomatic relative.

One should ask whether the patient has any difficulty seeing with dim illumination. Good questions to assess a patient's scotopic visual function include whether the patient has unusual difficulty finding his seat in a movie theater and whether they can see individual stars on a clear night. Strongly positive answers to these questions should suggest one of the photoreceptor disorders discussed in Chapter 5. One should also ask whether the patient has any other medical problems and in particular any unusual skin lesions, kidney problems, liver problems, or hearing difficulties. Strongly positive answers to these questions might suggest one of the systemic disorders associated with maculopathy such as Sjogren–Larsson syndrome, Alagille's syndrome, or Alport's syndrome (see Chapter 13). Last, it is important to ask the patient about exposure to medications. The most important of these are neuroleptics, medications for arthritis (especially chloroquine), oral tanning compounds, cancer drugs (tamoxifen), desferoxamine, and illicit intravenous drugs that might have been diluted with talc.

As with any complaint, one should determine the onset of the symptoms and whether it was associated with any other illness. For example, a sudden onset of visual dysfunction associated with a viral illness might suggest one of the inflammatory lesions discussed in Chapter 11. It is important to correctly identify toxic and inflammatory diseases for two reasons. First, one should not raise the specter of an inherited disease while considering an inflammatory or toxic etiology; and, if a toxic source can be identified, decreased exposure to the toxin may result in a stabilization or even improvement in vision.

If, after these questions, there is no history of systemic disease or drug exposure, no history of difficulty with night vision, and the time course is inconsistent with an inflammatory disease, there is a great likelihood that the patient is affected with a disorder falling in the first eight categories of Table 4-1. The specific diagnosis can usually be made with a combination of three procedures: (1) examination of other family members, (2) electro-oculography and/or electroretinography, and (3) fluorescein angiography. If there is any history of difficulty with night vision the situation can be further clarified by the addition of dark adaptometry and electroretinography (discussed further in Chapter 5). It is important to keep in mind that these disorders are heritable and that the patient may be more concerned with the chance of transmitting the disorder to future generations than with their own visual prognosis. Because the explanation of patterns of inheritance and risk of recurrence can be difficult for a patient to fully understand on a single visit, it is a good idea to send a follow-up letter to the patient stating one's opinion of the diagnosis and the recurrence risk. The patient will find such a letter very helpful when explaining the condition to other family members or other physicians involved in their care. Fortunately, the most common diseases in this group (drusen, the pattern dystrophies, and Best's disease) have a fairly good prognosis for good central vision into the sixth decade. As discussed more fully here, Stargardt's disease has the poorest prognosis for central vision but is usually inherited in an autosomal recessive fashion. Thus, a patient with Stargardt's disease usually has a very small risk of having an affected child.

Last, it should be mentioned that although the pathophysiological processes that result in visual loss in these diseases cannot at the present time be arrested or reversed, it is certainly not true that these diseases are untreatable. At the very least, patients can use an Amsler grid to help detect sudden changes in vision that could herald a treatable choroidal neovascular membrane. There is some evidence that certain patients with retinal degenerations may benefit from vitamin supplementation and reduction in ultraviolet light exposure. In addition, patients can be referred to a low vision specialist when appropriate to maintain their visual function at its highest possible level. Children with 20/100 or 20/200 vision can often do very well in regular schools, especially if the ophthalmologist takes the time to communicate with a child's teacher about the child's abilities and limitations.

STARGARDT'S DISEASE

Stargardt's disease is a familial maculopathy that was first described in 1909.[67] It is a rare condition that most general ophthalmologists will encounter only a few times during their career. The natural history of the disease is a progressive loss of central vision, usually to the level of legal blindness. A natural history study by Fishman and coworkers[22] showed that once a patient's visual acuity falls to 20/40, progression to the 20/200 level usually occurs within about 5 years. It is important to realize that such information is a population average because Stargardt's disease can behave quite differently in different families and among different individuals within the same family. At one extreme, a patient may present within the first decade of life complaining of decreased visual acuity. Ophthalmoscopic evaluation may reveal no discernible abnormality, and many such patients are initially thought to be malingerers. The presenting visual acuity may be as poor as 20/60 or 20/80 without overt ophthalmoscopic abnormalities (Figs. 4-2, 4-3). In many

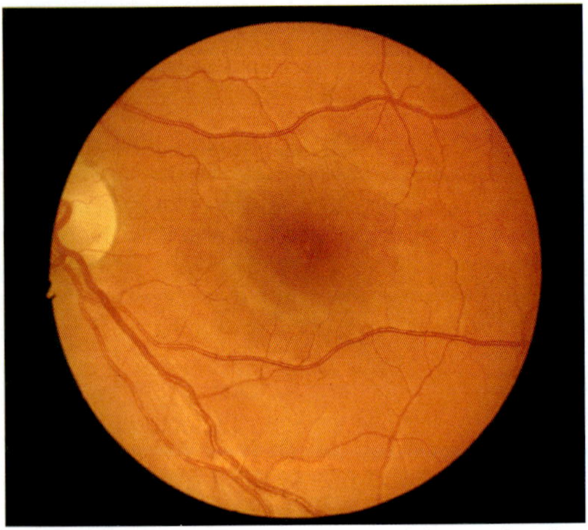

FIGURE 4-2. Early Stargardt's disease with subtle maculopathy. Color photograph reveals subtle yellow deposits at the level of the retinal pigment epithelium. The visual acuity in this eye is 20/80.

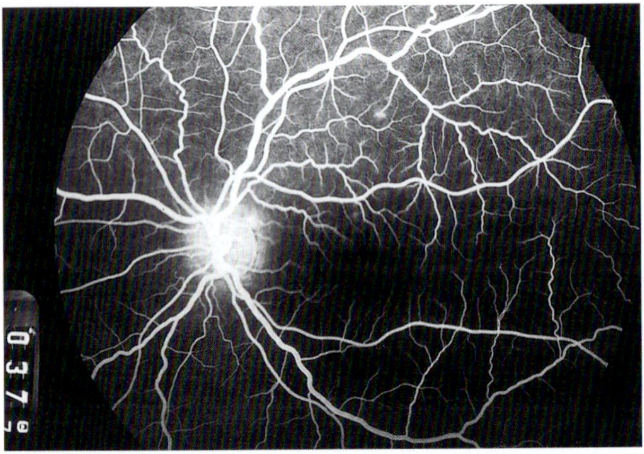

FIGURE 4-3. Fluorescein angiogram from patient shown in Figure 4-2 shows the retinal vasculature to be brightly fluorescent against the background of a dark choroid. This patient illustrates the value of a fluorescein angiogram for making the diagnosis of Stargardt's disease in its early stages.

cases, yellowish "pisciform" flecks and dots eventually appear in the macula and near the periphery (Fig. 4-4). Patches of geographic atrophy may develop and coalesce to form a "beaten bronze" appearance in the macula, which may occur in the absence of flecks in some cases (Figs. 4-5, 4-6). Patients with an early-onset variety of Stargardt's disease can have a visual acuity of 20/200 at the beginning of their second decade. At the other extreme, some patients present with an ophthalmoscopic appearance consistent with Stargardt's disease in mid- or late adult life. These patients often have near-normal visual acuity when first seen even though the macular abnormality is easily visible. These patients may retain good vision for many years but it seems that, even in these late-onset cases, once the visual acuity drops to 20/40 or so a more precipitous visual loss will occur within the next 5 years.[22] Some patients have only peripheral flecks, with little macular involvement. This pattern has been termed fundus flavimaculatus and has been considered by some authors to be a distinct disease. However, pedigrees have been described in which some patients have a *fundus flavimaculatus* appearance whereas other family members have a pronounced maculopathy.[1] Thus, at least in some families, the two

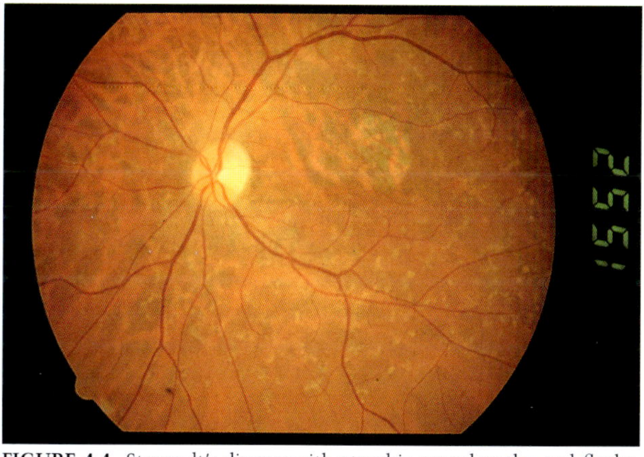

FIGURE 4-4. Stargardt's disease with atrophic maculopathy and flecks. The visual acuity in this eye is 20/500. The peripheral flecks have often been described as "pisciform" because of their resemblance to a fish tail. The individual elements of the yellowish deposits meet one another at acute angles. The maculopathy in this patient is atrophic without the "beaten metal" appearance seen in some patients.

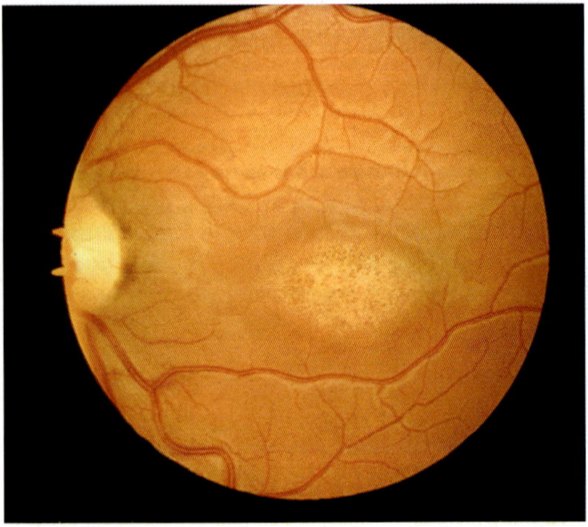

FIGURE 4-5. Stargardt's maculopathy without flecks. Note the "beaten metal" appearance of the macula without noticeable peripheral flecks. The visual acuity in this left eye is 20/100.

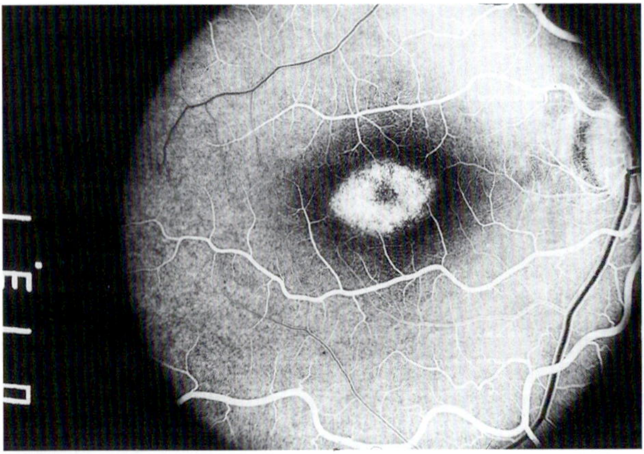

FIGURE 4-6. Fluorescein angiogram of the right eye of the patient shown in Figure 4-5. Filling of the choriocapillaris is normal in this midvenous phase angiogram. The area of the maculopathy is hyperfluorescent, reflecting the loss of retinal pigment epithelial cells in this zone. This patient illustrates that the absence of a "masked choroid" does not rule out the diagnosis of Stargardt's disease.

patterns are simply different clinical manifestations of the same heritable disorder.

It is important to recognize that Stargardt's disease can affect fairly young children or adults. Figure 4-7 is a cumulative age distribution of a series of Stargardt's patients reported by Aaberg,[1] which shows that a sizeable proportion of patients are first diagnosed in each of the first three decades of life. It is interesting that one patient included in this series was first diagnosed at age 71, which illustrates the potential overlap between the heritable dystrophies and "age-related" macular disease.

The most common presenting symptom in Stargardt's disease is decreased central vision. In those cases in which the macular lesions are subtle, it is important to remember that the juvenile form of ceroid lipofuscinosis can also present in a similar fashion. Thus, some questions should be asked about other neurological functions when this presentation is encountered.

There are no known systemic manifestations of Stargardt's disease. The condition is usually inherited in an autosomal recessive fashion, although autosomal dominant pedigrees cer-

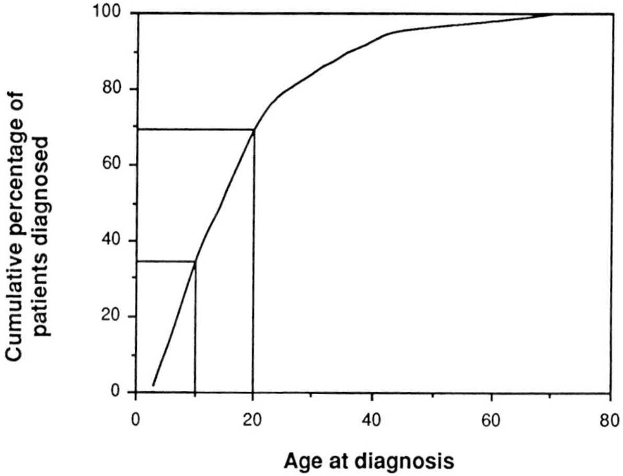

FIGURE 4-7. Cumulative distribution of the age at first diagnosis for a series of Stargardt's disease patients reported by Aaberg.[1] Age in years is given on the X axis; percentage of patients diagnosed at or before that age is given on the Y axis. Approximately one-third of the patients came to attention in each of the first two decades of life whereas the remaining third were diagnosed later. The oldest patient in this series was first diagnosed at age 71.

tainly do exist.[12,21,40] The autosomal dominant disease can be as severe as early-onset recessive Stargardt's or a mild condition that is difficult to distinguish from the pattern dystrophies.

As with Best's disease, the pathophysiology of Stargardt's disease is poorly understood. Several pathological studies have demonstrated lipofuscin accumulation within the retinal pigment epithelium. Mutations in the retina-specific ATP-binding cassette transporter gene (ABCR) cause recessive Stargardt's disease.[2] Most families with autosomal dominant Stargardt-like macular dystrophy have mapped to a locus on chromosome 6q[70] and appear to share a common ancester.[18]

The most helpful laboratory test for Stargardt's disease is a fluorescein angiogram. Between 50% and 80% of patients with Stargardt's disease exhibit a phenomenon known as a dark or masked choroid.[21,72] In such cases, the retinal circulation is seen in sharp contrast against a hypofluorescent choroid (see Fig. 4-3). The most likely explanation for this phenomenon is a blockage of choroidal fluorescence by lipofuscin-laden retinal pigment epithelial cells. The absence of this sign does not rule out Stargardt's disease (see Fig. 4-6), but its presence is quite helpful.

Stargardt's disease can be difficult to differentiate from early-onset progressive cone–rod dystrophies in children. Although the former usually stabilizes at 20/200 vision, the latter may progress to almost complete blindness. Some systemic disorders, such as neuronal ceroid lipofuscinosis, may have as the presenting sign a maculopathy that appears like Stargardt's, but the visual and systemic prognosis are much worse. Thus, it is wise to follow children closely for 6 months to a year after the initial diagnosis before giving a definitive prognosis. As genetic testing becomes more standard, it will be easier to distinguish phenocopies from each other.

There is no medical treatment for Stargardt's disease but, because many of these patients are relatively young when they lose vision, they are often highly motivated to use various low-vision aids. Prompt referral to a low-vision specialist can be very helpful for some patients.

BEST'S DISEASE

Best's vitelliform dystrophy[7] was first described in 1905 by Friedrich Best. The disorder is rare, and a general ophthalmologist may encounter only one or two affected families in an entire career. The natural history of the disease is variable. Vitelliform lesions may be observed shortly after birth in some affected individuals but they can also appear after 50 years of age. In most cases, affected patients retain reading and driving vision in at least one eye well into the seventh decade. Nonetheless, patients who can read the Snellen chart at the 20/30 to 20/50 level still complain that the distortion of their vision and small paracentral scotomas make reading and driving difficult in some situations. Choroidal neovascularization seems to occur in about 5% of affected eyes. Unfortunately, when such membranes do occur, they are often obscured by the lipofuscin pigment, which makes laser treatment difficult if not impossible. Moreover, the visual acuity in affected patients can drop several lines rather suddenly, suggesting the presence of a choroidal neovascular membrane, but a few weeks later return to near-normal levels.

The most common presenting symptom is decreased visual acuity and metamorphopsia. The ocular manifestations can range from a classic vitelliform lesion (Fig. 4-8) to smaller lesions more typical of one of the pattern dystrophies (Fig. 4-9). Late in the disease, geographic atrophy may be present at the site of the original macular lesion (Fig. 4-10). In a few patients, small

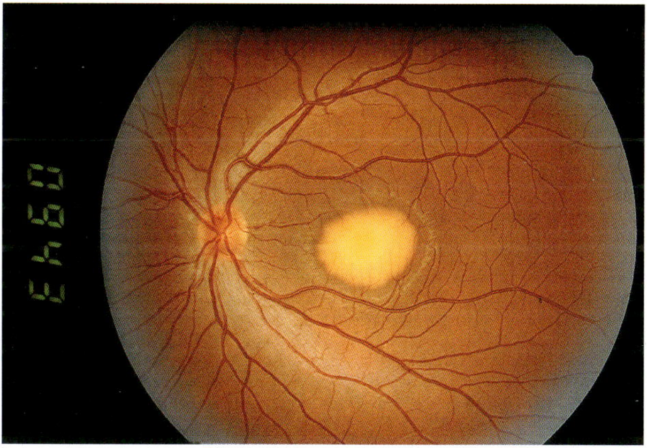

FIGURE 4-8. Best's vitelliform dystrophy with a classic "egg yolk" deposit of lipofuscin material beneath the retinal pigment epithelium (RPE) of the central macula. The vitelliform lesions were first noted in this patient at age 12; this photograph was taken at age 18. The visual acuity in this eye remains 20/20.

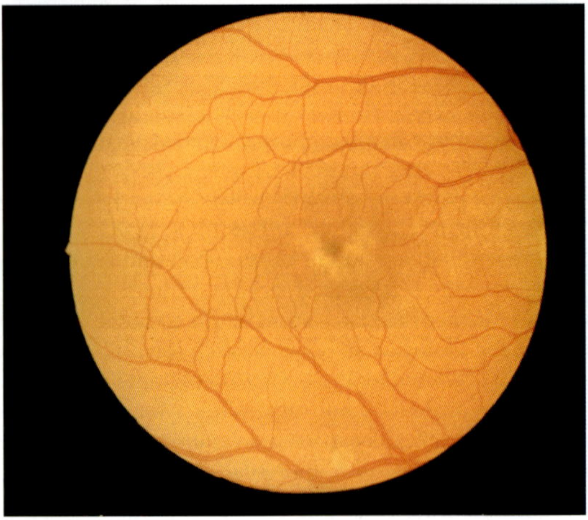

FIGURE 4-9. Dot and halo lesion in a patient with Best's disease, showing the right eye of a 34-year-old woman who is a cousin of the patient shown in Figure 4-8. The visual acuity in this eye is 20/40. The central hyperpigmentation surrounded by a halo of lipofuscin and atrophy is frequently seen in the pattern dystrophies. This patient illustrates that this finding is somewhat nonspecific and can be seen in Best's disease as well.

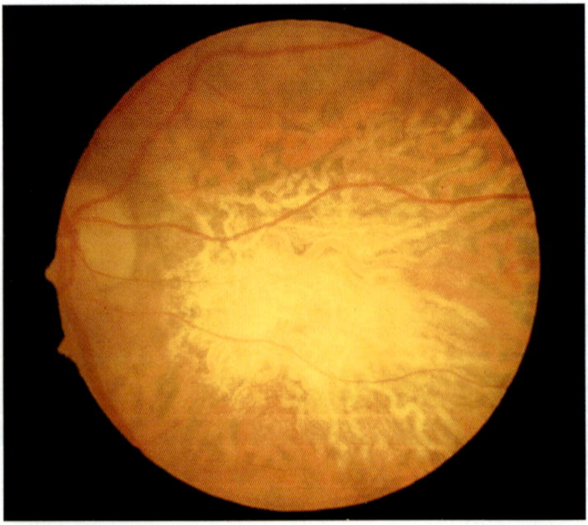

FIGURE 4-10. Choroidal sclerosis in Best's disease showing the left eye of a 78-year-old woman who is the great-aunt of the patient shown Figure 4-9. The visual acuity in the eye is 20/400. The patient is an obligate carrier of the Best's gene. There is total absence of the retinal pigment epithelium centrally with an associated loss of the choriocapillaris. The large choroidal vessels appear "sclerotic" against a background of almost bare sclera. This appearance can be seen as the end stage of several maculopathies including Best's disease, the pattern dystrophies, Stargardt's disease, and age-related macular degeneration.

pisciform deposits of lipofuscin reminiscent of Stargardt's disease can be seen late in the disease course (Fig. 4-11).

There are no systemic manifestations of Best's disease. The condition is inherited as an autosomal dominant trait with variable expressivity and incomplete penetrance. However, it is important to realize that the degree of penetrance of any disorder is dependent on the method used to diagnose it. That is, there are patients at 50% risk for Best's disease who have an absolutely normal fundus but later have children affected with the disease, which occurs in about 5% of patients in our experience. Thus, the penetrance of ophthalmoscopically visible disease at age 35 is 90% to 95%. In contrast, we have never observed a patient with a normal electro-oculogram (EOG) who had children affected with classic Best's disease. Thus, if the EOG is used for diagnosis, the penetrance of the disease is nearly 100%. Mutations in the VMD2 (vitelliform macular dystrophy) gene on chromosome 11 are responsible for Best's disease.[51,71] Ferrell and colleagues linked an atypical vitelliform dystrophy

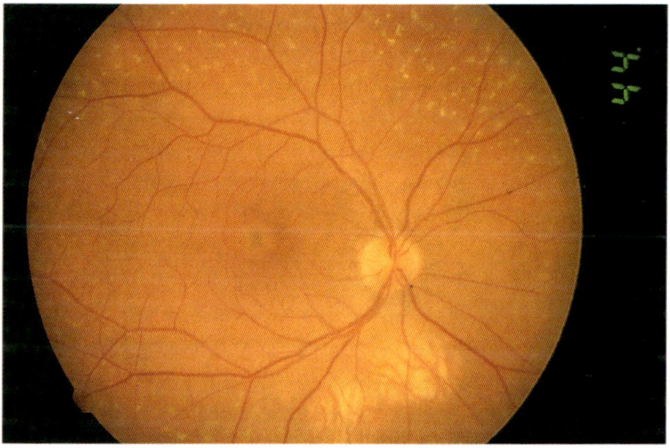

FIGURE 4-11. Pigmented vitelliform lesion, atrophy, and peripheral flecks in a patient with Best's disease. The left eye is shown of an 80-year-old patient with Best's disease who has children and nieces who are affected with classic vitelliform lesions. When first seen at age 52, his macula was found to be completely normal. When reexamined 28 years later, small pigmented vitelliform lesions were discovered. Later, he developed eccentric patches of retinal pigmented epithelium (RPE) atrophy and "pisciform" flecks reminiscent of fundus flavimaculatus or Stargardt's disease. This patient illustrates that abnormal lipofuscin-like accumulations can occur very late in patients with Best's disease.

to the classical genetic marker GPT-1, which was localized to the long arm of chromosome 8.[20] Their family had some clinical features that were not typical of classic Best's disease. Specifically, some affected individuals had normal or near-normal EOG ratios, and none of the patients had vitelliform lesions larger than one disk diameter in size.[33] Bestrophin, the product of the VMD2 gene, localizes to the basolateral plasma membrane of the retinal pigment epithelium.[43] The function remains unknown.

Without question, the best laboratory study to establish the presence of Best's disease is the electro-oculogram (Fig. 4-12). This test is based on the measurement of an electrical potential that is generated at or near the interface between the retinal pigment epithelial cells and the photoreceptors. In a normal eye, this potential responds to changes in illumination in the following way. If an eye is light adapted, and the lights are subsequently turned off, the resting potential falls gradually to a "dark trough" 10 to 15 min later. When the light is switched on again, this potential rises over the next 10 to 12 minutes to a value that is roughly twice the magnitude of the dark trough. The EOG test result is usually expressed as the *Arden ratio*[3] of the light peak to dark trough. This ratio is insensitive to variations in skin conductivity and other variables that do affect the magnitudes of the individual voltages. The exact magnitude of the Arden ratio is dependent on the size and intensity of the light stimulus but is fairly reproducible with a given instrument. In a patient with Best's disease, there is little change in this resting voltage regardless of the light condition. Thus, when the lights are turned off the voltage falls very little and when the lights are turned on again the voltage rises little if at all. Thus, patients with Best's disease have a light peak to dark trough ratio of less than 1.5. This electrical abnormality is probably present at birth and can precede the development of ophthalmoscopically visible lesions by several decades. Figure 4-12 shows the EOG patterns from two siblings from a family affected with Best's disease. One can see that the affected brother has a diminished Arden ratio (1.2–1.3) whereas the unaffected brother has ratios greater than 2.0.

Our understanding of the pathophysiology of Best's disease is limited. The few specimens that have been studied histopathologically have revealed lipofuscin accumulations within retinal pigment epithelial cells and in the sub-RPE space.[24,50,77] Some material has also been described within the

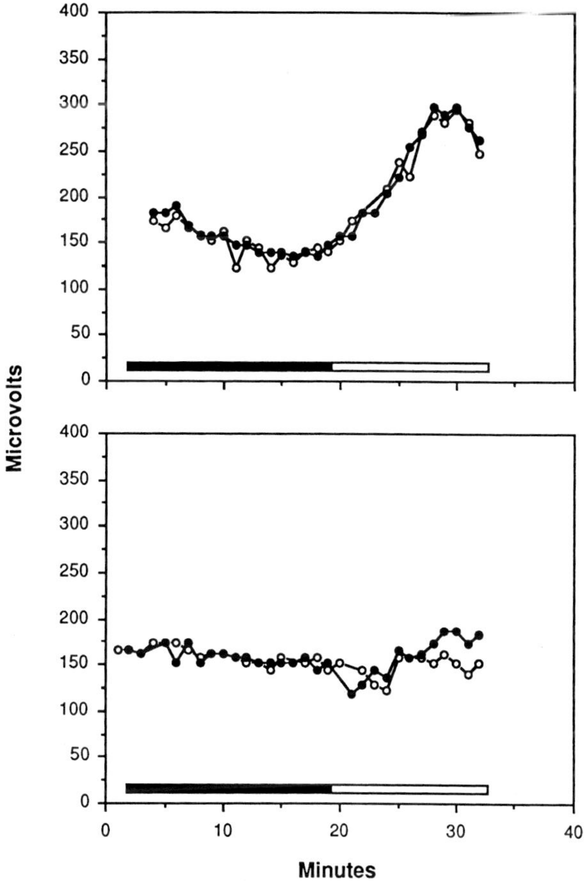

FIGURE 4-12. Electro-oculograms of two brothers from a family affected with Best's disease. *Closed circles*, measurements from the right eye; *open circle*, measurements from the left eye. The *bar* beneath each recording depicts the state of retinal illumination (*closed*, dark; *open*, light). *Top:* recordings from the eyes of the unaffected patient. The voltage recorded at the peak of the light response in this patient is twofold higher than that recorded in the dark. *Bottom:* abnormal recordings from the affected patient. The average ratio of the "light peak" to "dark trough" voltages in this patient is 1.2.

retina itself. Unfortunately, no pathological specimen of an early vitelliform lesion has been studied. Thus, we do not have any direct knowledge of the exact configuration of the vitelliform lesion. It seems likely that the "egg yolk" lies beneath the retinal pigment epithelium because patients with such lesions can still have normal visual acuity. Thus, it is unlikely that this material is between the retinal pigment epithelial cells and the photoreceptors. Some authors believe that the material is confined to the retinal pigment epithelial cells themselves, but the pseudohypopyon appearance of some lesions (Fig. 4-13) argues for an extracellular location of this material. It is not known whether this material accumulates because of a defect in macular metabolism, or whether the lipofuscin is a normal metabolic by-product that simply has difficulty transiting Bruch's membrane to reach the circulation of the choriocapillaris. The autosomal dominant nature of the disorder would be

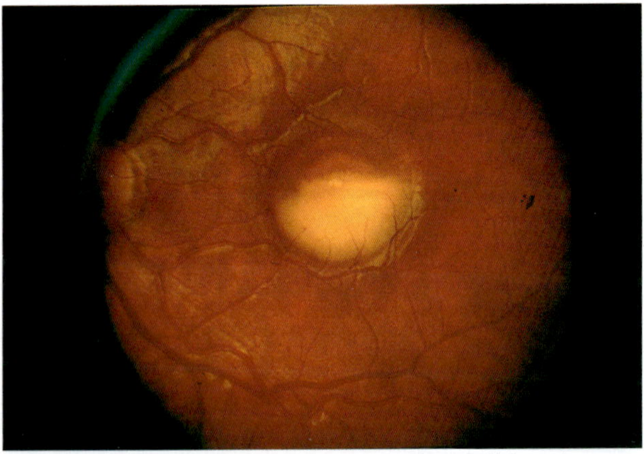

FIGURE 4-13. Pseudohypopyon appearance of a vitelliform lesion in Best's disease, showing the left eye of a 12-year-old patient who is the grandson of the patient shown in Figure 4-10. The visual acuity in this eye was 20/50 at the time of this photograph but improved to 20/20 before age 20. Note that the lipofuscin material has "layered out" with a thicker component below and a serous component above. This figure suggests that the vitelliform collection of lipofuscin is in the sub-RPE space. If it were confined to the retinal pigment epithelial cells, it would not be able to layer gravitationally. If it were present in the subretinal space, the visual acuity would not be 20/50.

more compatible with a structural abnormality than an enzymatic one.

There is no medical treatment for Best's disease. As already mentioned briefly, choroidal neovascular membranes occur in a few percent of affected eyes and in some cases might be amenable to laser photocoagulation. Such treatment would be complicated by the fact that the membranes would most likely develop beneath the lipofuscin pigment, which would make visualization difficult. It is also important to recognize that these patients rarely have aggressive disciform processes evolving from such membranes. Thus, it is probably hazardous to extrapolate the laser treatment benefits obtained in age-related macular degeneration to patients with Best's disease.

THE PATTERN DYSTROPHIES

Between 1950 and 1977, at least eight different hereditary maculopathies were reported in the ophthalmic literature as new and distinct entities (Fig. 4-14). As a group, these disorders are characterized by relatively good vision in the first five decades of life, a striking pattern of yellow or black pigmentation at the level of the retinal pigment epithelium, and a relative absence of typical drusen. Most of the *pattern dystrophies* have normal or near-normal findings on psychophysical and electrophysiological tests. The notable exception is that affected individuals in some pedigrees have a moderately abnormal EOG.[16]

Sjogrens's reticular dystrophy[15,58] is an autosomal recessive disease characterized by a network of pigmented lines surrounding the macula that resembles a fishnet with knots at the intersections of the lines. Autosomal dominant pedigrees of reticular dystrophies have also been reported. The EOG is abnormal.[38] Fundus pulverulentus[60] is a presumably autosomal dominant condition with RPE mottling in the posterior pole and near periphery. Slezak and Hommer considered that this disorder was distinguishable from Sjogren's dystrophy by the absence of reticular lines. Benedikt and Werner[6] reported a family affected with an autosomal dominant condition that shared features of reticular dystrophy and fundus pulverulentus. One affected patient had the classic reticular lines, whereas others had granular pigmentation without definite lines. *Mesker's macroreticular dystrophy*[45] is characterized by a reticular pigmentation in which the mesh size of the "net" is approximately one disc diameter

	a	b	c	d
Reticular Autosomal Recessive Sjogren, 1950	●	●	●	●
Grouped Pigmentary Dystrophy Autosomal Dominant Forgacs and Bozin, 1966			●	
Fundus Pulverulentus Autosomal Dominant Slezak and Hommer, 1969	●		●	●
Macro-Reticular Autosomal Recessive Mesker, et al. 1970	●	●	●	●
Butterfly Autosomal Dominant Deutman, et al. 1970	●	●	●	●
Reticular Autosomal Dominant Benedikt and Werner, 1971	●			
Adult Foveo-Macular Autosomal Dominant Gass, 1974			●	
Pattern Dominant Marmor and Byers, 1977	●			●

FIGURE 4-14. Four different definitions of pattern dystrophy. The individual disorders that are commonly considered as one of the pattern dystrophies are listed at the *left*. Four of the many publications in the literature that discuss the concept of grouping these as a single clinical entity are indicated by lowercase letters across the top of the figure: *a*, Marmor and Byers 1977;[42] *b*, Hseih, Fine, and Lyons 1977;[35] *c*, Watzke, Folk, and Lang 1982;[74] *d*, de Jong and Delleman 1982.[14] *Black dots* indicate the component dystrophies that each group included in their definition of pattern dystrophy.

in size (at least twice as large as that in Sjogren's cases). *Butterfly dystrophy*[16] is an autosomal dominant disorder in which yellow deposits are seen in the macula at the level of the RPE, radiating from the fovea in a pattern reminiscent of a butterfly's wings (Fig. 4-15). In 1974, Gass[27] described a *peculiar foveomacular dystrophy* characterized by symmetrical, round or oval, yellow lesions in the fovea, approximately one-third disc diameter in size, with a central hyperpigmented spot (Fig. 4-16). Singerman et al.[57] reported a large family with a similar condition that they termed *dominant progressive macular dystrophy*.

Benign concentric annular macular dystrophy[17] is an extremely rare autosomal dominant disorder characterized by a fairly stationary bull's-eye maculopathy that resembles chloroquine toxicity. Some affected patients have electroretinographic, color vision, and dark adaptation abnormalities and some

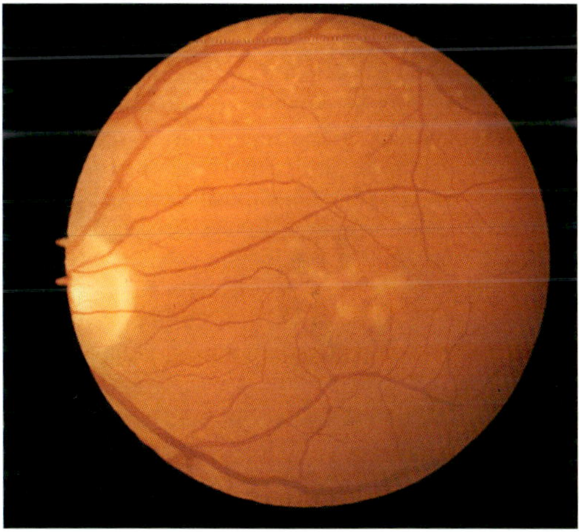

FIGURE 4-15. Butterfly pattern dystrophy, showing the left eye of a 65-year-old patient with 20/50 vision. Butterfly lesions typically have three to five "arms" of yellow sub-RPE material extending from a central collection that may be pigmented.

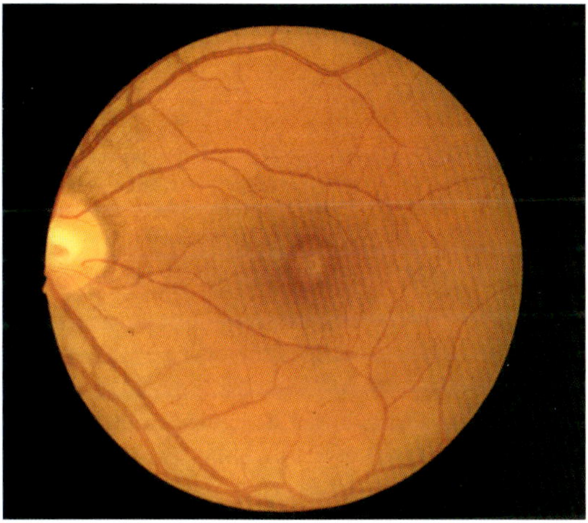

FIGURE 4-16. Peculiar foveomacular dystrophy, showing the left eye of a 41-year-old woman with 20/40 vision. There is a small "one-third disc diameter" vitelliform lesion centered on the foveola. These small lesions can occasionally be seen in families with classic Best's disease. Note the absence of typical drusen.

authors would classify this among the cone dystrophies. However, its good visual prognosis (20/25 at age 68 in one reported patient), coupled with the ophthalmoscopic and angiographic evidence of a macular RPE injury, makes it clinically similar to the other pattern dystrophies discussed here.

The ophthalmoscopic similarity of some of these entities, coupled with their similar clinical course, led several authors[14,35,42,74] to propose grouping these entities under the term pattern dystrophy. Unfortunately, there have been nearly as many different groupings of the component entities as there are entities themselves (see Fig. 4-14). It is curious that none of the authors who proposed pattern dystrophy groupings included dominant Stargardt's disease or the dominant slowly progressive macular dystrophy of Singerman et al.[57] as the clinical and electrophysiological findings in the latter conditions overlap those of the entities they chose to include. The existence of these different classification schemes in the literature has rendered the term pattern dystrophy fairly nonspecific. Nonetheless, it is important to recognize that there are a number of heritable maculopathies that are distinct from familial drusen and from early-onset Stargardt's disease and which in general, have a better prognosis than the latter two disorders.

The most common presenting symptom of one of the pattern dystrophies is a slightly diminished visual acuity or metamorphopsia in a patient in their twenties or thirties. Almost as often, the patients are asymptomatic and come to attention because of the discovery of unusual macular lesions during routine ophthalmoscopy. Individuals affected with one of these disorders will often have relatively young children, nieces, or nephews whom they will ask their ophthalmologist to examine for evidence of the disease. The latter situation is the usual way a pediatric ophthalmologist will encounter these conditions. Some of the pattern dystrophies can definitely be manifest in the first decade of life.[11,15,54]

The most important entity in the differential diagnosis of pattern dystrophy is early-onset Stargardt's disease, which has a much poorer visual prognosis. The finding of a masked choroid on fluorescein angiography (see Fig. 4-3) can help establish the latter diagnosis but the absence of this sign does not rule it out. The presence of a dot or flecklike maculopathy with reduced vision in a patient less than 20 years of age should always be considered to be Stargardt's disease (and a somewhat guarded visual prognosis should be given) unless a number of older family members (a parent, a grandparent, aunts, or uncles) can be shown to have similar lesions with good vision. Another entity that can be distinguished fairly readily from the pattern dystrophies is Best's disease. One can usually find classic vitelliform lesions in at least one family member with the latter disease and, although the EOG Arden ratio can be depressed in pattern dystrophy, it is rarely 1.1 or 1.2 whereas it is usually that low in Best's. It has been my experience that the moderately depressed EOGs in pattern dystrophy occur in older patients with more advanced disease, whereas in Best's disease the EOG ratio can be very low even in ophthalmoscopically normal affected patients in their first decade of life.

With the exception of Sjogren's original family in which spherophakia, iris abnormalities, and deafness were associated with the reticular dystrophy, pattern dystrophies are rarely associated with systemic disorders. Anecdotal association with Crohn's disease has been reported. One important association is with *maternally inherited diabetes and deafness* (MIDD), a mitochondrial disorder in which approximately 85% of adult patients have been reported to exhibit a linear pigmentary maculopathy. The maculopathy appears to be rare in childhood.[44] The pathophysiology of these disorders is largely unknown. One interesting observation is that the distribution of the abnormal pigment in the pattern dystrophies seems to correspond in size and shape with the margins of the choriocapillaris lobules.[42] Such a pattern is fairly nonspecific and can be seen in other retinal disorders,[5] including Best's disease (Fig. 4-17).

Many of the remarks made at the opening of this chapter concerning the genetic heterogeneity of the RPE dystrophies apply directly to the "pattern dystrophies"; that is, nearly every author who has studied one of these families has remarked that certain individuals in the family have ophthalmoscopic appearances compatible with one of the individual dystrophies while other family members appear to have another. Occasionally this occurs in two eyes of one patient.[30,31] One interesting paper reports a 10-year follow-up of a single patient whose lesions evolved through a series of stages, each mimicking one of the individually described pattern dystrophies.[52]

We and others have identified mutations in the *RDS/peripherin gene* in some patients with pattern dystrophies.[46,47,79] However, linkage analysis has excluded the RDS/peripherin gene from involvement in the pattern dystrophy of other large families,[76] indicating that at least two genes must exist that are

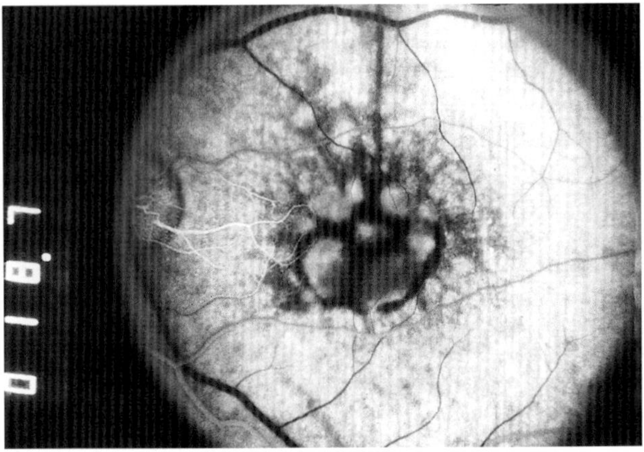

FIGURE 4-17. Reticular pigmentation in a patient with Best's disease, shown in fluorescein angiogram from the right eye of a 49-year-old man who is the father of the patient shown in Figure 4-13. The orientation and periodicity of the hyperpigmentation are similar to that seen in the reticular dystrophies. This distribution has been previously noted to correspond to the interfaces between choriocapillaris lobules.

capable of causing this phenotype. There are reports of the same peripherin/RDS mutations causing clinical presentations appearing such as retinitis pigmentosa, pattern dystrophy, and fundus flavimaculatus in different members of the same family[78]; this reinforces the concept that different genetic defects can produce identical clinical pictures while the same defect can produce different clinical appearances in different people and even in the same person over time.

The treatment of pattern dystrophy is similar to that of other conditions in this chapter. Choroidal neovascular membranes occur in a few percent of affected eyes and may be amenable to laser treatment. Patients should monitor their vision with an Amsler grid and report any sudden changes immediately. However, because the natural history of the disease is fairly benign, and the pattern lesions can stain with fluorescein even in the absence of neovascularization, laser treatment should probably be reserved for patients with discrete, well-visualized, juxta- or extrafoveal membranes. Indocyanine green videoangiography may be useful in some cases.[41]

DRUSEN

Typical *drusen* are small accumulations of lipofuscin within and beneath the retinal pigment epithelium. They are much more common in Caucasians than in darkly pigmented individuals and are more common with increasing age. Visual loss from these lesions is rare before the age of 50, which has led to the use of the term age-related macular degeneration. This term tends to obscure the fact that most drusen are probably inherited in an autosomal dominant fashion.[28] Drusen can range from small, very discrete lesions, (Fig. 4-18) to accumulations of cellular debris and macromolecules that are so large they might better be termed retinal pigment epithelial detachments (Fig. 4-19). Drusen can occasionally be observed in asymptomatic individuals in their third decade. Thus, there is some overlap between this very prevalent entity and the less common pattern dystrophies that were discussed in the previous section.

It is worthwhile to distinguish a second form of drusen that are thought to result from a nodular thickening of the basement membrane of the RPE.[29] These "cuticular" or "basal laminar" drusen (Fig. 4-20) are more commonly seen in younger

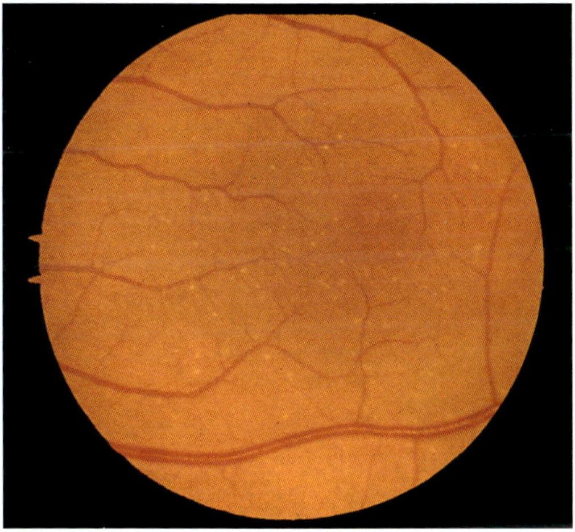

FIGURE 4-18. Small drusen in the left eye of an asymptomatic 35-year-old woman. Visual acuity is 20/25.

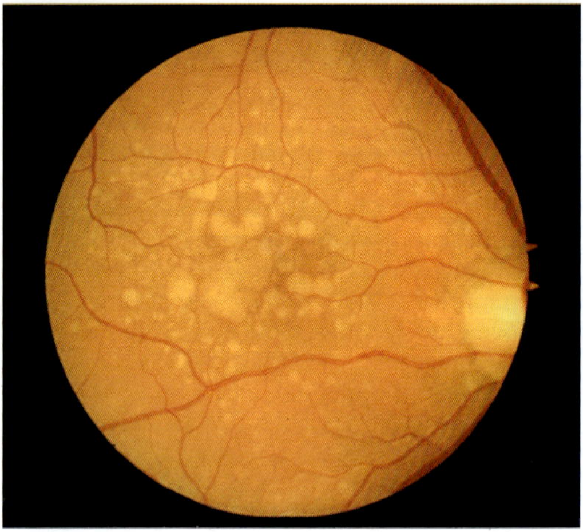

FIGURE 4-19. Large drusen in the left eye of a 60-year-old patient with 20/40 vision. Most of the retinal pigment epithelial abnormality is confined to an area two by three disc diameters in size. At the periphery of this zone, the drusen are rather small; near the center, they coalesce into larger accumulations that may be more appropriately termed retinal pigment epithelial detachments.

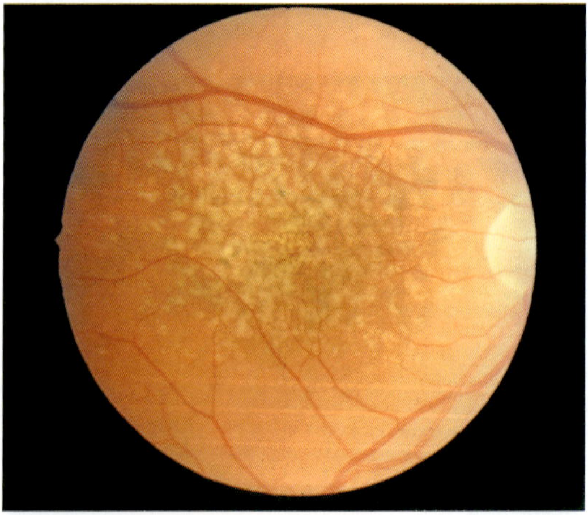

FIGURE 4-20. Cuticular drusen in the right eye of a 42-year-old patient with 20/15 vision. Note the uniformly sized yellow deposits at the level of the retinal pigment epithelium, believed to be nodular thickenings of Bruch's membrane. With time, more typical drusen can become admixed with these cuticular drusen, as is beginning to occur centrally in this patient. In some cases, a vitelliform pigment epithelial detachment can occur. (From Ref. 26, with permission.)

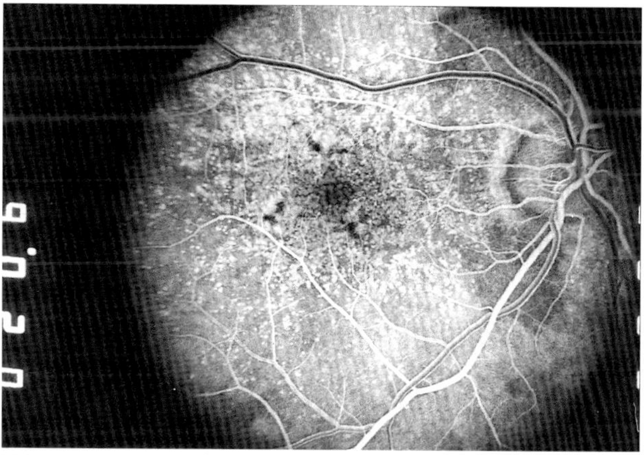

FIGURE 4-21. Cuticular drusen in a midvenous-phase fluorescein angiogram of the patient in Figure 4-20. The drusen hyperfluoresce early and stain in later frames of the study (not shown). The lesions are often more dramatically seen on the angiogram than by ophthalmoscopy.

individuals and are most easily recognized as a myriad of equal-sized hyperfluorescent dots in the early phase of a fluorescein angiogram (Fig. 4-21). With increasing age, typical drusen are often admixed with the cuticular ones, and in late stages even a vitelliform RPE detachment can occur.[26]

The natural history of drusen is variable. Some patients experience a progressive loss of central vision while others have essentially normal vision for many years. The most common presenting symptom is decreased central visual acuity or a recent onset of metamorphopsia. In the latter case, a choroidal neovascular membrane is often found. There are no known systemic manifestations of macular drusen. The most important laboratory test is a fluorescein angiogram for the detection of choroidal neovascularization. As are the other disorders discussed in this chapter, typical drusen are characterized histopathologically by abnormalities of Bruch's membrane and an accumulation of organelles and macromolecules within and beneath the RPE.[19,48,56,73] This appearance could be the result of a defect in metabolism of the RPE or macular retina, but the autosomal dominant nature of the condition would be more compatible with a structural abnormality in Bruch's membrane.

Basal laminar drusen are even more likely to result from a structural abnormality in Bruch's membrane.

The drusen seen in *Malattia Levetinese* and *Doyne honeycomb retinal dystrophy* are autosomal dominant and occur in children as well as adults. Mutations in the EFEMP1 gene on chromosome 2 are the cause.[69] Another form of autosomal dominant drusen has been reported that may present as early as 3 years of age with fine drusen, most conspicuous in the macula, with or without atrophic maculopathy. This form has been mapped to chromosome 6q14.[68] It is of interest that *Alport's syndrome,* which is associated with fine drusen-like deposits at the level of the RPE, has been shown to be caused by a defect in type IV collagen.[4]

The treatment of drusen consists of identifying choroidal neovascular membranes as early as possible and treating them with laser photocoagulation. Many of these patients also benefit from referral to low-vision specialists as the disease progressively affects their central visual acuity.

NORTH CAROLINA MACULAR DYSTROPHY

North Carolina macular dystrophy was initially described by Lefler et al. in 1971.[39] It was further described by Frank and coworkers in 1974,[25] who termed the disease *dominant progressive foveal dystrophy*. This condition has recently been shown to be the same as *central areolar pigment epitheliopathy*.[61] In fact, the individual illustrated in this chapter (Fig. 4-22) was initially reported as part of a series of central areolar pigment epitheliopathy,[32] but was later found to be related to the original large North Carolina dystrophy family.[61]

The most common presenting symptom in North Carolina macular dystrophy is decreased central vision. The onset of disease is very early in life, and the macular lesion probably stabilizes in most patients by 10 years of age. Visual acuity can range from 20/20 to 20/200. Small[63] reexamined 22 individuals originally reported by Frank and coworkers and found that only 1 patient showed evidence of progression of the disease during the two decades that separated the two reports.

The ocular manifestations of the more severe grades of North Carolina dystrophy are clear cut. The center of the lesion appears to be a staphyloma with little if any choroidal or retinal

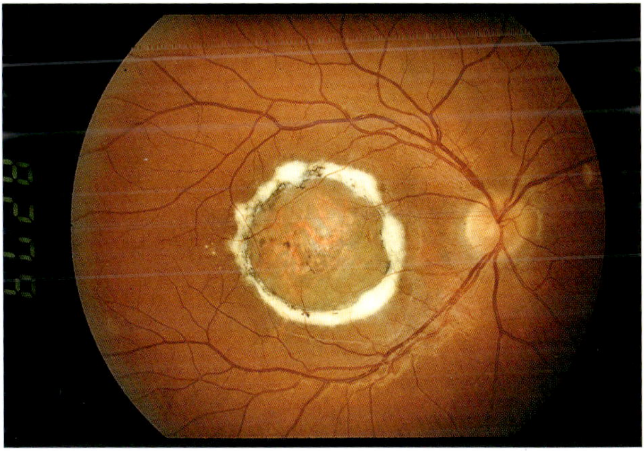

FIGURE 4-22. North Carolina macular dystrophy, showing the right eye of an 11-year-old patient with 20/200 vision. Photographs of this patient at age 9 have been previously published.[61] The lesion and the visual acuity has been stationary since early childhood. Typical features of the disease are the staphylomatous-appearing crater surrounded by a gliotic rim. The base has a shiny appearance similar to that seen in some patients with Stargardt's disease.

pigment epithelial tissue remaining at the base. There is a hypertrophic rim of tissue surrounding the lesion (see Fig. 4-22). Typical-appearing drusen may be observed in the periphery. There are no known systemic manifestations of the disease.

The disease is inherited in an autosomal dominant fashion. The gene that causes the disease was mapped to the long arm of chromosome 6 in 1992 by Small, and the locus has since been further refined. There is no evidence for genetic heterogeneity in this disease.[64] Electroretinography and electro-oculography are normal in North Carolina macular dystrophy. Despite the hypertrophic "disciform" appearance of the edge of these lesions, no active choroidal neovascular membrane has been demonstrated in these patients.[62] Thus, fluorescein angiography is probably not warranted in these patients unless other conditions are being considered.

The pathophysiology of the disease is unknown, but its very early onset, dominant inheritance, and slow progression suggest a structural abnormality at the level of the basement membrane of the RPE.

There is no treatment for North Carolina macular dystrophy. Fortunately, the disease is stable in most patients.

SORSBY'S FUNDUS DYSTROPHY

In 1949, Sorsby et al. reported an extensive study of four large English families affected with an autosomal dominant maculopathy.[66] Although some features of these families are common to dominant drusen and the pattern dystrophies, there are sufficient differences to warrant recognition as a specific entity.

The central feature of *Sorsby's fundus dystrophy* is the development of bilateral subfoveal choroidal neovascular membranes at about the age of 40 years. The macular lesions evolve into a picture of geographic atrophy with pronounced black pigmentation occurring in clumps around the central atrophic zone. Continued peripheral migration of the atrophy results in atrophic areas extending well beyond the temporal arcades with the loss of even ambulatory vision in many patients (Fig. 4-23).

The original families reported by Sorsby and coworkers were later reexamined and reported.[9,34,53] These papers reported an additional early feature of the disease, the appearance of numerous fine drusen or a confluent plaque of yellow material beneath the RPE of the posterior pole. A fluorescein angiographic abnormality was also identified that suggested a decreased perfusion of the choriocapillaris. An additional report described the histopathological features of the disease.[10] A confluent, lipid-containing deposit was seen between the basement membrane of the retinal pigment epithelium and the inner collagenous layers of Bruch's membrane. This deposit differed from that of age-related macular degeneration in that the abnormalities were almost totally limited to the vitreal side of the elastic lamina of Bruch's membrane.

In summary, the term Sorsby's dystrophy should be reserved for an autosomal dominant condition in which central choroidal neovascular membranes occur in the relative absence of typical drusen. It is distinguished from the pattern dystrophies by its relatively poor visual prognosis. That is, many of Sorsby's patients had vision of 20/200 or worse before reaching their sixth decade whereas most patients with pattern dystrophy maintain visual acuities of 20/50 or better in this age range. Moreover, choroidal neovascular membranes occur in only about 5% of patients with the pattern dystrophies. Most families with

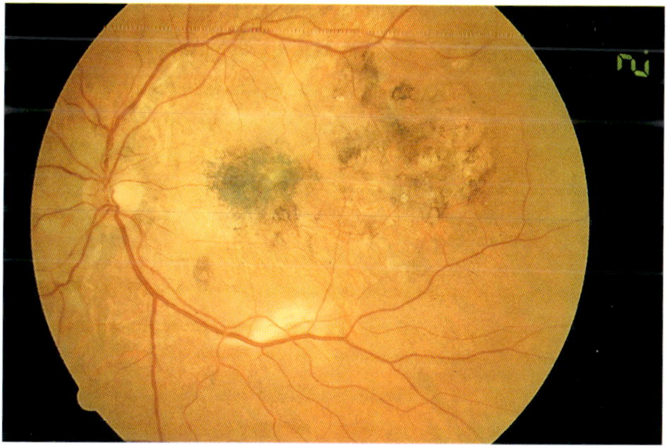

FIGURE 4-23. Sorsby's macular dystrophy, showing the right eye of a 69-year-old man with 20/2000 vision. His 95-year-old mother is similarly affected. Characteristic features include a large area of RPE atrophy extending beyond the temporal arcades. Clumps of hyperpigmentation are admixed with subretinal fibrosis. It is not uncommon for these patients to lose even ambulatory vision by the sixth decade.

Sorsby's fundus dystrophy have been found to harbor mutations in the TIMP3 gene.[75]

There is no curative medical treatment for Sorsby's fundus dystrophy, nor are there any data in the literature regarding the effectiveness of laser treatment for the choroidal neovascular membranes. However, the progressive centrifugal RPE atrophy that occurs even in the absence of overt neovascularization suggests that laser treatment would not be beneficial. There is some evidence that vitamin A supplementation may be beneficial in this disorder.[36]

FENESTRATED SHEEN MACULAR DYSTROPHY

Fenestrated sheen macular dystrophy is an extremely rare autosomal dominant macular dystrophy. Only four families have been described in the literature.[13,49,59,65] The disease is characterized by sharply demarcated small red lesions that are located in the outer retina (Fig. 4-24). No thickening or thinning of the

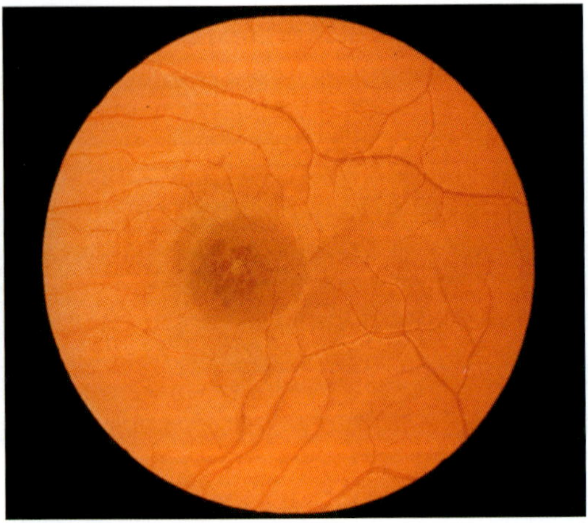

FIGURE 4-24. Fenestrated sheen macular dystrophy, showing the left eye of a 7-year-old patient originally reported by Sneed and Seiving.[65] The reddish discolorations have no associated elevation. With time, the redness fades and is replaced by a more atrophic RPE change. (Courtesy of Sneed and coworkers, used with permission.)

retina is associated with the lesions, only the abnormal color. The red lesions are most noticeable in the first decade of life. In older patients, the red lesions fade and a retinal pigment epithelial mottling appears in its place.

Most affected patients are asymptomatic and come to attention when the retinal lesions are noticed during routine ophthalmoscopy. Sneed and Sieving[65] reported significantly diminished photopic and scotopic ERGs in affected patients. There are no known systemic manifestations of this disease, and the visual prognosis is excellent.

CRYSTALLINE RETINAL DYSTROPHIES

In 1937, Bietti described patients with a disorder of the retinal pigment epithelium and choroid characterized by scattered yellow-white crystals in the posterior pole.[8] These patients also had superficial crystals in the cornea near the limbus. The disorder began in the third decade of life. The presence of *crystalline retinal dystrophy* in siblings suggested the possibility of autosomal recessive inheritance. More recently, histopathological examination of two such cases revealed crystals resembling cholesterol inclusions in the fibroblasts of the cornea and conjunctiva, as well as in circulating lymphocytes.[80] Abnormalities of fatty acid metabolism and absence of fatty acid binding by two cytosolic proteins have been noted. Patients have progressive night blindness and visual field loss. Autosomal recessive Bietti crystalline dystrophy has been linked to chromosome 4q35.[37]

In 1990, Richards and coworkers[55] reported an autosomal dominant family in which nine individuals were affected with a crystalline dystrophy indistinguishable from that described by Bietti (Fig. 4-25). The proband of that family had a subnormal ERG and pericentral scotomas with visual field testing. The proband also had crystal formation in the lysosomes of circulating lymphocytes.

The differential diagnosis of crystalline retinopathy includes *oxalosis*, exposure to methoxyflurane, *cystinosis*, and exposure to certain other drugs including *tamoxifen*, *canthaxanthine*, and talc. The crystalline retinopathy and keratopathy of *cystinosis* begin in childhood.

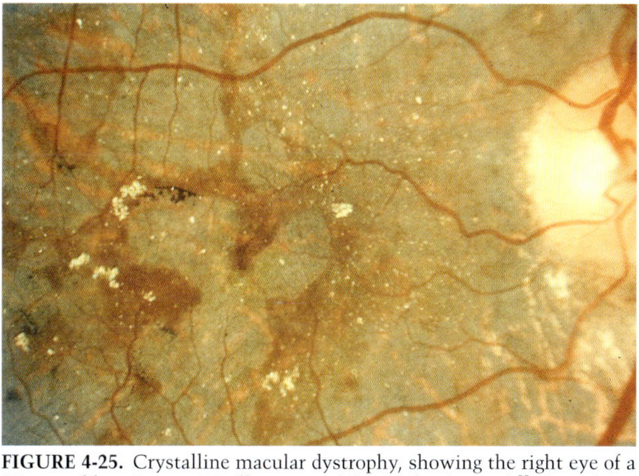

FIGURE 4-25. Crystalline macular dystrophy, showing the right eye of a 54-year-old patient originally reported by Richards et al.[55] Deposition of crystalline material is seen within the retina and associated areas of atrophy of the retinal pigment epithelium. (Courtesy of Richards and coworkers, used with permission.)

Acknowledgments. The text and figures in this chapter were derived largely from those prepared by Edwin M. Stone, MD, PhD, in the previous edition of this textbook. Dr. Drack is supported in part by the Georgia Lions Children's Eyecare Center and Research to Prevent Blindness.

References

1. Aaberg TM. Stargardt's disease and fundus flavimaculatus: evaluation of morphologic progression and intrafamilial co-existence. Trans Am Ophthalmol Soc 1986;84:453–487.
2. Allikmets R, Singh N, Sun H, et al. A photoreceptor cell-specific ATP-binding transporter gene (ABCR) is mutated in recessive Stargardt macular dystrophy. Nat Genet 1997;15(3):236–246.
3. Arden GB, Barrada A, Kelsey JH. New clinical test of retinal function based upon the standing potential of the eye. Br J Ophthalmol 1962;46:449–467.
4. Barker DF, Hostikka SL, Zhou J, et al. Identification of mutations in the COL4A5 collagen gene in Alport Syndrome. Science 1990;248: 1224–1227.
5. Bastiaensen LAK, Hoefnagels KLJ. Patterned anomalies of the retinal pigment epithelium: dystrophy or syndrome? Doc Ophthalmol 1983; 55:17–29.
6. Benedikt O, Werner W. Retikulare pigmentdystophie der Netzhaut. Klin Monatsbl Augenheilkd 1971;159:794–798.
7. Best F. Uber eine hereditare maculaaffektion: Bietrage zur vererbungslehre. Z Augenheilkd 1905;13:199–212.
8. Bietti GB. Ueber familiares Vorkommen von retinitis punctata albescense (verbunden mit'dystrophia marginalis cristallinea cornea'): Glitzern des Glaskorpers und anderen degenerativen Augenveranderungen. Klin Monatsbl Augenheilkd 1937;99:737–756.
9. Capon MRC, Polkinghorne PJ, Fitzke FW, Bird AC. Sorsby's pseudoinflammatory macula dystrophy—Sorsby's fundus dystrophies. Eye 1988;2:114–122.
10. Capon MRC, Marshall J, Krafft JI, Alexander RA, Hiscott PS, Bird AC. Sorsby's fundus dystrophy: a light and electron microscopic study. Ophthalmology 1989;96:1769–1777.
11. Chopdar A. Reticular dystrophy of retina. Br J Ophthalmol 1976;60: 342–344.
12. Cibis GW, Morey M, Harris DJ. Dominantly inherited macular dystrophy with flecks (Stargardt). Arch Ophthalmol 1980;98:1785–1789.
13. Daily MJ, Mets MB. Fenestrated sheen macular dystrophy. Arch Ophthalmol 1984;102:855–856.
14. de Jong PTVM, Delleman JW. Pigment epithelial pattern dystrophy; four different manifestations in a family. Arch Ophthalmol 1982; 100:1416–1421.

15. Deutman AF, Rumke AML. Reticular dystrophy of the retinal pigment epithelium. Arch Ophthalmol 1969;82:4–9.
16. Deutman AF, van Blommestein JDA, Henkes HE, Waardenburg PJ, Solleveld van Driest E. Butterfly-shaped pigment dystrophy of the fovea. Arch Ophthalmol 1970;83:558.
17. Deutman AF. Benign concentric annular macular dystrophy. Am J Ophthalmol 1974;78:384–396.
18. Donoso LA, Frost AT, Stone EM, et al. Autosomal dominant Stargardt-like macular dystrophy: founder effect and reassessment of genetic heterogeneity. Arch Ophthalmol 2001;119(4):564–570.
19. Feeney-Burns L, Ellersieck MR. Age-related changes in the ultrastructure of Bruch's membrane. Am J Ophthalmol 1985;100:686–697.
20. Ferrell RE, Mintz-Hittner H, Antoszyk JH. Linkage of atypical vitelliform macular dystrophy (VMD-1) to the soluble glutamate pyruvate transaminase (GPT1) locus. Am J Hum Genet 1983;35:78–84.
21. Fish G, Grey R, Sehmi KS, Bird AC. The dark choroid in posterior retinal dystrophies. Br J Ophthalmol 1981;65:359–363.
22. Fishman GA, Farber M, Patel DS, Derlacki DJ. Visual acuity loss in patients with Stargardt's macular dystrophy. Ophthalmology 1987;94:809–813.
23. Forgacs PJ, Bozin I. Manifestation familiale de pigmentations groupees de la region maculaire. Ophthalmologica 1966;152:364–368.
24. Frangieh GT, Green WR, Fine SL. A histopathologic study of Best's macular dystrophy. Arch Ophthalmol 1982;100:1115–1121.
25. Frank HR, Landers MB, Williams RJ, Sidbury JB. A new dominant progressive foveal dystrophy. Am J Ophthalmol 1974;78:903–916.
26. Gass JDM, Jallow S, Davis B. Adult vitelliform macular detachment occurring in patients with basal laminar drusen. Am J Ophthalmol 1985;99:445–459.
27. Gass JDM. A clinicopathologic study of a peculiar foveomacular dystrophy. Trans Am Ophthalmol Soc 1974;72:138–156.
28. Gass JDM. Stereoscopic atlas of macular diseases. St. Louis: Mosby, 1987:60–91.
29. Gass JDM. Stereoscopic atlas of macular diseases. St. Louis: Mosby, 1987:92–97.
30. Giuffre G, Lodato G. Vitelliform dystrophy and pattern dystrophy of the retinal pigment epithelium: concomitant presence in a family. Br J Ophthalmol 1986;70:526–532.
31. Gutman I, Walsh JB, Henkind P. Vitelliform macular dystrophy and butterfly-shaped epithelial dystrophy: a continuum? Br J Ophthalmol 1982;66:170–173.
32. Hermsen VM, Judisch GF. Central areolar pigment epithelial dystrophy. Ophthalmologica 1984;189:69–72.
33. Hittner HM, Ferrell RE, Borda RP, Justice J. Atypical vitelliform macular dystrophy in a five-generation family. Br J Ophthalmol 1984;68:199–207.

34. Hoskin A, Bird AC, Sehmi K. Sorsby's pseudoinflammatory macular dystrophy. Br J Ophthalmol 1981;65:859–865.
35. Hsieh RC, Fine BS, Lyons JS. Patterned dystrophies of the retinal pigment epithelium. Arch Ophthalmol 1977;95:429–435.
36. Jacobson SG, Cideciyan AV, Regunath G, Rodriguez FJ, Vandenburgh K, Sheffield VC, Stone EM. Night blindness in Sorsby's fundus dystrophy reversed by vitamin A. Nat Genet 1995;11(1):27–32.
37. Jiao X, Munier FL, Iwata F, et al. Genetic linkage of Bietti crystallin corneoretinal dystrophy to chromosome 4q35. Am J Hum Genet 2000;67(5):1309–1313.
38. Kingham JD, Fenzl RE, Willerson D, Aaberg TM. Reticular dystrophy of the retinal pigment epithelium. A clinical and electrophysiologic study of three generations. Arch Ophthalmol 1978;96(7):1177–1184.
39. Lefler WH, Wadsworth JAC, Sidbury JB Jr. Hereditary macular degeneration and aminoaciduria. Am J Ophthalmol 1971;78:224–230.
40. Lopez PF, Maumenee IH, delaCruz Z, Green WR. Autosomal-dominant fundus flavimaculatus. Ophthalmology 1990;97:798–809.
41. Marano F, Deutman AF, Leys A, Aandekerk AL. Hereditary retinal dystrophies and choroidal neovascularization. Graefe's Arch Clin Exp Ophthalmol 2000;238(9):760–764.
42. Marmor MF, Byers B. Pattern dystrophy of the pigment epithelium. Am J Ophthalmol 1977;84:32–44.
43. Marmorstein AD, Marmorstein LY, Rayborn M, Wang X, Hollyfield JG, Petrukhin K. Bestrophin, the product of the Best vitelliform macular dystrophy gene (VMD2), localizes to the basolateral plasma membrane of the retinal pigment epithelium. Proc Natl Acad Sci USA 2000;97(23):12758–12763.
44. Massin P, Virally-Monod M, Vialettes B, et al. Prevalence of macular pattern dystrophy in maternally inherited diabetes and deafness. GEDIAM Group. Ophthalmology 1999;106(9):1821–1827.
45. Mesker RP, Oosterhuis JA, Delleman JW. A retinal lesion resembling Sjogren's dystrophy reticularis laminae pigmentosae retinae. In: Perspectives in ophthalmology, vol 2. Amsterdam: Excerpta Medica, 1970:40–45.
46. Nichols BE, Sheffield VC, Vandenburgh K, Drack AV, Kimura AE, Stone EM. Butterfly-shaped pigment dystrophy of the fovea is caused by a point mutation in codon 167 of the RDS gene. Nat Genet 1993; 3:202–207.
47. Nichols BE, Drack AV, Vandenburgh K, Kimura AE, Sheffield VC, Stone EM. A 2 base pair deletion in the RDS gene associated with butterfly-shaped pigment dystrophy of the fovea. Hum Mol Genet 1993;2:601–603.
48. Newsome DA, Hewitt T, Huh W, Robey PG, Hassell JR. Detection of specific extracellular matrix molecules in drusen, Bruch's membrane and ciliary body. Am J Ophthalmol 1987;104:373–381.
49. O'Donnell FE, Welch RB. Fenestrated sheen macular dystrophy. Arch Ophthalmol 1979;97:1292–1296.

50. O'Gorman S, Flaherty WA, Fishman GA, Berson EL. Histopathologic findings in Best's vitelliform macular dystrophy. Arch Ophthalmol 1988;106:1261–1268.
51. Petrukhin K, Koisti MJ, Bakall B, et al. Identification of the gene responsible for Best macular dystrophy. Nat Genet 1998;19(3):241–247.
52. Piccolino FC, Zingirian M. Pattern dystrophy of the retinal pigment epithelium with vitelliform macular lesion: evolution in ten years. Int Ophthalmol 1988;11:207–217.
53. Polkinghorne PJ, Capon MRC, Berninger T, Lyness AL, Sehme K, Bird AC. Sorsby's fundus dystrophy. Ophthalmology 1989;96:1763–1768.
54. Prensky JG, Bresnick GH. Butterfly-shaped macular dystrophy in four generations. Arch Ophthalmol 1983;101:1198–1203.
55. Richards BW, Brodstein DE, Nussbaum JJ, Ferencz JR, Meada K, Weiss L. Autosomal dominant crystalline dystrophy. Ophthalmology 1991;98:658–665.
56. Sarks SH. Ageing and degeneration in the macular region: a clinicopathological study. Br J Ophthalmol 1976;60:324–341.
57. Singerman LJ, Berkow JW, Patz A. Dominant slowly progressive macular dystrophy. Am J Ophthalmol 1977;83:680–693.
58. Sjogren H. Dystrophia reticularis laminae pigmentosae retinae. Acta Ophthalmol 1950;28:279–295.
59. Slagsvold JE. Fenestrated sheen macular dystrophy. A new autosomal dominant maculopathy. Acta Ophthalmol 1981;59:683–688.
60. Slezak H, Hommer K. Fundus pulverulentus. Albrecht Von Graefe's Arch Klin Exp Ophthalmol 1969;178:177–182.
61. Small KW, Hermsen V, Gurney N, Fetkenhour CL, Folk JC. North Carolina macular dystrophy and central areolar pigment epithelial dystrophy. Arch Ophthalmol 1992;110:515–518.
62. Small KW, Killian J, McLean WC. North Carolina's dominant progressive foveal dystrophy: how progressive is it? Br J Ophthalmol 1991;75:401–406.
63. Small KW. North Carolina macular dystrophy, revisited. Ophthalmology 1989;96:1747–1754.
64. Small KW, Udar N, Yelchits S, et al. North Carolina macular dystrophy (MCDR1) locus: a fine resolution genetic map and haplotype analysis. Mol Vision 1999;5:38.
65. Sneed SR, Sieving PA. Fenestrated sheen macular dystrophy. Am J Ophthalmol 1991;112:1–7.
66. Sorsby A, Joll Mason ME, Gardener N. A fundus dystrophy with unusual features. Br J Ophthalmol 1949;33:67–97.
67. Stargardt K. Ueber familiare, progressive degeneration in der makulagegend des auges. Albrecht Von Graefe's Arch Klin Exp Ophthalmol 1909;71:534–550.
68. Stefko ST, Zhang K, Gorin MB, Traboulsi EI. Clinical spectrum of chromosome 6-linked autosomal dominant drusen and macular degeneration. Am J Ophthalmol 2000;130(2):203–208.

69. Stone EM, Lotery AJ, Munier FL, et al. A single EFEMP1 mutation associated with both Malattia Leventinese and Doyne honeycomb retinal dystrophy. Nat Genet 1999;22(2):199–202.
70. Stone EM, Nichols BE, Kimura AE, Weingeist TA, Drack A, Sheffield VC. Clinical features of a Stargardt-like dominant progressive macular dystrophy with genetic linkage to chromosome 6q. Arch Ophthalmol 1994;112(6):765–772.
71. Stone EM, Nichols BE, Streb LM, Kimura AE, Sheffield VC. Genetic linkage of vitelliform macular degeneration (Best's disease) to chromosome 11q13. Nat Genet 1992;1(4):246–250.
72. Uliss AE, Moore AT, Bird AC. The dark choroid in posterior retinal dystrophies. Ophthalmology 1987;94:1423–1427.
73. van der Schaft TL, Mooy CM, deBruijn WC, Oron FG, Mulder PGH, deJong PTVM. Histologic features of the early stages of age-related macular degeneration. Ophthalmology 1992;99:278–286.
74. Watzke RC, Folk JC, Lang RM. Pattern dystrophy of the retinal pigment epithelium. Ophthalmology 1982;89:1400–1406.
75. Weber BHF, Vogt G, Pruett RC, et al. Mutations in the tissue inhibitor of metalloproteinases-3 (TIMP3) in patients with Sorsby's fundus dystrophy. Nat Genet 1994;8:352–356.
76. Weigell-Weber M, Kryenbuhl C, Buchi ER, Spiegel R. Genetic heterogeneity in autosomal dominant pattern dystrophy of the retina. Mol Vision 1996;2:6.
77. Weingeist TA, Kobrin JL, Watzke RC. Histopathology of Best's macular dystrophy. Arch Ophthalmol 1982;100:1103–1114.
78. Weleber RG, Carr RE, Murphey WH, Sheffield VC, Stone EM. Phenotypic variation including retinitis pigmentosa, pattern dystrophy, and fundus flavimaculatus in a single family with a deletion of codon 153 or 154 of the peripherin/RDS gene. Arch Ophthalmol 1993;111(11):1531–1542.
79. Wells J, Wroblewski J, Keen J, et al. Mutations in the human retinal degeneration slow (RDS) gene can cause either retinitis pigmentosa or macular dystrophy. Nat Genet 1993;3:213–218.
80. Wilson DJ, Weleber RG, Klein ML, Welch RB, Green R. Bietti's crystalline dystrophy. A clinicopathologic correlative study. Arch Ophthalmol 1989;107:213–221.

5

Retinitis Pigmentosa and Associated Disorders

Arlene V. Drack and Alan E. Kimura

Retinitis pigmentosa (RP) is a general term used to refer to a group of related inherited diseases typically characterized by poor vision in dim light, constricted visual fields, bone spicule-like pigmentation of the fundus, and electroretinographic evidence of photoreceptor cell dysfunction. These diseases can be inherited as an autosomal dominant, autosomal recessive, or X-linked recessive trait. Mitochondrial inheritance has also been described, often as part of a syndrome. It has been estimated that RP affects approximately 1 in 3700 people in the United States. Inherited retinopathies affect approximately 1 in 2000 individuals worldwide.[131] Approximately 20% of these cases are autosomal dominant, and 6% to 9% are X-linked.[22,23] The remaining 71% to 84% are either autosomal recessive or isolated "simplex" cases. The latter may represent autosomal recessive disease, a new autosomal dominant mutation, or an environmental phenocopy. In the United Kingdom, X-linked RP appears to be more common than in the United States.[70]

This chapter summarizes the clinical and electrophysiological features of various types of retinitis pigmentosa and other related photoreceptor disorders. The organization of the chapter is summarized in Table 5-1. First, some general features of these disorders and the approach to working up patients suspected to have one of them are presented. Next, the three hereditary types of "classic" RP and the rare congenital form (Leber's congenital amaurosis) are discussed. Systemic disorders associated with retinitis pigmentosa are only briefly summarized because they are discussed fully in Chapter 13. Last, three additional forms of heritable photoreceptor dysfunction are discussed: congenital

TABLE 5-1. Varieties of Retinitis Pigmentosa and Associated Disorders.

Retinitis pigmentosa (RP)
Clinical features
Workup
Treatment
Hereditary subtypes of typical RP
Autosomal dominant
Autosomal recessive
X-linked
Leber's congenital amaurosis
RP and systemic diseases
Usher syndrome
Alstrom disease
Bardet–Biedl syndrome
Retinal renal syndromes
Ceroid lipofuscinoses
Mitochondrial diseases
Other photoreceptor disorders
Congenital stationary night blindness
Cone dystrophies
Dyschromatopsias
Other RP-like retinal disorders
Unilateral pigmentary retinopathy
X-linked juvenile retinoschisis
Goldmann–Favre syndrome
Gyrate atrophy
Choroideremia

stationary night blindness, cone dystrophies, and congenital dyschromatopsias.

RETINITIS PIGMENTOSA (PROGRESSIVE ROD/CONE DYSTROPHY)

Clinical descriptions of night blindness consistent with the diagnosis of retinitis pigmentosa (RP) were made as early as 1744 by Ovelgun. Donders first used the phrase "retinitis pigmentosa" in 1855. Karpe is credited with developing clinical electroretinography (ERG) in 1945. He detected abnormally low ERGs in patients with RP and noted that these abnormalities could precede the onset of ophthalmoscopically visible changes. Gouras and Carr subsequently identified preferential rod photoreceptor dysfunction in patients with early autosomal dominant retinitis pigmentosa.[57] In 1989, McWilliam et al.[98] reported linkage of the disease phenotype in a large family with autosomal dominant RP (ADRP) to a genetic marker on the long arm of chromosome three. The proximity of this marker to the rhodopsin gene led Dryja and his co-workers[34–39] to examine the rhodopsin gene in patients with ADRP, and in 1990 they identified the first rhodopsin mutations in such patients. In 1991, two groups identified ADRP-causing mutations in the peripherin/RDS gene.[40,74] Subsequently, retinitis pigmentosa has been proven to be a very genetically heterogeneous group of disorders.[20,68,71,135] Of interest, genotype–phenotype correlations are rarely strong. In fact, for the inherited retinopathies the rule has been that disorders that look clinically similar may have different genetic causes, whereas those with identical gene defects may present with very different clinical findings. Because of this, arguments can be made for discarding the existing clinically based nomenclature in favor of one that describes the genetic subtype of the disorder. In reality, however, most diagnoses still must be made clinically at this writing.

Clinical Features

The earliest symptom of RP and related disorders is often night blindness. Young children may not be capable of articulating this, and some patients may not give a history of subjective night blindness even when objective difficulty with dark adaptation can be documented. Parents should be asked whether their child clings to them or guides himself or herself along walls or furniture in dimly lit rooms or movie theaters. A child's activity in the exam room can also be evaluated after dimming the lights. Older children and adults may describe themselves as clumsy or admit to difficulty seeing the stars at night or finding their seat in a dark theater. Often children with RP are referred because of decreased visual acuity or the discovery of abnormal fundus pigmentation on routine ocular examination. Some children come to an ophthalmologist because of a positive family history without any symptoms themselves. Fundus findings include arteriolar narrowing, waxy pallor of the disc, cystoid macular edema and bone spicule-like pigment changes (Figs. 5-1, 5-2, 5-3). Vitreous cells and posterior subcapsular cataracts are also commonly observed.

Pigmentary changes in the fundus are variable and may even be absent (retinitis pigmentosa sine pigmento), making

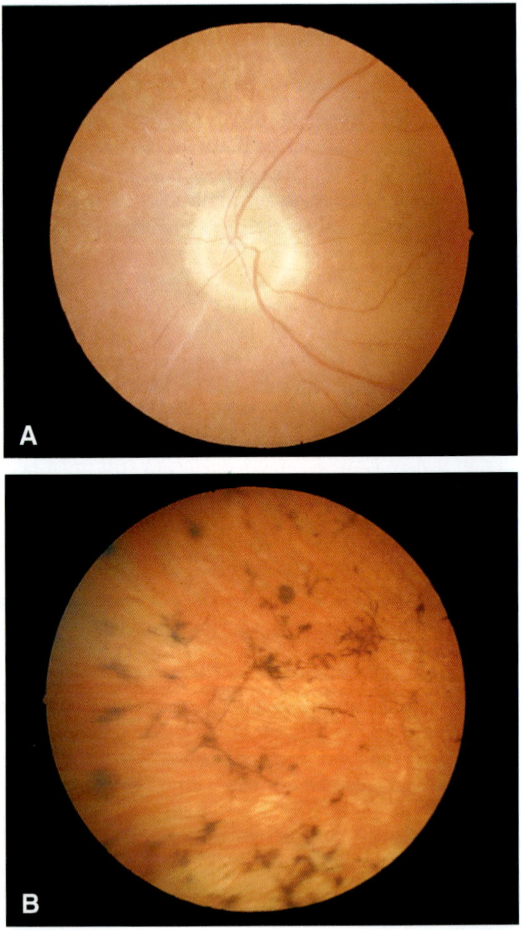

FIGURE 5-1A,B. Fundus photographs of a patient with late-stage rhodopsin-associated retinitis pigmentosa (Pro-23-His). **(A)** Optic disc and major retinal vessels. Note "waxy pallor" and significant arteriolar attenuation. **(B)** A more peripheral view of the same patient showing classic bone spicule-like hyperpigmentation. The visual fields from this patient are shown in Figure 5-6.

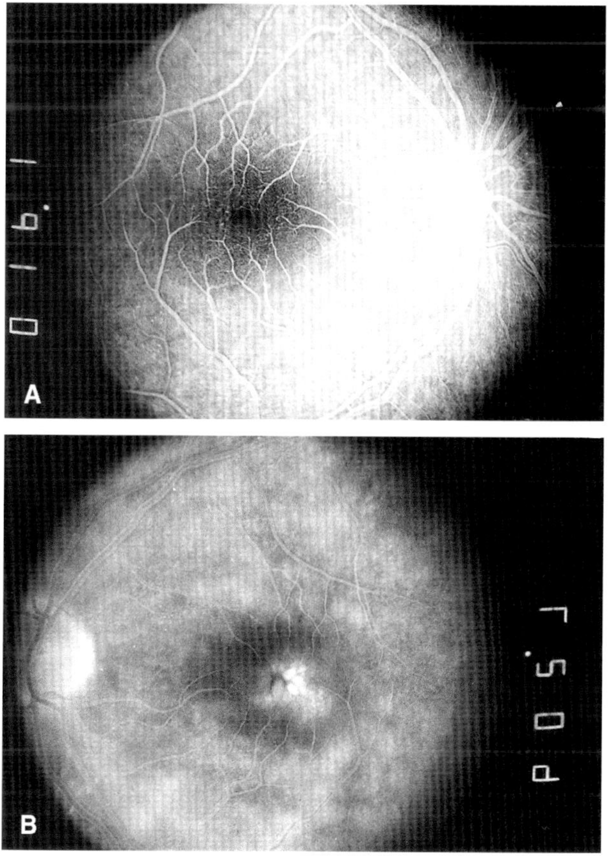

FIGURE 5-2A,B. Fluorescein angiogram of a patient with Usher syndrome. **(A)** Early phase of the angiogram. Subtle abnormalities of the foveal avascular zone are visible. **(B)** Late phase of the angiogram. Pronounced cystoid macular edema and deep retinal pigment epithelial leakage are evident.

symptoms and family history especially important in the decision to proceed with further evaluation. White dots may also be observed deep in the retina; when marked, this appearance is known as retinitis punctata albescens (RPA). Fundus albipunctatus (FAP) has similar white dots, but is associated with a

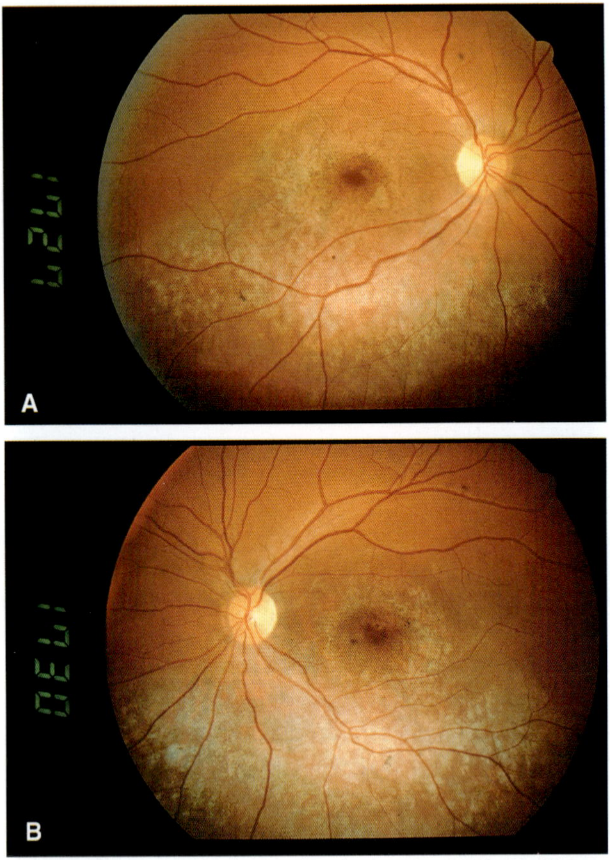

FIGURE 5-3A,B. Fundus photographs of a patient with rhodopsin-associated retinitis pigmentosa (Val-87-Asp). The retinal degeneration is more pronounced in the inferior quadrants than the superior quadrants and involves the macula as well. The visual fields from this patient are shown in Figure 5-5.

stationary night blindness, not progressive RP. Historically, the uniqueness of retinitis pigmentosa sine pigmento and retinitis punctata albescens has been argued, because both have been observed in affected patients from ADRP and ARRP pedigrees in which other family members demonstrate bone spicules and typical fundus changes characteristic of retinitis pigmentosa. RP sine pigmento is believed by most investigators to be an early stage of RP before the bone spicule-type of hyperpigmentation and atrophy are manifest.[116] RPA has been seen in various subtypes of early stages of RP.[100] One family with an RPA appearance was found to have a heterozygous mutation of the RDS/peripherin gene.[75] A consanguineous pedigree from Saudi Arabia with ARRP with a RPA phenotype was found to be caused by homozygous mutations in the RLBP1 gene and was slowly progressive.[79]

Workup

A standard clinical evaluation for a patient suspected to have an inherited retinal dystrophy includes a history and physical examination directed toward the signs and symptoms of rod and cone photoreceptor dysfunction. In addition to refraction, retinal biomicroscopy, and indirect ophthalmoscopy, we usually include three laboratory tests in the workup as well: visual field evaluation, dark adaptometry, and electroretinography. The purpose of these three tests is to determine the presence or absence of retinal disease, to confirm and refine the diagnosis, and to establish a baseline level of visual function. In at least one patient per family, DNA screening for known retinal dystrophy mutations may be offered.

Visual field loss is progressive in the rod and cone dystrophies and may demonstrate variability as the disease progresses. Early in the course of retinitis pigmentosa, paracentral scotomas and, later, a complete ring scotoma may be seen (Fig. 5-4). Some patients with rhodopsin-associated retinitis pigmentosa show a preferential superior visual field loss[65,133] (Fig. 5-5). Late in the course of retinitis pigmentosa, the ring scotomas break out into the periphery and there is progressive constriction of the peripheral isopters. Typically, only a small central island remains, occasionally accompanied by another temporal island in the periphery (Fig. 5-6). Legal blindness in many states is defined by less than 20° of a central island to a III4e isopter. RP patients may be legally blind on the basis of constricted visual fields even though they have relatively good central vision. Visual field loss is generally symmetrical between both eyes, and marked asymmetry may suggest a nonhereditary basis for poor vision.

Dark adaptometry measures the patient's threshold for detecting a test spot of light as they progressively adapt to darkness.

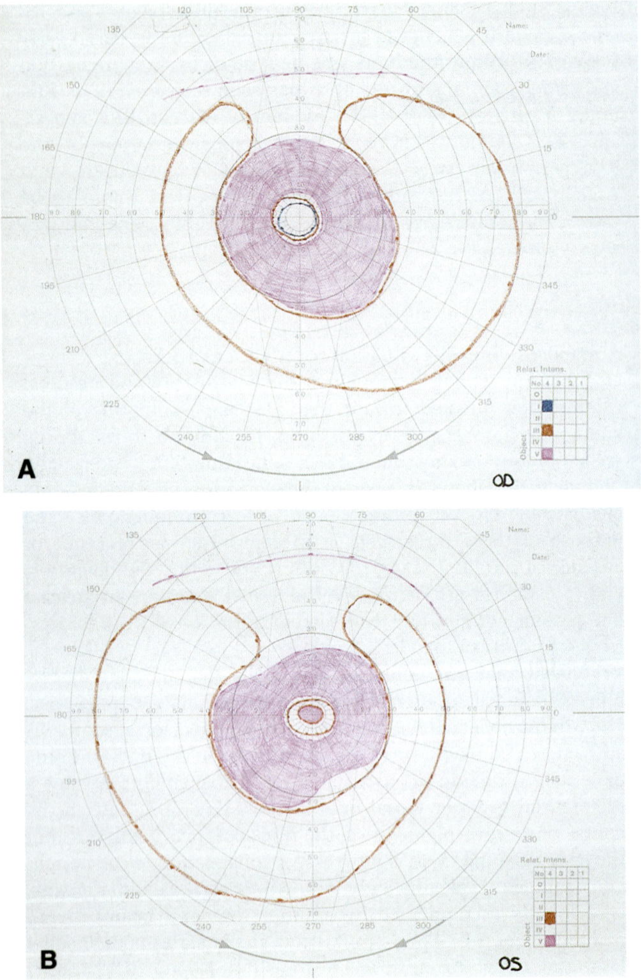

FIGURE 5-4A,B. Ring scotomata in a patient with retinitis pigmentosa.

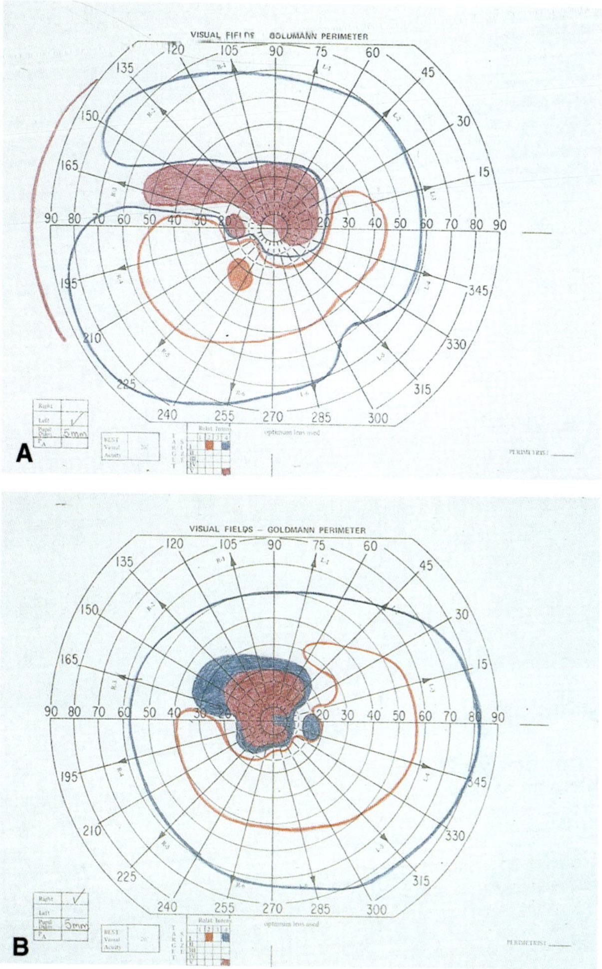

FIGURE 5-5A,B. Goldmann visual fields of a patient with rhodopsin-associated retinitis pigmentosa. These visual fields are those of the patient whose fundus photographs are shown in Figure 5-3. Note the selective loss of field superiorly that corresponds to the retinal degeneration in the inferior quadrants.

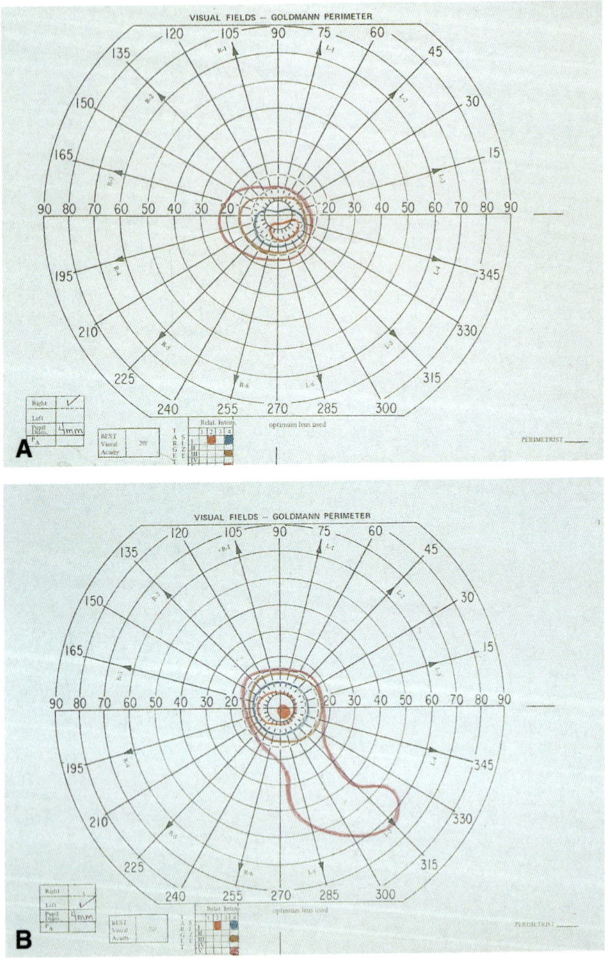

FIGURE 5-6A,B. Visual fields of a patient with late-stage rhodopsin-associated retinitis pigmentosa (fundus photographs shown in Figure 5-1). In the right eye (**A**), only a small central island of vision remains; in the left eye (**B**), an inferotemporal island is also present.

Like perimetry, this psychophysical test requires good patient cooperation. The clinical dark-adaptation curve shows that sensitivity is initially determined by cones, followed by a cone–rod break around 9 to 11 min after the preadapting bleaching light is turned off (Fig. 5-7). Sensitivity continues to improve as the rods begin to determine the threshold sensitivity. The threshold generally is reached after about 30 min in darkness. RP patients may demonstrate several abnormalities, including a delayed cone–rod break, an elevated final threshold, and an abnormally prolonged recovery to final threshold over many hours. Late-stage RP patients typically have a final threshold elevated over 3 log units (Fig. 5-7). Subjective complaints of nyctalopia are not universal, particularly in early phases of RP, or if patients have a regional loss of sensitivity as opposed to a generalized loss.

Electroretinography (ERG) is essential in the workup of inherited retinal dystrophies. The variety of protocols in use today limits the ability to compare ERG results between laboratories. In 1989, the International Society for Clinical Electrophysiology of Vision (ISCEV) Standardization Committee published criteria for a standardized ERG.[69] With a standard flash luminance and rod-suppressing background, five standard responses are recorded (Fig. 5-8). Use of this protocol allows

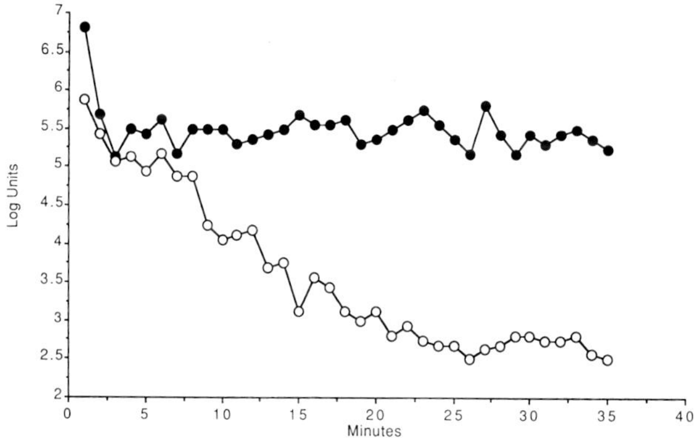

FIGURE 5-7. Dark adaptation curves. The dark adaptation of a normal patient (*open symbols*) shows a normal cone–rod break before 10 min with final threshold reached at just over 25 min. A patient with retinitis pigmentosa (*closed symbols*) does not show a cone–rod break and has a final threshold that is 3 log units greater than that of the normal patient.

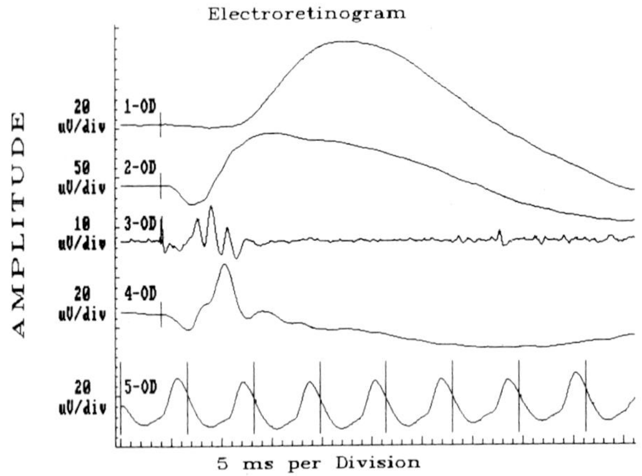

FIGURE 5-8. Standardized electroretinogram from normal patient. *Top to bottom*: selective rod response; maximal combined rod–cone response; oscillatory potentials; selective cone response; 30-Hz flicker (cone) response.

investigators from different laboratories to compare selective rod and cone responses, as well as the maximal, combined response of the rods and cones, oscillatory potentials, and 30-Hz flicker. Cone dystrophy patients demonstrate preferential cone dysfunction early in the course of the disease (Fig. 5-9), whereas typical RP patients show predominantly abnormal rod responses (Fig. 5-10). Progressive reductions in amplitude and prolongation of implicit time are features of rod–cone and cone–rod dystrophies. Later in the course of many types of RP, the ERG may become nonrecordable. Nonhereditary pigmentary retinopathies show no change in the ERG over time. Congenital stationary night blindness has been classified into a Schubert–Bornschien type (Fig. 5-11) and a Riggs type,[121,124] based on the ERG and dark adaptation. Miyake et al.[105] further subclassified the former into a complete and incomplete type.

The ERG can also be useful in helping to diagnose the carrier state of X-linked recessive RP. B-wave amplitude reductions in the maximal, combined response of the rods and cones are often diagnostic. A loss of oscillatory potentials may help diagnose the carrier state in X-linked CSNB. A pattern of hyperpigmentation resembling "cracked mud" is probably more useful than the ERG in diagnosing the carrier state of choroideremia.

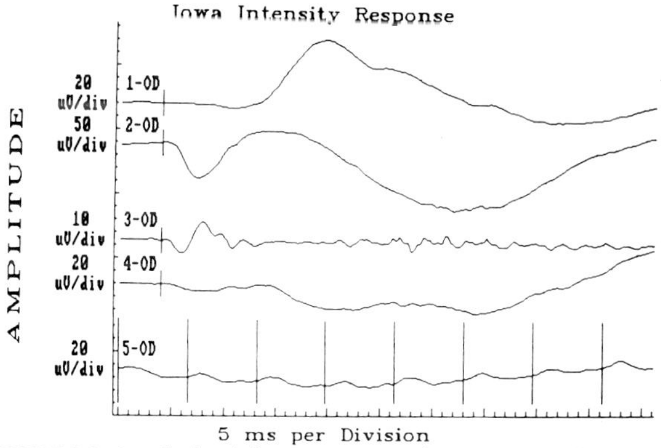

FIGURE 5-9. Standardized electroretinogram from patient with cone dystrophy. *Top* to *bottom*: normal selective rod response; mildly subnormal combined rod–cone response; oscillatory potentials; nonrecordable cone response; a barely recordable and markedly delayed 30-Hz flicker (cone) response.

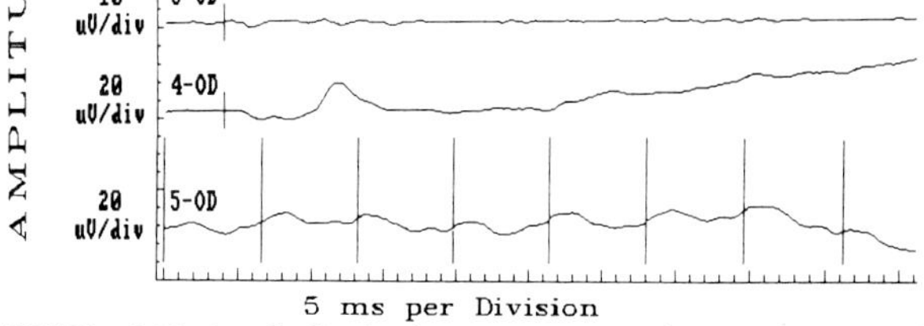

FIGURE 5-10. Standardized electroretinogram from patient with rhodopsin-associated retinitis pigmentosa (Pro-23-His). *Top* to *bottom*: nonrecordable selective rod response; low-amplitude maximal combined rod–cone response; nonrecordable oscillatory potentials; low-amplitude, delayed cone response; a barely recordable and markedly delayed 30-Hz flicker (cone) response.

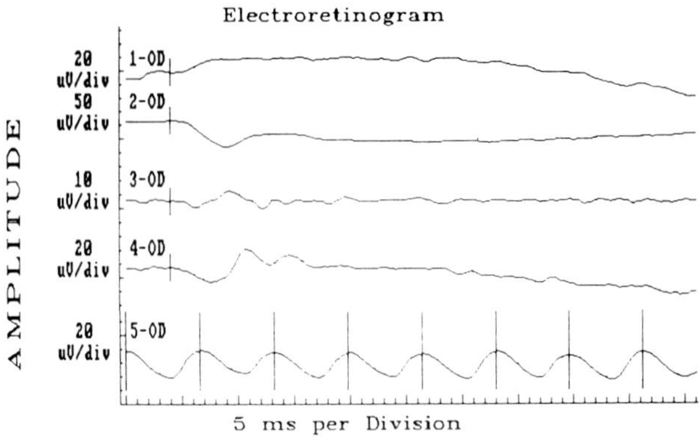

FIGURE 5-11. Standardized electroretinogram from patient with autosomal recessive congenital stationary night blindness. *Top* to *bottom*: nonrecordable selective rod response; markedly subnormal combined rod–cone response with preferential loss of the b-wave; minimal oscillatory potentials; subnormal cone response; delayed 30-Hz flicker (cone) response.

ERG testing of infants may be performed with the aid of the parents positioning the child, using a standard protocol; this allows results to be comparable to later ERGs when the patient is older. The ERG response may change over the first 6 months of life; some infants having nonrecordable ERGs as infants later develop negative-wave ERGs typical of CSNB. Therefore, a definitive diagnosis should be withheld until confirmed with repeat testing. Children from approximately 1 year to 6 or 7 years of age may find it difficult or impossible to cooperate with ERG testing. In these cases, a filament electrode may be used. If the diagnosis is of sufficient urgency, ERG under general anesthesia, or with chloral hydrate sedation with continuous monitoring of vital signs, may be indicated. These latter methods may not be comparable to standard ERG but can give a general idea of whether retinopathy is present.

Electro-oculography (EOG) is most often reserved for patients suspected of having Best disease.

Molecular testing is currently available for RP patients through several tertiary care centers as a part of ongoing research programs. Such testing will undoubtedly become more widely available in the coming years. Molecular testing has several potential benefits to patients as well as to the research community. Such testing is capable of reliably identifying affected individuals before overt symptoms are present. Also, it allows one to reassure some family members at risk for disease that they will not develop it and to identify molecularly affected children who will benefit from closer follow-up. Moreover, molecular diagnosis provides a mechanism for different research centers to compare and pool results from patients with identical mutations, making it possible to evaluate correlations between genotype and phenotype. As these correlations are established in the literature, molecular testing may also be useful prognostically.

Treatment

Although the photoreceptor cell death of retinitis pigmentosa cannot at present be arrested or reversed, some vision-threatening complications can be successfully managed. Cataracts can be extracted when they become visually significant.[9] However, visual acuity loss in retinitis pigmentosa is more likely to result from macular disease than from cataracts.[44] A trial of systemic carbonic anhydrase inhibitors for RP patients with cystoid macular edema is indicated, particularly when associated with diffuse retinal pigment epithelial leakage on fluorescein angiography.[45] Grid photocoagulation has also been suggested for macular edema in retinitis pigmentosa.[62] An ophthalmologist should not overlook the potential benefit of refraction and referral to a low-vision clinic to optimize the RP patient's visual function. It has been noted that, once vision drops below 20/40, further decline is often rapid.[96] Therefore, children with RP require close follow-up to document changes in vision and to allow educators to tailor the school environment accordingly. Many children have adequate vision to attend regular school for many years, but should be counseled about the need to consider their progressive loss of acuity and color vision when making career choices.

Several rare syndromes have RP as an associated finding, and some of these disorders are caused by metabolic derangements that can be reversed or retarded with drugs, dietary manipulation, or plasmapheresis. In addition, vitamin A deficiency and certain drug toxicities, such as desferoxamine (desferal), can mimic RP but have a much better prognosis if diagnosed early in their course. Desferoxamine should be stopped immediately if vision drops and/or the ERG becomes abnormal. All patients with newly diagnosed retinitis pigmentosa should have a history taken and undergo a physical examination to rule out these treatable diseases. A list of some treatable causes of retinal degeneration can be found in Chapter 13.

High-dose vitamin A palmitate may be helpful for some patients with retinal degenerations; there is evidence that central vision remains stable longer. Vitamin A can be toxic in high doses and should only be used after liver function and baseline fat-soluble vitamin levels have been evaluated. Because the optimal safe dose for children is not known, caution is advised in prescribing for this age group.[13] Neurotrophic growth factors delivered by subretinal injection of adenovirus-associated vectors has been shown to rescue photoreceptors in rats.[59] In dogs, a viral vector has been used to reverse vision loss and ERG changes in RPE65 retinal degeneration, which is similar to human Leber's congenital amaurosis (LCA).[1] Daily injections of melatonin delay photoreceptor degeneration in the *rds/rds* mouse.[90] Lutein dietary supplementation improved macular pigmentation in patients with Usher syndrome and RP, although central vision did not improve during 6 months of study.[2] A retinal computer chip has shown early promise in restoring at least some light perception, but results are preliminary.

Because the advances in diagnosis and treatment of RP are increasing at such a rapid rate, consideration should be given to referring affected patients to centers that are actively participating in RP research for at least one visit. This step not only allows patients to personally contribute to the study of their disease but will also provide them with an ongoing source of current information about their condition.

MAJOR TYPES OF HEREDITARY RP

Retinitis pigmentosa has typically been classified according to inheritance type. However, investigators have further subclassified the diseases with various electrophysiological and psychophysical tests.

Autosomal Dominant RP

Twenty-two percent of all RP was found to be autosomal dominant (ADRP) in one large study.[23] There are often no symptoms in childhood, but children may come to an ophthalmologist to rule out ADRP if they have an affected parent or other relative. The most common forms of ADRP in North American and European pedigrees appear to have a later onset and less severe clinical course than X-linked and recessive forms. Although some patients report the onset of nyctalopia in the first decade,[43] Tanino and Ohba found the onset of symptoms such as nyctalopia at a median age of 10.7 years in autosomal recessive disease and 23.4 years in autosomal dominant disease.[136] Berson et al. found that older patients with ADRP are more likely to retain recordable ERG amplitudes than age-matched patients with ARRP.[14]

Massof and Finkelstein[97] recognized two distinct types of RP among AD and simplex patients, and Lyness et al.[93] also concluded that rod photoreceptor involvement appeared to be either diffuse or regionalized. Massof and Finkelstein type 1 patients have diffuse loss of rod sensitivity with patchy cone loss, absent rod ERG, and night blindness from infancy or childhood, whereas type 2 patients have a regionalized loss of both rod and cone function with adult-onset night blindness and some recordable rod ERG until late in life. Fishman et al. used a combination of ophthalmoscopy, electroretinography, visual fields, and central vision to further subdivide the regional ADRP patients into three groups with decreasing severity of symptoms.[43]

Rhodopsin gene mutations account for about 25% to 30% of cases of ADRP in North America (Fig. 5-12).[34,131] Rhodopsin is the predominant protein contained within the discs of the rod photoreceptor outer segments. It plays a pivotal role in initiating the cascade of phototransduction that ultimately leads to the perception of light. There are at least nine different loci where dominant mutations cause RP. At this writing, the following genes have been identified: rhodopsin (RHO), retinal degeneration slow (RDS), leucine zipper motif protein (NRL), an oxygen-regulated photoreceptor protein (RP1),[12] and the retinal fascin gene (FSCN2) in Japanese patients.[139] RDS mutations account for about 2% of cases[36] whereas NRL are responsible for 5.6%.[12] Mutations in the gene for peripherin/RDS cause ADRP[40,74] as well as the more benign pattern macular dystrophy. The human peripherin gene has sequence homology with the murine RDS (retinal degeneration slow) gene. Peripherin is a protein present in the peripheral aspect of the rod and cone photoreceptor discs. It may play a role in disc assembly or in maintaining the stability of the disc shape.[31]

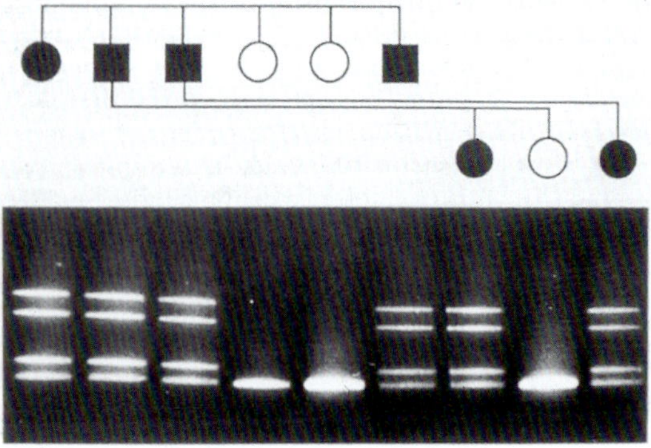

FIGURE 5-12. Denaturing gradient gel analysis of a family afflicted with rhodopsin-associated retinitis pigmentosa (Thr-17-Met). Individuals heterozygous for the mutation have four bands on the gel whereas normal individuals have a single band. *Closed pedigree symbols* indicate clinically affected individuals. There is perfect segregation of the disease phenotype with the molecular genotype. (From Sheffield et al. Am J Hum Genet 1991;49:699–706, with permission.)[126]

Autosomal Recessive RP

Autosomal recessive RP (ARRP) is probably the most common form of retinitis pigmentosa, although only about 9% of RP patients can be definitely confirmed to have this type of inheritance.[23] Many simplex cases are undoubtedly AR. Up to 40% of recessive cases are associated with other systemic pathology or syndromes and 18% have associated hearing loss. Autosomal recessive inheritance of retinitis pigmentosa is suggested when both parents of an affected individual are normal, especially if there is consanguinity. The existence of an affected female (e.g., the patient, a cousin, or sibling), or of male-to-male transmission, helps differentiate this entity from X-linked RP. The clinical course varies widely in age of onset from infancy to the age of 50 or 60[143] but may be more severe than most AD cases. A homozygous null mutation in the rhodopsin gene has been demonstrated to cause ARRP in one family.[123] Mutations in the RLBP1 gene cause ARRP of the Bothnia type, a childhood-onset RP that may present with intraretinal white dots and has a high prevalence in Northern Sweden.[25] Slowly progressive retinitis punctata albescens has been associated with different mutations of this same gene.[79] Mutations in the CNGB1 gene have been implicated in a French family with severe ARRP.[7] Six genetic loci have been identified for Usher syndrome, an autosomal recessive form of RP associated with deafness.[21,77,81,82,130] Bardet–Biedl syndrome, which presents with ARRP and obesity, polydactyly, and renal abnormalities, has also been mapped.[85a,129] Alstrom syndrome, which includes obesity RP, insulin resistant diabetes, as well as other variable associations, is caused by mutations of the ALMS1 gene.[30a] Neurological evaluation, genetic workup, and careful physical examination may be indicated in children presenting with ARRP to rule out associated abnormalities.

X-linked Recessive RP

Significantly reduced visual function usually occurs at a younger age in X-linked recessive RP (XLRP) (Fig. 5-13) than in other forms of retinitis pigmentosa. Most patients with X-linked RP are legally blind (acuity <20/200) by age 30.[16,42,70] There is also an increased incidence of myopic refractive errors in X-linked

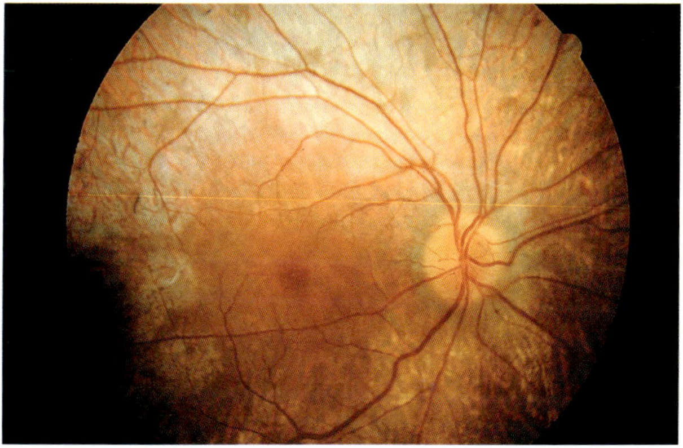

FIGURE 5-13. Fundus photograph of a 10-year-old boy with X-linked retinitis pigmentosa. Note the extensive retinal degeneration by the end of the first decade.

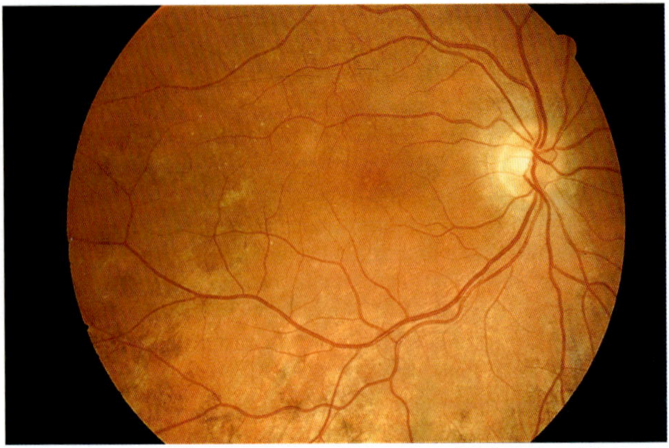

FIGURE 5-14. Fundus photograph of a carrier of X-linked retinitis pigmentosa, from the mother of the patient in Figure 5-13. Note the islands of affected retina that may represent the effect of unfavorable lyonization of clones of retinal cells. This patient is asymptomatic even though she is 20 years older than her son.

RP patients.[127] Examination of obligate female carriers (Fig. 5-14) occasionally reveals electroretinographic dysfunction and ophthalmoscopically visible pigmentary degeneration.[115] Lyonization may be unfavorably skewed, causing symptoms in some female carriers. A unique, golden metallic reflex is seen in one form of X-linked RP carriers.[114]

Two distinct loci on the X chromosome are associated with XLRP: RP2 at Xp11[19] and RP3 at Xp21.[107] The RPGR gene at XP21.1 is mutated in about 20% of families with XLRP.[60]

DIGENIC RP

With the ability to genotype patients with RP has come the understanding that some patients have mutations of more than one gene causing their disorder. Are these cases autosomal dominant or recessive? Although some phenotypes require mutations of two different genes to cause pathology and mutation of either of these genes alone causes no disorder, others manifest as one type of retinal dystrophy when one gene is mutated and another when a second genetic mutation is added. These forms are termed digenic. An example is retinitis pigmentosa caused by co-inheritance of a peripherin mutation and a ROM1 mutation.[92]

LEBER'S CONGENITAL AMAUROSIS

Leber's congenital amaurosis (LCA) is a group of ocular diseases characterized by severely reduced vision from birth associated with nystagmus or roving eye movements. Most of these children also have high hyperopia,[49,140] although a subgroup have myopia.[66] Affected infants are often referred to an ophthalmologist when a parent or pediatrician notices that the child does not respond to faces, or when nystagmus or strabismus is noted. Most cases are autosomal recessive; however, autosomal dominant pedigrees have been reported.

Many patients with LCA, as well as other types of infantile blindness, rub or poke their eyes. This phenomenon is called the oculodigital sign of Franceschetti[50] and has been purported to cause enophthalmos. Although the apparent cause is an attempt at retinal stimulation, other poorly understood factors contribute, making this behavior a difficult one to stop. Cataracts and keratoconus may be seen in older children. The reported prevalence of neurological abnormalities in LCA varies from 17% to 37%.[4,51] Most children with LCA have normal intelligence, and the psychomotor retardation that has been described may have been secondary to sensory deprivation in some cases.[111]

Rare systemic associations with LCA include deafness, cardiomyopathy, polycystic kidney disease, and osteopetrosis.[86a] Mutations of at least seven genes can cause LCA. At this writing, 15% to 28% of patients could be genotyped.[131] One causative gene is RPGRIP1 on chromosome 14q11, which encodes a protein that interacts with the protein product of the RPGR gene on the X chromosome[35]; this accounts for approximately 6% of cases of LCA.[55] Mutations of the latter cause X-linked RP. Another is the RPE65 gene, for which gene therapy has restored vision in a dog model of LCA.[1] RPE65 mutations account for about 5% of human LCA.

An ophthalmologist confronted with an infant with congenital nystagmus must rule out a sensory disturbance as the cause. In one study, 74 of 81 prospectively studied patients (91%) with congenital nystagmus were eventually found to have one of the following diagnoses: albinism, LCA or "early-onset RP," achromatopsia, or CSNB.[141] Albinism and LCA were the most commonly observed. All these diagnoses, as well as idiopathic congenital nystagmus, are consistent with very poor visual responses in infancy. All but LCA/early-onset RP usually show improvement in visual responses with age. Fundus examination often does not aid in diagnosis. As many as one-half of patients with LCA retain a normal fundus appearance at least until 1 year of age, with arteriolar attenuation and optic nerve pallor more prevalent by age 2 to 3 years. Unusual ophthalmoscopic variants include the presence of a macular "coloboma-like lesion,"[66,95] yellow flecks or white dots, a "marbleized" pattern, salt-and-pepper pigmentary changes, and a nummular pattern.

Electrophysiological testing is essential to establishing the proper diagnosis. The ERG is typically extinguished in LCA/early-onset RP, differentiating these from syndromes with similar initial presentation. One caveat is that, because the ERG may be normally reduced in early infancy,[53] one should repeat the ERG at a later time, especially if vision seems to be improving. For example, congenital stationary night blindness has been reported to present as blindness in infancy with a nonrecordable ERG that improves with age along with acuity.[88,145] Children with CSNB are often myopic rather than hyperopic, whereas the reverse is true for most LCA patients.

Joubert syndrome can also mimic LCA. This syndrome is characterized by neonatal tachypnea, mental retardation, agenesis of the cerebellar vermis, oculomotor apraxia, brainstem malformation, and a congenital retinal dystrophy.[72,83,87] The correct diagnosis can be made by demonstrating hypoplasia of the cerebellar vermis with neuroimaging. Patients with oculomotor apraxia (OMA) cannot make voluntary horizontal saccades, which leads to the impression the child cannot fix and follow. Following objects with the use of head thrusts differentiates this condition from true vision loss. Patients who do not have pigmentary retinopathy, but only OMA, may have good vision.

Delayed visual maturation is another challenging clinical problem that may present similar to LCA. Infants with delayed visual maturation have normal eyes without nystagmus, but they do not exhibit appropriate fixation responses for age. The visual evoked potential (VEP) may be attenuated but the ERG is normal. Many of these children have a good prognosis for development of normal vision.[41,88,142]

Multisystem metabolic syndromes such as infantile phytanic acid storage disease and infantile neuronal ceroid lipofuscinosis should also be considered in the differential of a young child with poor vision and an abnormal ERG. Most, but not all, of these children have neurological abnormalities at the time of presentation. Intrauterine infections should also be considered (see Congenital Retinal Disease section in Chapter 13).

RETINITIS PIGMENTOSA ASSOCIATED WITH SYSTEMIC DISEASES

A more detailed and systematic approach to RP associated with systemic disease can be found in Chapter 13. Only the most common examples of RP associated with major systemic syndromes are discussed here.

Usher Syndrome

When retinitis pigmentosa is associated with sensorineural hearing loss, the disorder is termed *Usher syndrome*. This condition is the most common cause of combined deaf-blindness in the United States, and represents a heterogeneous group of autosomal recessively inherited diseases. Of children born with hearing impairment, 3% to 6% have Usher syndrome. Lack of recognition of the coexistence of RP in deaf children may lead to years of frustration, with visual field decrease mistaken as clumsiness. For this reason, all deaf children should have a screening ERG at about age 7 or 8 years, earlier if there are any symptoms of RP. Studies by Merin et al. and Fishman et al. have suggested two common types, and a third rarer subtype; these subtypes are termed USH1, USH2, and USH3.[47,99]

Type I Usher's patients have profound congenital sensorineural hearing loss, usually resulting in unintelligible speech, and mild nonprogressive ataxia associated with absent vestibular function. Slowly progressive retinal degeneration is often noted in early adolescence, with severe impairment of vision around the age of 40. Type II patients have a moderate to profound, nonprogressive, congenital sensorineural impairment, generally intelligible speech, and normal vestibular responses. Visual deficits tend to occur in later adolescence, and good vision is likely to be preserved until 50 to 60 years of age.[117]

Visual fields and dark adaptation are abnormal in Usher's syndrome, often by adolescence. The ERG is typically extinguished or very reduced at presentation in type I. In Type II the ERG is usually recordable. Consultation with otolaryngology is essential because vestibular dysfunction is the best way to distinguish between the two types of Usher syndrome. A rapid initial screen may be performed in the office by having the child or an affected relative attempt toe-to-heel walking. Patients with type I Usher's syndrome usually have difficulty with this maneuver. The differential diagnosis of Usher syndrome includes Alstrom disease, Bardet–Biedl syndrome, Refsum disease, Cogan syndrome, retinal-renal syndromes, and Leber's congenital amaurosis, as well as the mitochondrial myopathies and mucopolysaccharidoses. There are at least six different genetic loci for USH1; one of the common causative genes is MYO7A. One of the genes causing USH2 is the USH2A gene.[4a,18,91] Cochlear implant surgery can restore hearing to many children with Usher syndrome.

Alstrom Syndrome

Alstrom disease[103] presents with impaired vision from the first year of life with nystagmus, photoaversion, and an atypical pigmentary retinopathy, which progresses to bare light perception by the second decade. Bull's-eye maculopathy may be present, and the cone portion of the ERG is abnormal before the rods. Childhood obesity, insulin-resistant diabetes mellitus, sensorineural deafness, and normal mentation are characteristically present. Variably present associations include acanthosis nigricans, baldness, hypogonadism, and life-threatening renal failure. Alstrom syndrome has been mapped to chromosome 2p and is autosomal recessive.[30]

Bardet–Biedl Syndrome

Bardet–Biedl syndrome is an autosomal recessive, multisystem disease characterized by obesity, polydactyly, hypogenitalism, mental retardation, and pigmentary retinopathy. Macular pigment mottling is present with relatively little of the typical bone spicule-like hyperpigmentation. When recordable, a rod–cone dystrophy appears to be most common. Postaxial polydactyly, brachydactyly, and syndactyly, which are common in Bardet–Biedl patients, may be subtle and easily overlooked, particularly if surgery was performed early in life. Diagnosis requires examination of feet and hands and may require radiography. Various authors have argued for distinguishing Bardet–Biedl from the entity of Laurence–Moon syndrome. Patients with the latter develop spastic paresis and extensive choroidal atrophy but lack polydactyly and obesity.[26] Mutations in the MKKS gene cause Bardet–Biedl syndrome.[78,129]

Retinal-Renal Syndromes

Retinitis pigmentosa may be associated with renal failure. Juvenile nephronophthisis or Senior–Loken syndrome is an autosomal recessively inherited disease that features a retinal pigmentary degeneration which may be sectoral, and juvenile-onset renal failure, often requiring renal transplant.[125] The Saldino–Mainzer syndrome features congenital blindness and renal disease.[94]

Neuronal Ceroid Lipofuscinosis

The *neuronal ceroid lipofuscinoses* or *lipopigment storage diseases* (e.g., Batten's disease) are lysosomal storage diseases that are associated with retinal degeneration and neurological deterioration. The infantile form (Haltia–Santavuori) is an autosomal recessive disorder characterized by delayed mental and motor development after a normal first 6 months of life. Patients have nonrecordable ERGs and are totally blind by 2 to 3 years of age. The mean age of death is 6.5 years. The late infantile form (Jansky–Bielschowsky) generally occurs between 2 to 4 years of age and begins with seizures, followed by ataxia, delayed mental and motor development, and decerebrate rigidity before death. Optic atrophy and pigmentary retinopathy accompany the visual loss. Unlike the first two forms, the juvenile type (Batten's, or Spielmeyer–Batten–Vogt) begins with visual loss before the onset of neurological deterioration. Central visual loss begins between the ages of 3 and 7, with death from neurological complications by 20 years.[119,132] The diagnosis of infantile ceroid lipofuscinosis may be aided by the finding of electron-dense bodies within neurons from a rectal biopsy or sural nerve, lymphocytes, brain, or conjunctiva. However, these changes are somewhat nonspecific.[24] Mutations in the CLN1, CLN2, and CLN3 genes cause infantile NCL, late infantile NCL, and juvenile NCL, respectively.[148]

OTHER PHOTORECEPTOR DISORDERS

Congenital Stationary Night Blindness

Congenital stationary night blindness (CSNB), similar to RP, is characterized by abnormal scotopic vision. Three main forms of CSNB have been described: (1) X-linked, the most common; (2) autosomal dominant, typified by the large French Nougaret pedigree; and (3) autosomal recessive, which is rare. Most cases of the latter have been in consanguineous or Jewish families. Snellen visual acuities of CSNB patients range from normal to 20/200, with most cases of severely decreased vision associated with myopia.[64,101] Khouri and colleagues reported a family of X-linked CSNB and hyperopia.[80] Unlike RP patients, the visual function remains stable throughout life, with rare reports of slowly progressive loss of vision.[5] With the exception of myopic changes, the fundus appearance of CSNB patients is normal. Although dark adaptometry curves are typically 2 to 3 log units above normal, some CSNB patients do not complain of nyctalopia.[118] The most common reasons for presentation in childhood are nystagmus, decreased vision, and myopia. Patients with the latter signs invariably have the X-linked or autosomal recessive forms of the disease, because in the autosomal dominant or Nougaret form of CSNB the vision is normal and there is no nystagmus.

Electroretinography is important in the diagnosis of CSNB, and there are several classifications of patients based on these studies. The negative ERG in X-linked and autosomal recessive CSNB, characterized by a selective loss of the b-wave amplitude, is called the Schubert–Bornschein type.[124] The photopic a-wave may also be squared off secondary to a lesser contribution of the early components of the oscillatory potentials. The much rarer Riggs type[121] appears to be associated with autosomal dominant forms of CSNB and has a relatively normal a- and b-wave configuration, with absent rod responses and subnormal cone responses.

Miyake et al. classified the more prevalent Schubert–Bornschein patients into "complete" and "incomplete" types.[105] Patients with the "complete" type of CSNB have poor rod function and absolute psychophysical thresholds that are mediated by cones. Rod responses are selectively diminished on the electroretinogram. Patients with the "incomplete" type of CSNB still have rods mediating threshold but the threshold is elevated.

Interestingly, the ERG reveals marked cone dysfunction in incomplete CSNB, whereas in the complete type cone function is not as severely affected. The validity of Miyake's subtyping is indirectly supported by the lack of any reports finding both subtypes within the same pedigree.

The rate of rhodopsin turnover following a bright light bleach is normal in AD CSNB.[27] Alpern and associates studied pupillary responses and found that rod bleaching signals were normal in spite of poor rod vision, further suggesting that the defect in CSNB is postreceptoral.[3] X-linked CSNB has been mapped to Xp11.[108] Mutations in the NYX gene cause X-linked complete congenital stationary night blindness.[11] Mutations in the CACNA1F gene on Xp11.23 cause another, incomplete form.[10] Autosomal dominant CSNB of the Nougaret type has been attributed to mutations in the GNAT1 gene on 3p22.[37] Various forms of CSNB have been shown to be caused by a number of genes including those which encode rhodopsin, the alpha subunit of rod transducin, the beta subunit of rod cGMP phosphodiesterase, rhodopsin kinase, arrestin, 22 cis retinol dehydrogenase, and a retinal L-type calcium channel.[34] In these disorders the rods are present and function, but abnormally.

There are several rare forms of autosomal recessive CSNB which feature very prolonged recovery of absolute threshold of light sensitivity. These forms differ from the more typical types discussed previously in that they do not have a normal fundus appearance. Fundus albipunctatus is characterized by fine yellow-white dots scattered throughout the retina except for the fovea. There are no other gross abnormalities of the optic nerve, retinal vessels or pigment. Mutations in the RDH5 gene on chromosome 12q13–q14 have been reported in this disorder.[147] Patient's with Oguchi disease may exhibit the Mizuo-Nakamura phenomenon under the proper circumstances. This phenomenon is the appearance of an unusual yellow iridescent sheen in the retina following light exposure which gradually resolves in the dark.[106] Mutations of the SAG(arrestin) and RHOK (Rho kinase) genes cause Oguchi disease.[52,147] The fleck retina of Kandori is a very rare condition which features larger, more irregular yellow flecks than seen in fundus albipunctatus. Electrophysiologic and psychophysical findings are similar to fundus albipunctatus.[76] Although Oguchi disease and fundus albipunctatus are considered stationary, some patients lose vision in late adulthood.

Cone Dystrophies

The cone dystrophies, like the rod-cone dystrophies, represent a heterogeneous group of diseases. Cone dystrophies and cone-rod dystrophies can be inherited in an autosomal dominant, autosomal recessive fashion, or X-linked fashion.

The diagnosis of cone dystrophy is suggested by a history of central acuity loss and poor color discrimination, often accompanied by nystagmus, severe photophobia, and photoaversion. Cone–rod dystrophies are essentially the reverse of rod–cone dystrophies or RP in that they are progressive retinal dystrophies but begin with central vision loss and cone dysfunction rather than peripheral loss and dark adaptation difficulties. Ophthalmoscopy may show a symmetrical "bull's-eye" pattern of macular atrophy, particularly in the autosomal dominant form, although this clinical picture is not specific (see Chapter 13 for the differential diagnosis of "bull's-eye" macula). A more diffuse atrophy of the retina and retinal pigment epithelium in the macula may be seen in the autosomal recessive forms.[48] Electroretinography shows selective loss of cone function, which helps distinguish macular pigmentary changes in cone dystrophy from Stargardt's disease and fundus flavimaculatus.

Rod involvement may eventually become evident on ERG, and perimetry may show constricted visual fields or ring scotoma.[84,122] Ophthalmoscopy at later stages often shows bone spicule-like hyperpigmentation and atrophy in the periphery similar to typical rod–cone degenerations. If severe, symptoms of nyctalopia may be found. The latter are often called cone–rod dystrophies to describe the predominant cone involvement with accompanying rod dysfunction.

Other patterns of cone dysfunction have been reported in which full-field ERG results appear normal. Selective central or peripheral cone involvement has been documented.[85,112,122] The more typical cone dystrophies described previously may also show telangiectasias of the optic nerve head and temporal disc pallor as well.[63] Early in the course of the disease, cone–rod dystrophy may appear to resemble Stargardt disease. The former is progressive whereas the latter is not; therefore, documentation of a stable ERG is necessary for a definitive clinical diagnosis of Stargardt disease.

Autosomal dominant cone–rod dystrophy is caused by mutations in the guanylate cyclase 2D gene (GUCY2D) on chromosome 17p, the RDS/peripherin gene on 6p12, GUCA1A on 6p21, CRX on 19q, and three other loci on 6q and 17q.[33]

Dyschromatopsias (Color Blindness)

Normal males have one normal red pigment gene and one to three green pigment genes in a tandem array on their single X chromosome. Unequal homologous recombination during meiosis can give rise to a variable number of green pigment genes yet still produce a complement with normal color vision. Congenital dyschromatopsias (inherited disorders of color vision) result from either a complete loss of red or green pigment genes or a hybrid red-green pigment gene whose spectral characteristics are anomalous.[109] Acquired dyschromatopsias (disorders of color vision caused by disease) are probably related to selective loss of function of cone photoreceptors or their associated higher-order neurons.[61]

The ophthalmologist is often asked to evaluate a child's color vision because of poor performance on certain color-related tasks, or positive family history, or to aid in diagnosing an ocular condition. *Color vision testing* in children is a challenge. Many children misname colors early in life despite normal vision (this is a common cause of requests for color vision testing). The standard Ishihara plates can be used to screen children on a routine basis. Even if a child cannot yet identify numbers, he or she can be asked to trace the numbers on the plates. The Ishihara plates only test for red-green deficiency and may therefore miss patients with blue-yellow defects. For this reason, they are most useful for detecting congenital dyschromatopsia. The Hardy Rand Rittler plates detect yellow-blue defects and utilize shapes instead of numbers. The D-15 test detects a broad range of color defects but may be more difficult for younger children because it involves matching similar colors. A gross evaluation of color vision may be obtained by having children match pieces of colored yarn or other objects.

The most common cause of defective color vision in childhood is a congenital dyschromatopsia. These disorders are classified according to the types of cone pigments present. Trichromats possess all three types: red, green, and blue. Dichromats have only two of the three pigments and monochromats only one. The terminology becomes complex when naming the associated color vision defects; protanomaly (a "defect of the first type") is a loss of red sensitivity, deuteranomaly ("defect of the second type") a loss of green, and tritanomaly ("defect of the third type") a loss of blue. If the loss of sensitivity is complete, the suffix changes to "opia," for example, from protanomaly (partial loss of red sensitivity) to protanopia (complete loss of red sensitivity). Sophisticated testing is often necessary to exactly categorize a given defect. The most common types are X-linked deuteranomaly, deuteranopia, and protanopia. Approximately 6% of Caucasian males have this form of dyschromatopsia, which can often be diagnosed by Ishihara plates. Inherited tritanomaly and tritanopia are much more rare (0.005% of the population) and are autosomal dominant. Visual acuity is normal in these entities.

Complete achromatopsia (rod monochromatism) is a rare autosomal recessive condition. Individuals are truly "colorblind," interpreting the world in shades of gray. The Sloan achromatopsia test is a good test to aid in this diagnosis but may be difficult to perform in children. This condition usually presents with nystagmus and marked photophobia in early childhood, with color vision defects demonstrated later in life when the child can cooperate. Visual acuity is poor, usually in the 20/200 range. Darkly tinted lenses may improve visual function, even indoors. Achromatopsia is caused by mutations in the CNGA2 gene, which encodes the alpha-subunit of the cone photoreceptor cGMP-gated channel,[146] and in the CNGB3 gene, which encodes the beta-subunit of the cone cyclic nucleotide-gated cation channel that generates the light-evoked electrical responses of the cones.[134] The latter is the cause of achromatopsia in the Pingelapese islands.

Incomplete achromatopsia (blue cone monochromatism) is a condition in which patients have only short-wavelength, blue cones that function normally. There are nonhomologous deletions near the beginning of the red and green genes, which inactivates production of these two pigments.[110] Deletions of the locus control region upstream of the red and green pigment genes, deletions of red pigment exons, and point mutations in isolated pigment genes caused by rearrangements have all been reported.[6,86] It is inherited as an X-linked recessive condition and features males with poor vision from birth, ranging from 20/60 to 20/200 vision. Retinal pigmentary changes and a slow decrease in visual acuity may be seen over time in adulthood. The Berson color vision test may be used to distinguish blue cone monocromatism from complete achromatopsia.[17] Carrier females may have subtle ERG and eye movement abnormalities.[15,56] The differential diagnosis for these conditions includes albinism, CSNB, and congenital motor nystagmus. The latter may be X linked, but maps to a different locus.[79a] Acquired color vision loss may be caused by seizure medication such as vigabatrin and carbamazepine, toxins such as styrene, and combinations of substances such as melatonin, zoloft, and high-protein diet.[89,113,137]

OTHER RP-LIKE RETINAL DISORDERS

Unilateral Pigmentary Retinopathy

Most investigators believe that the concept of unilateral retinitis pigmentosa is flawed and favor the term unilateral pigmentary degeneration. Unlike classic RP, there is usually no family history, and the onset of the disease is relatively late. Although a few cases of rhodopsin-associated ADRP may present with a falsely negative family history, mild functional involvement, and very asymmetrical retinal changes, unilateral retinal pigmentary degeneration in a child should not be considered RP unless all other possible diagnoses have been excluded. Although typical retinitis pigmentosa may exhibit some degree of asymmetrical involvement, both eyes manifest the disease. Strict criteria for the diagnosis of unilateral pigmentary degeneration demand that the fellow eye have a normal ophthalmoscopic appearance, as well as psychophysical and electroretinographic function that does not deteriorate over time.[28]

Reported causes for unilateral pigmentary degeneration include trauma, a transient ophthalmic artery occlusion,[28] longstanding serous detachment of the neurosensory retina from an optic pit,[120] asymmetrical Toxoplasmosis, Rubella, Cytomegalovirus, Herpes simplex virus (TORCH) infections, and retained intraocular foreign body.[8,29] The inflammatory response to a subretinal parasite known as the diffuse unilateral subacute neuroretinitis (DUSN) syndrome[54] could be added to the differential diagnosis of unilateral disease. A careful birth and prenatal history should be taken, because retinopathy of prematurity is often asymmetrical and may leave retinal pigmentary changes in one eye as a result of either the disease or the treatment.

X-Linked Juvenile Retinoschisis

The diagnosis of X-linked juvenile retinoschisis is usually made on the basis of ophthalmoscopy and an X-linked recessive pattern of inheritance. Children with this disease usually come to attention because of decreased vision on school screening or acute vision loss from vitreous hemorrhage. Foveal retinoschisis is found in nearly all cases, with peripheral retinoschisis present in 50% of cases. Atrophic macular lesions are rarely seen. The vitreous body is optically empty or contains dense bands. Red-free photographs are often useful to diagnose foveal retinoschisis, and a lack of dye leakage on fluorescein angiography can help make the correct diagnosis if cystoid macular edema is erroneously suspected as the cause of poor vision. Electroretinography should be performed and generally shows a selective loss of the b-wave amplitude. In spite of an apparent selective foveal involvement by ophthalmoscopy in 50% of cases, involvement of the full-field electroretinogram suggests panretinal disease. In addition to predominant b-wave loss, dysfunction of the inner retinal layers is suggested by markedly reduced oscillatory potentials.[104] The XLRS1 gene on Xp22 has been found to harbor mutations in this disorder.[18]

OTHER SYNDROMES

The Goldman–Favre syndrome is a very rare autosomal recessive condition, reported mainly in the European literature. Affected patients typically complain of nyctalopia and have an "optically empty" vitreous with a nonrecordable ERG.[46] It is the most severe form of enhanced S-cone syndrome caused by mutation of the nuclear receptor gene, NR2E3.[60a] Patients with gyrate atrophy present with nyctalopia at 20 to 30 years of age and have poorly recordable rod and cone ERGs with constricted visual fields. They are usually myopic, with cataracts and characteristic nummular areas of chorioretinal atrophy. Pedigree analysis suggests autosomal recessive inheritance. Biochemical studies reveal hyperornithemia and a reduction in ornithine alpha-aminotransferase activity. Dietary modifications ameliorate the disease.[138,144] Affected males with the X-linked disorder choroideremia usually complain of nyctalopia between 20 and 30 years of age and may have a fundus appearance at some stages of the disease similar to patients with gyrate atrophy. Deterioration of the RPE and choroid is progressive and does not feature extensive pigmentary clumping, as is typical in RP. ERGs are markedly affected early in life as are the visual fields.[128] The preponderance of male involvement within the pedigree and the characteristic radial, "splattered mud" pattern of hyperpigmentation in the periphery of carrier females helps distinguish this X-linked recessive disease from gyrate atrophy. The choroideremia gene (CHM) has been identified and maps to Xq21.2.[32] Gyrate atrophy is AR and is caused by mutations of the ornithine aminotransferase gene on 10q26.[102] Spinocerebellar ataxia type 7 (SCA7), also called olivopontocerebellar atrophy type III, may present as a retinal degeneration in infancy or childhood. It is usually accompanied by ophthalmoplegia, ataxia, and progressive neurological deterioration. This disorder is autosomal dominant and maps to chromosome 3p. Expansions of CAG repeats in the gene affect the protein product, ataxin 7. Normal alleles have from 7 to 16 repeats whereas abnormal alleles have more than 41.[58] The more repeats present, the worse the disease, and because repeats tend to increase with succeeding generations, especially if transmitted by the father, the disorder may be worse with each generation. Parents should be examined closely for subtle maculopathy or mild ataxia.

SUMMARY

The application of molecular biology to clinical medicine is a relatively recent development but has already had great impact upon our understanding of disease processes. It has improved our ability to care for RP patients by allowing us to establish a diagnosis of ADRP, even when clinical suspicion may be low, as well as to remove the fear of disease from unaffected relatives. Refinement in the diagnosis of simplex cases, where no family history is available, is now possible for many retinal dystrophies using molecular genetic techniques to identify abnormal candidate genes. Early success in treating retinal degenerations in animals give us hope that advances in the molecular understanding of retinal degenerations can soon be translated into more effective treatments for these diseases.

Acknowledgments. The text and figures in this chapter were derived largely from those prepared by Alan E. Kimura, MD,

Arlene Drack, MD, and Edwin M. Stone, MD, PhD, in the previous edition of this textbook. Dr. Drack is supported by the Georgia Lions Children's Eyecare Center.

References

1. Acland GM, Aguirre GD, Zhang Q, et al. Gene therapy restores vision in a canine model of childhood blindness. Nat Genet 2001; 28(1):92–95.
2. Aleman TS, Duncan JL, Bieber ML, et al. Macular pigment and lutein supplementation in RP and Usher syndrome. Investig Ophthalmol Vis Sci 2001;42(8):1873–1881.
3. Alpern M, Holland MG, Oba N. Rhodopsin bleaching signals in essential nightblindness. J Physiol 1972;225:457–476.
4. Alstrom CH, Olson OA. Heredoretinopathia congenitalis monohybrida recessiva autsomalis. Hereditas 1957;43:1–177.

4a. Astuto LM, Weston MD, Carner, CA, et al. Genetic heterogeneity of Usher syndrome. Am J Hum Genet 2000;67(6):1569–1574.

5. Auerbach E, Godel V, Rowe H. An electrophysiological and psychophysical study of two forms of congenital night blindness. Investig Ophthalmol 1969;8:332–345.
6. Ayyagari R, Kakuk LE, Coats CL, et al. Bilateral macular atrophy in blue cone monochromacy with loss of the locus control region (LCR) and part of the red pigment gene. Mol Vis 1999;5:13.
7. Bareil C, Hamel CP, Delague V, Arnaud B, Demaille J, Claustres M. Segregation of a mutation in CNGB1 encoding the beta-subunit of the rod cGMP-gated channel in a family with autosomal recessive retinitis pigmentosa. Hum Genet 2001;108(4):328–334.
8. Bastek JV, Foos RY, Heckenlively J. Traumatic pigmentary retinopathy. Am J Ophthalmol 1981;92:621–624.
9. Bastek JV, Heckenlively JR, Straatsma BR. Cataract surgery in retinitis pigmentosa patients. Ophthalmology 1982;89:880–884.
10. Bech-Hansen NT, Naylor MJ, Maybaum TA, et al. Loss of function mutations in a calcium-channel alpha 1-subunit gene in Xp11.23 cause incomplete X-linked congenital stationary night blindness. Nat Genet 1998;19(3):264–267.
11. Bech-Hansen NT, Naylor MJ, Maybaum TA, et al. Mutations in NYX, encoding the leucine-rich proteoglycan nyctalopin, cause X-linked complete stationary night blindness. Nat Genet 2000; 26(3):319–323.
12. Berson EL, Grimsby JL, Adams SM, et al. Clinical features and mutations in patients with dominant retinitis pigmentosa-1(RP1). Investig Ophthalmol Vis Sci 2001;42(10):2217–2224.
13. Berson EL. Nutrition and retinal degenerations. Int Ophthalmol Clin 2000;40:93–111.
14. Berson EL. Retinitis pigmentosa and allied disease: applications of electroretinographic testing. Int Ophthalmol 1981;4:7–22.

15. Berson EL, Sandberg MA, Maguire A, Bromley WC, Roderick TH. Electroretinograms in carriers of blue cone monochromatism. Am J Ophthalmol 1986;102(2):254–261.
16. Berson EL, Sandberg MA, Rosner B, Birch DG, Hanson AH. Natural course of retinitis pigmentosa over a three year interval. Am J Ophthalmol 1985;99:240–251.
17. Berson EL, Sandberg MA, Rosner B, Sullivan PL. Color plates to help identify patients with blue cone monochromatism. Am J Ophthalmol 1983;95(6):741–747.
18. Bessant DA, Ali RR, Bhattacharya SS. Molecular genetics and prospects for therapy of the inherited retinal dystrophies. Curr Opin Genet Dev 2001;11(3):307–316.
19. Bhattacharya SS, Wright AF, Clayton JF, et al. Close genetic linkage between X-linked retinitis pigmentosa and a restriction fragment length polymorphism identified by recombinant DNA probe L1.28. Nature (Lond) 1984;309:253–255.
20. Blanton SH, Heckenlively JR, Cottingham AW, et al. Linkage mapping of autosomal dominant retinitis pigmentosa (RP1) to the pericentric region of human chromosome 8. Genomics 1992;11: 857–869.
21. Bolz H, von Brederlow B, Ramirez A, et al. Mutation of CDH23 encoding a new member of the cadherin family, causes Usher syndrome type 1D. Nat Genet 2001;2791:108–112.
22. Boughman JA, Coneally PM, Nance WE. Population genetics studies of retinitis pigmentosa. Am J Hum Genet 1980;32:223–235.
23. Boughman JA, Fishman GA. A genetic analysis of retinitis pigmentosa. Br J Ophthalmol 1983;67:449–454.
24. Brod RD, Packer AJ, Van Dyck HJL. Diagnosis of neuronal ceroid lipofuscinosis by ultrastructural examination of peripheral blood lymphocytes. Arch Ophthalmol 1987;105:1388–1393.
25. Burstedt MS, Forsman-Semb K, Golovleva I, Janunger T, Wachtmeister L, Sandgren O. Ocular phenotype of bothnia dystrophy, an autosomal recessive retinitis pigmentosa associated with an R234W mutation in the RLBP1 gene. Arch Ophthalmol 2001;119(2): 260–267.
26. Campo RV, Aaberg TM. Ocular and systemic manifestations of the Bardet-Biedl syndrome. Am J Ophthalmol 1982;94:750–756.
27. Carr RE, Ripps H, Siegel IM, Weale RA. Rhodopsin and the electrical activity of the retina in congenital night blindness. Investig Ophthalmol 1966;5:497–507.
28. Carr RE, Siegel IM. Unilateral retinitis pigmentosa. Arch Ophthalmol 1973;90:21–26.
29. Cogan DG. Pseudoretinitis pigmentosa. Arch Ophthalmol 1969;81: 45–53.
30. Collin GB, Marshall JD, Cardon LR, Nishina PM. Homozygosity mapping at Alstrom locus to chromosome 2p. Hum Mol Genet 1997; 6(2):213–219.

30a. Collin GB, Marshall JD, Ikeda A, et al. Mutations in ALMS1 cause obesity, type 2 diabetes and neurosensory degeneration in Alstrom syndrome. Nat Gent 2002;31(1):74–78.
31. Connell G, Bascom R, Molday L, Reid D, McInnes RR, Molday RS. Photoreceptor peripherin is the normal product of the gene responsible for retinal degeneration in the rds mouse. Proc Natl Acad Sci USA 1991;88:723–726.
32. Cremers FPM, van de Pol TJR, van Kerhoff LPM, Wieringa B, Ropers HH. Cloning of a gene that is rearranged in patients with choroideraemia. Nature (Lond) 1990;347:674–677.
33. Downes SM, Payne AM, Kelsell RE, et al. Autosomal dominant cone-rod dystrophy with mutations in the guanylate cyclase 2D gene encoding retinal guanylate cyclase-1. Arch Ophthalmol 2001;119:1667–1673.
34. Dryja TP. Molecular genetics of Oguchi disease, fundus albipunctatus, and other forms of stationary night blindness. Am J Ophthalmol 2000;130(5):547–563.
35. Dryja TP, Adams SM, Grimsby JL, et al. Null RPGRIP1 alleles in patients with Leber congenital amaurosis. Am J Hum Genet 2001;68(5):1295–1298.
36. Dryja TP, Hahn LB, Kajiwara K, Berson EL. Dominant and digenic mutations in the peripherin/RDS and ROM1 genes in retinitis pigmentosa. Investig Ophthalmol Vis Sci 1997;38:1972–1982.
37. Dryja TP, Hahn LB, Reboul T, Arnaud B. Missense mutation in the gene encoding the alpha subunit of rod transducin in the Nougaret form of congenital stationary night blindness. Nat Genet 1996;13(3):358–360.
38. Dryja TP, McEvoy JA, McGee TL, Berson EL. Novel ghodopsin mutations Gly114Val and Gln184Pro in dominant retinitis pigmentosa. Investig Ophthalmol Vis Sci 2000;41:3124–3127.
39. Dryja TP, McGee TL, Reichel E, et al. A point mutation of the rhodopsin gene in one form of retinitis pigmentosa. Nature (Lond) 1990;343:364–366.
40. Farrer GJ, Kenna P, Jordan SA, et al. A three base-pair deletion in the peripherin-RDS gene in one form of retinitis pigmentosa. Nature (Lond) 1991;354:478–480.
41. Fielder AR, Russell-Eggitt IR, Dodd KL, Mellor DH. Delayed visual maturation. Trans Ophthalmol Soc UK 1985;104:653–661.
42. Fishman GA. Retinitis pigmentosa. Visual loss. Arch Ophthalmol 1978;96:1185–1188.
43. Fishman GA, Alexander KR, Anderson RJ. Autosomal dominant retinitis pigmentosa: a method of classification. Arch Ophthalmol 1985;103:366–374.
44. Fishman GA, Fishman M, Maggiano J. Macular lesions associated with retinitis pigmentosa. Arch Ophthalmol 1977;95:798–803.
45. Fishman GA, Gilbert LD, Fiscella RG, Kimura AE, Jampol LM. Acetazolamide for treatment of chronic macular edema in retinitis pigmentosa. Arch Ophthalmol 1989;107:1445–1452.

46. Fishman GA, Jampol LM, Goldberg MF. Diagnostic features of the Favre–Goldmann syndrome. Br J Ophthalmol 1976;60:345–353.
47. Fishman GA, Kumar A, Joseph ME, Torok, Anderson RJ. Usher's syndrome: ophthalmic and neuro-otologic findings suggesting genetic heterogeneity. Arch Ophthalmol 1983;101:1367–1374.
48. Fishman GA, Sokol S. Electrophysiologic testing in disorders of the retina, optic nerve, and visual pathway. San Francisco: American Academy of Ophthalmology, 1990.
49. Foxman SG, Wirtschafter FD, Letson RD. Leber's congenital amaurosis and high hyperopia: a discrete entity. In: Henkind P (ed) Acta XXIV International Congress of Ophthalmology, vol 1. Philadelphia: Lippincott, 1983:55–85.
50. Franceschetti A. Rubeola pendant la grossesse et cataracte congenitale chez l'enfant, accompagnee du phenomene digito-oculaire. Ophthalmologica 1947;114:332–339.
51. Francois J. Leber's congenital tapetoretinal degeneration. Int Ophthalmol Clin 1968;8:929–947.
52. Fuchs S, Nakazawa M, Maw M, Tamai M, Oguchi Y, Gal A. A homozygous 1 base pair deletion in the arrestin gene is a frequent casue of Oguchi disease in Japanese. Nat Genet 1995;10(3):360–362.
53. Fulton AB, Hansen RM. Electroretinography: application to clinical studies of infants. J Pediatr Ophthalmol 1985;22:251–255.
54. Gass JDM, Braunstein RA. Further observations concerning the diffuse unilateral subacute neuroretintis syndrome. Arch Ophthalmol 1983;101:1689–1697.
55. Gerber S, Perrault I, Hanein S, et al. Complete exon–intron structure of the RPGR-interacting protein (RPGRIP1) gene allows the identification of mutations underlying Leber's congenital amaurosis. Eur J Hum Genet 2001;9(8):561–571.
56. Gottlob I. Eye movement abnormalities in carriers of blue-cone monochromatism. Investig Ophthalmol Vis Sci 1994;35(9):3556–3560.
57. Gouras P, Carr RE. Electrophysiological studies in early retinitis pigmentosa. Arch Ophthalmol 1964;72:104–110.
58. Grattan-Smith PJ, Healey S, Grigg JR, Christodoulou J. Spinocerebellar ataxia type 7: a distinctive form of autosomal dominant cerebellar ataxia with retinopathy and marked genetic anticipation. J Paediatr Child Health 2001;37(1):81–84.
59. Green ES, Rendahl KG, Zhou S, et al. Two animal models of retinal degeneration are rescued by recombinant adeno-associated virus-mediated production of FGF-5 and FGF-18. Mol Therapy 2001;3(4): 507–515.
60. Guevara-Fujita M, Fahrner S, Buraczynska K, et al. Five novel RPGR mutations in families with X-linked retinitis pigmentosa. Hum Mutat 2001;17(2):151.
60a. Haider NB, Jacobsen SG, et al. Mutation of a nuclear receptor gene, NR2E3, causes enhanced S cone syndrome, a disorder of retinal cell fate. Nat Genet 2000;24(2):99–100.

61. Hart WM. Acquired dyschromatopsias. Surv Ophthalmol 1987;32: 10–31.
62. Heckenlively JR. Grid photocoagulation for macular edema in patients with retinitis pigmentosa. Am J Ophthalmol 1987;104: 94–95.
63. Heckenlively JR, Martin DA, Rosales TO. Telangiectasia and optic atrophy in cone-rod degenerations. Arch Ophthalmol 1981;99: 1983–1991.
64. Heckenlively JR, Martin DA, Rosenbaum AL. Loss of electroretinographic oscillatory potentials, optic atrophy, and dysplasia in congenital stationary night blindness. Am J Ophthalmol 1983;96: 526–534.
65. Heckenlively JR, Rodriguez JA, Daiger SP. Autosomal dominant sectoral retinitis pigmentosa. Two families with transversion mutation in codon 23 of rhodopsin. Arch Ophthalmol 1991;109:84–91.
66. Heher KL, Traboulsi EI, Maumenee IA. The natural history of Leber's congenital amaurosis. Age-related findings in 35 patients. Ophthalmology 1992;99:241–245.
67. Hirose E, Inoue Y, Morimura H, et al. Mutations in the 11-*cis* retinol dehydrogenase gene in Japanese patients with fundus albipunctatus. Investig Ophthalmol Vis Sci 2000;41(12):3933–3935.
68. Inglehearn CF, et al. A new locus for autosomal dominant retinitis pigmentosa on chromosome 7p. Nat Genet 1993;4:51–53.
69. International Society for the Clinical Electrophysiology of Vision. International Standardization Committee. Standard for clinical electroretinography. Arch Ophthalmol 1989;107:816–819.
70. Jay B, Bird A. X-linked retinitis pigmentosa. Trans Am Acad Ophthalmol Otolaryngol 1973;77:641–651.
71. Jordan SA, Farrar GJ, Kenna P, et al. Localization of an autosomal dominant retinitis pigmentosa gene to chromsome 7q. Nat Genet 1993;4:54–58.
72. Joubert M, Eisenring J, Robb JP, Andermann F. Familial agenesis of the cerebellar vermis. A syndrome of episodic hyperpnea, abnormal eye movements, ataxia, and retardation. Neurology 1969;19:813–825.
73. Judisch GF, Anderson S, Bell WE. Chloral hydrate sedation as a substitute for examination under anesthesia in pediatric ophthalmology. Am J Ophthalmol 1980;89:560–563.
74. Kajiwara K, Hahn LB, Mukai S, Travis GH, Berson EL, Dryja TP. Mutations in the human retinal degeneration slow gene in autosomal dominant retinitis pigmentosa. Nature (Lond) 1991;354:480–483.
75. Kajiwara K, Sandberg MA, Berson EL, Dryja TP. A null mutation in the human peripherin/RDS gene in a family with autosomal dominant retinitis punctata albescans. Nat Genet 1993;3:208–212.
76. Kandori F, Setogawa T, Tamai A. Electroretinographic studies on fleck retina with congenital nonprogressive night blindness. Yonago Acta Med 1966;10:98–108.

77. Kaplan J, Gerber S, Bonneau D, et al. A gene for Usher syndrome type 1 (USH1A) maps to chromosome 14q. Genomics 1992;14:979–987.
78. Katsanis N, Beales PL, Woods MO, et al. Mutations in MKKS cause obesity, retinal dystrophy and renal malformations associated with Bardet-Biedl syndrome. Nat Genet 2000;26(1):67–70.
79. Katsanis N, Shroyer NF, Lewis RA, et al. Fundus albipunctatus and retinitis punctata albescens in a pedigree with an R150Q mutation in RLBP1. Clin Genet 2001;59(6):424–429.
79a. Kerrison JB, Giorda R, Lenart TD, Drack AV, Maumenee IH. Clinical and genetic analysis of a family with X-linked nystagmus. Ophthalmol Genet 2001,22(4):241–248.
80. Khouri G, Mets MB, Smith VC, Wendell M, Pass A. X-linked congenital stationary night blindness. Review and report of a family with hyperopia. Arch Ophthalmol 1988;106:1417–1422.
81. Kimberling WJ, Moller CG, Davenport S, et al. Linkage of Usher syndrome type 1 gene (USH1B) to the long arm of chromsome II. Genomics 1992;14:988–994.
82. Kimberling WJ, Weston MD, Moller C, et al. Localization of Usher syndrome type II to chromosome 1q. Genomics 1990;7:245–249.
83. King MD, Dudgeon J, Stephenson JBP. Joubert's syndrome with retinal dysplasia; neonatal tachypnoea as the clue to a genetic brain-eye malformation. Arch Dis Child 1984;59:709–718.
84. Krauss HR, Heckenlively JR. Visual field changes in cone-rod degenerations. Arch Ophthalmol 1982;100:1784–1790.
85. Krill AE, Deutman AF, Fishman M. The cone degenerations. Doc Ophthalmol 1973;35:1–80.
85a. Kwitek-Black AE, Carmi R, Duyk GM, et al. Linkage of Bardet–Biedl syndrome to chromosome 16q and evidence for no allelic genetic heterogeneity. Nat Genet 1993;5(4):392–396.
86. Ladekjaer-Mikkelsen AS, Rosenberg T, Jorgensen AL. A new mechanism in blue cone monochromatism. Hum Genet 1996;98(4):403–408.
86a. Lambert SR, Kriss A, Taylor D, Coffey R, Pembrey M. Follow-up and diagnostic reappraisal of 75 patients with Leber's congenital amaurosis. Am J Ophthalmol 1989;107:624–631.
87. Lambert SR, Kriss AT, Gresty M, Benton, S, Taylor, D. Joubert syndrome. Arch Ophthalmol 1989;107:709–713.
88. Lambert SR, Kriss A, Taylor D. Delayed visual maturation: a longitudinal clinical and electrophysiological assessment. Ophthalmology 1989;96:524–528.
89. Lehman NL, Johnson LN. Toxic optic neuropathy after concomitant use of melatonin, zoloft, and a high protein diet. J Neuro-Ophthalmol 1999;19(4):232–234.
90. Liang FQ, Aleman TS, Zaixian Yang, et al. Melatonin delays photoreceptor degeneration in the rds/rds mouse. NeuroReport 2001; 12(5):1011–1014.

91. Liu XZ, Blanton SH, Bitner-Glindzicz M, et al. Haplotype analysis of the USH1D locus and genotype-phenotype correlations. Clin Genet 2001;60(1):58–62.
92. Loewen CJ, Moritz OL, Molday RS. Molecular characterization of peripherin-2 and rom-1 mutants responsible for digenic retinitis pigmentosa. J Biol Chem 2001;276(25):22388–22396.
93. Lyness AL, Ernst W, Quinlan MP, et al. A clinical, psychophysical, and electroretinographic survey of patients with autosomal dominant retinitis pigmentosa. Br. J Ophthalmol 1985;69:326–339.
94. Mainzer F, Saldino RM, Ozononoff M, Minagitt M. Familial nephropathy associated with retinitis pigmentosa, cerebellar ataxia and skeletal abnormalities. Am J Med 1970;49:556–562.
95. Margolis S, Scher BM, Carr RE. Macular colobomas in Leber's congenital amaurosis. Am J Ophthalmol 1977;83:27–31.
96. Marmor MF. Visual loss in retinitis pigmentosa. Am J Ophthalmol 1980;89:692–698.
97. Massof RW, Finkelstein D. Subclassifications of retinitis pigmentosa from two-color scotopic static perimetry. Doc Ophthalmol Proc Ser 1981;26:219–225.
98. McWilliam P, Farrar GJ, Kenna P, et al. Autosomal dominant retinitis pigmentosa (ADRP): localization of an ADRP gene to the long arm of chromosome 3. Genomics 1989;5:619–622.
99. Merin S, Abraham FA, Auerbach E. Usher's and Hallgren's syndromes. Acta Genet Med Gemellol (Roma) 1974;23:49–55.
100. Merin S, Auerbach E. Retinitis pigmentosa. Surv Ophthalmol 1976;20:303–346.
101. Merin S, Rowe H, Auerbach E, Landau J. Syndrome of congenital high myopia with nyctalopia. Report of findings in 25 families. Am J Ophthalmol 1970;70:541–547.
102. Michaud J, Thompson GN, Brody LC, et al. Pyridoxine responsive gyrate atrophy of the choroid and retina: clinical and biochemical correlates of the mutation A226V. Am J Hum Genet 1995;56(3):616–622.
103. Millay RH, Weleber RG, Heckenlively JR. Ophthalmologic and systemic manifestations of Alstrom's disease. Am J Ophthalmol 1986;102:482–490.
104. Miyake Y, Kawase Y. Reduced amplitude of oscillatory potentials in female carriers of X-linked recessive congenital stationary night blindness. Am J Ophthalmol 1984;98:208–215.
105. Miyake Y, Yagasaki K, Horiguchi M, Kawase Y, Kanda T. Congenital stationary night blindness with negative electroretinogram. A new classification. Arch Ophthalmol 1986;104:1013–1020.
106. Mizuo G. On a new discovery in the dark adaptation on Oguchi's disease. Acta Soc Ophthalmol Jpn 1913;17:1148.
107. Musarella MA, Anson-Cartwright CL, McDowell C, et al. Physical mapping at a potential X-linked retinitis pigmentosa locus (RP3) by pulsed-field gel electrophoresis. Genomics 1991;11(2):263–273.

108. Musarella MA, Weleber RG, Murphey WH, et al. Assignment of the gene for complete X-linked congenital stationary night blindness (CSNB1) to Xp11.3. Genomics 1989;5:727–737.
109. Nathans J. The genes for color vision. Sci Am 1989;260:42–49.
110. Nathans J, Davenport CM, Maumenee IH, et al. Molecular genetics of human blue cone monochromacy. Science 1989;245:831–838.
111. Nickel B, Hoyt CS. Leber's congenital amaurosis: is mental retardation a frequent associated defect? Arch Ophthalmol 1982;100:1089–1092.
112. Noble KG, Siegel IM, Carr RE. Progressive peripheral cone dysfunction. Am J Ophthalmol 1988;106:557–560.
113. Nousiainen I, Kalvainen R, Mantyjarvi M. Color vision in epilepsy patients treated with vigabatrin or carbamazepine monotherapy. Ophthalmology 2000;107(5):884–888.
114. Nussbaum RL, Lewis RA, Lesko JG, Ferrell R. Mapping X-linked ophthalmic disease. II. Linkage relationship of X-linked retinitis pigmentosa to X chromosomal short arm markers. Hum Genet 1985;70:45–50.
115. Peachey NS, Fishman GA, Derlacki DJ, Alexander KR. Rod and cone dysfunction in carriers of X-linked retinitis pigmentosa. Ophthalmology 1988;95:677–685.
116. Pearlman JT, Flood TP, Seiff SR. Retinitis pigmentosa without pigment. Am J Ophthalmol 1976;81:417–419.
117. Piazza L, Fishman GA, Farber M, Derlacki D, Anderson RJ. Visual acuity loss in patients with Usher's syndrome. Arch Ophthalmol 1986;104:1336–1339.
118. Price MJ, Judisch, Thompson HS. X-linked congenital stationary night blindness with myopia and nystagmus without clinical complaints of nyctalopia. J Pediatr Ophthalmol Strabismus 1988;25:33–36.
119. Raitta C, Santavouri P. Ophthalmologic findings in infantile type of so-called neuronal ceroid lipofuscinosis. Acta Ophthalmologica 1973;51:755–763.
120. Regenbogen L, Stein R, Lazar M. Macular and juxtapapillary serous retinal detachment associated with pit of optic disc. Ophthalmologica 1964;148:247–251.
121. Riggs LA. Electroretinography in cases of night blindness. Am J Ophthalmol 1954;38:70–78.
122. Ripps H, Noble KG, Greenstein VC, et al. Progressive cone dystrophy. Ophthalmology 1987;94:1401–1409.
123. Rosenfeld PJ, Cowley GS, McGee TL, Sandberg MA, Berson EL, Dryja TP. A null mutation in the rhodopsin gene causes rod photoreceptor dysfunction and autosomal recessive retinitis pigmentosa. Nat Genet 1992;1(3):209–213.
124. Schubert G, Bornschein H. Beitrag zur Analyse des menschlichen Elektroretinograms. Ophthalmologica 1952;123:396–413.
125. Senior B, Friedmann A, Braudo JL. Juvenile familial nephropathy with tapetoretinal degeneration. Am J Ophthalmol 1961;52:625–633.

126. Sheffield VC, Fishman GA, Beck JS, Kimura AE, Stone EM. Identification of novel rhodopsin mutations associated with retinitis pigmentosa by GC-clamped denaturing gradient gel electrophoresis. Am J Hum Genet 1991;49:699–706.
127. Sieving PA, Fishman GA. Refractive errors of retinitis pigmentosa patients. Br J Ophthalmol 1978;62:163–167.
128. Sieving PA, Niffennegger, Berson E. ERG findings in selected pedigrees with choroideremia. Am J Ophthalmol 1986;101:361–367.
129. Slavotinek AM, Stone EM, Myktyn K, et al. Mutations in MKKS cause Bardet–Biedl syndrome. Nat Genet 2000;26(1):15–16.
130. Smith RJH, Lee EC, Kimberling WJ, et al. Localization of two genes for Usher syndrome type 1 to chromosome 11. Genomics 1992;14:995–1002.
131. Sohocki MM, Daiger SP, Bowne SJ, et al. Prevalence of mutations causing retinitis pigmentosa and other inherited retinopathies. Hum Mutat 2001;17(1):42–51.
132. Spalton DJ, Taylor DS, Sanders MD. Juvenile Batten's disease: an ophthalmological assessment of 26 patients. Br J Ophthalmol 1980;64:726–732.
133. Stone EM, Kimura AE, Nichols BE, Khadivi P, Fishman GA, Sheffield VC. Regional distribution of retinal degeneration in patients with the proline to histidine mutation in codon 23 of the rhodopsin gene. Ophthalmology 1991;98:1806–1813.
134. Sundin OH, Yang JM, Li Y, et al. Genetic basis of total colourblindness among the Pingelapese islanders. Nat Genet 2000;25(3):289–293.
135. Sung CH, Davenport CM, Hennessey JC, et al. Rhodopsis mutations in autosomal dominant retinitis pigmentosa. Proc Natl Acad Sci USA 1991;88:6481.
136. Tanino T, Ohba N. Studies on pigmentary retinal dystrophy. I. Age of onset of subjective symptoms and the mode of inheritance. Jpn J Ophthalmol 1976;20:474–481.
137. Triebig G, Stark T, Ihrig A, Dietz MC. Intervention study on acquired color vision deficiences in styrene exposed workers. J Occup Environ Med 2001;43(5):494–500.
138. Valle D, Walser M, Brusilow SW, et al. Gyrate atrophy of the choroid and retina. Amino acid metabolism and correction of hyperornithinemia with an arginine deficient diet. J Clin Invest 1980;65:371–378.
139. Wada Y, Abe T, Takeshita T, Sato H, Yanashima K, Tamai M. Mutation of human retinal fascin gene (FSCN2) causes dominant retinitis pigmentosa. Investig Ophthalmol Vis Sci 2001;42(10):2395–2400.
140. Wagner RS, Caputo AR, Nelson LB, Zanoni D. High hyperopia in Leber's congenital amaurosis. Arch Ophthalmol 1985;103:1507–1509.
141. Weiss AH, Biersdorf WR. Visual sensory disorders in congenital nystagmus. Ophthalmology 1989;96:517–523.

142. Weiss AH, Kelly JP, Phillips JO. The infant who is visually unresponsive on a cortical basis. Ophthalmology 2001;108(11):2076–2087.
143. Weleber RG. Retinitis pigmentosa and allied disorders. In: Ryan SJ (ed) Retina. St. Louis: Mosby, 1989:299–420.
144. Weleber RG, Kennaway NG. Clinical trial of vitamin B_6 for gyrate atrophy of the choroid and retina. Ophthalmology 1981;88:316.
145. Weleber RG, Tongue AAT. Congenital stationary night blindness presenting as Leber's congenital amaurosis. Arch Ophthalmol 1987;105:360–365.
146. Wissinger B, Gamer D, Jagle H, et al. CNGA3 mutations in hereditary cone photoreceptor disorders. Am J Hum Genet 2001;69(4):L722–L737.
147. Yamamoto S, Sippel KC, Berson El, Dryja TP. Defects in the rhodopsin kinase gene in the Oguchi form of stationary night blindness. Nat Genet 1997;15(2):175–178.
148. Zhong N, Moroziewicz DN, Ju W, et al. Heterogeneity of late-infantile neuronal ceroid lipofuscinosis. Genet Med 2000;2(6):312–318.

6

Disorders of the Vitreous and Vitreoretinal Interface

David M. Brown and Thomas A. Weingeist

The human vitreous is a complex extracellular matrix composed of 98% water and 2% solid material. The basic structure of the vitreous matrix is a scaffold of cross-linked collagen fibrils with hyaluronic acid molecules within the scaffold. Hyaluronic acid is very hydrophilic, and water molecules are attracted to the scaffold providing turgor and rigidity to the matrix. The vitreous is primarily a solid gel in children's eyes but becomes progressively more liquid with aging. Liquefaction of the vitreous occurs when the hyaluronic acid depolymerizes, freeing the bound water and allowing the collagen scaffold to collapse. The collagen filaments then coalesce to form collagen fibers, causing the "floaters" seen by patients with aging of the vitreous.

Several hereditary degenerative conditions are characterized by an abnormal appearance of the vitreous gel structure and associated retinal changes. Because of the intimate relationship between the vitreous and the retina, it is often difficult to identify which tissue is primarily affected. Some of these diseases may arise from abnormal formation or accelerated degenerative changes of the vitreous body that lead to secondary retinal changes. Other entities are most likely caused by abnormal development of retinal vasculature, which leads to secondary vitreous degeneration in the areas of avascular retina.

Many of the vitreoretinopathies discussed in this chapter have similar findings with only a few differentiating points. Table 6-1 provides an introduction to these disorders and demonstrates the overlapping clinical findings in many of the diseases.

TABLE 6-1. Vitreoretinopathy Review.

	Lattice degeneration	*Wagner syndrome*	*Stickler syndrome*	*Erosive*	*Goldmann–Favre syndrome*	*X-linked retinoschisis*	*Snowflake*	*ADViRC*	*ADNIV*	*FEVR*
Vitreous syneresis	Focal	++	++	++	++	+	+	+	+	±
Cataract		+	+	+	+		+	+	+	
Risk of retinal detachment	2%	<5%	50%	50%	<5%	5%–10%	33%	<2%	20%	4%–30%
Foveal changes	–	–	–	RPE "erosion"	Foveal schisis	Foveal schisis	– –	CME	CME	Ectopic fovea
Prominent pigmentary retinopathy	–	+	–	+	+	–		+	+	–
ERG changes	–	b-wave → extinguished	–	b-wave → extinguished	Extinguished	b-wave	b-wave		b-wave	
Inflammation/ neovascularization	–	–	–	–	–	–	–	+	++	+
Inheritance pattern	Polygenic	AD	AD	AD	AR	XL	AD	AD	AD	AD/AR/XL
Systemic manifestations	–	–	Orofacial and orthopedic	–	–	–	–	–	–	– 11q131AD
Genetic Locus	Unknown	5q13	COL2A1 COL11A1	5q13	NR2E3	XLRS1	–		11q13	Norrie disease gene (XL)

ADViRC, autosomal dominant vitreoretinochoroidopathy; ADNIV, autosomal dominant neovascular inflammatory vitreoretinopathy; FEVR, familial exudative vitreoretinopathy; RPE, retinal pigment epithelium; CME, cystoid macular edema; AR, autosomal recussive; XL, X-linked; RD, retinal detachment.

LATTICE DEGENERATION

Lattice degeneration is the most common vitreoretinal abnormality and occurs in 6% to 8% of the population. It is asymptomatic unless complicated by retinal tears or detachment. Lattice degeneration is an important clinical entity in this regard because it is responsible for 20% to 30% of all rhegmatogenous retinal detachments. It is more common in patients with myopia, and is found in both sexes and all races.

Ocular findings in lattice degeneration are limited to the vitreous and retinal changes. The lesions consist of a localized thinning of the inner retinal layers, an overlying adjacent zone of liquified vitreous surrounded by a sheath of condensed vitreous fibrils, and a firm attachment of the vitreous sheath to the edges of the retinal lesion.[7] Other retinal changes are observed in some cases: pigmentation (seen to some degree in 82%) (Fig. 6-1); whitish-yellow surface flecks; round, oval, or linear white patches or red craters; small atrophic round holes; branching white lines; yellow atrophic spots (depigmentation of the pigment epithelium); and, rarely, tractional tears at the ends or posterior margins of the lesions.[8] The characteristic white lines are blood vessels coursing through the lattice lesion and are not required for the diagnosis (Fig. 6-2). Retinal detachments occur

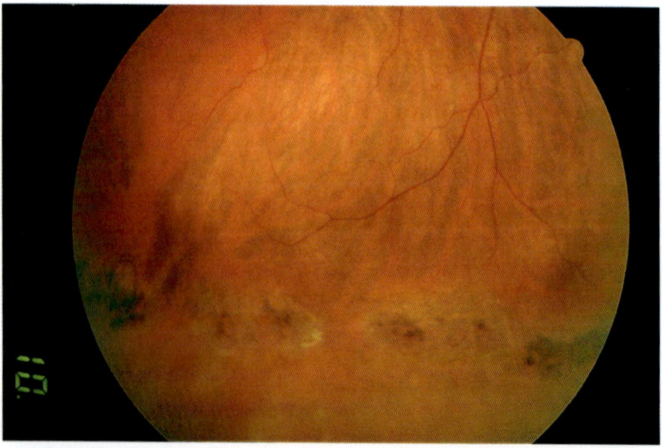

FIGURE 6-1. Pigmented oval lattice degeneration lesions in the midperiphery in an asymptomatic patient.

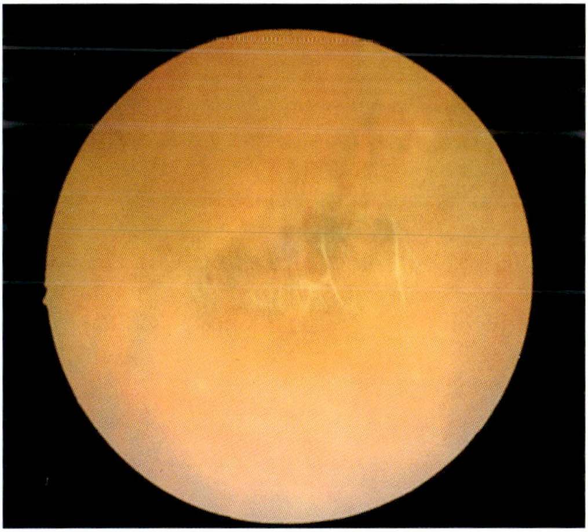

FIGURE 6-2. Retinal detachment associated with retinal break in lattice degeneration. The characteristic white lines are blood vessels coursing through the lattice lesion.

in 2% of patients with lattice degeneration by two distinct pathogenetic mechanisms. The most common type usually occurs in patients over age 50 and is initiated by a sudden posterior vitreous detachment that in turn leads to a tractional retinal tear in a lattice lesion or at a vitreoretinal adhesion in a clinically normal area.[9] The other type of detachment, which occurs in younger patients without posterior vitreous detachments, is caused by atrophic holes present in the lattice lesions. These detachments are often asymptomatic and limited in nature.

The prevalence of lattice degeneration is essentially unchanged throughout life, and new lesions are generally not seen after the second decade.[15] Thus, lattice degeneration is presumed to be a localized developmental lesion of the vitreoretinal juncture. Although the vitreous overlying the clinical lattice lesions is liquefied, there are no central vitreous changes (liquefaction or synchysis senilis) or premature posterior vitreous detachment in patients with lattice degeneration. Likewise, there are no known systemic associations. Inheritance is probably polygenic, although pedigrees with autosomal dominant inheritance have been reported.[8]

Most lattice lesions are asymptomatic and are never associated with retinal detachments. Similarly, only about 1 in 365 patients with atrophic holes in lattice actually develops retinal detachments. Thus, prophylactic treatment of lattice lesions is not recommended. Tractional tears associated with lattice degeneration are an indication for demarcation with laser photocoagulation or cryotherapy because 10% to 27% of these will progress to retinal detachment. New holes and tears may develop in lattice with time. All patients with lattice degeneration should have a yearly indented peripheral retina exam. They should also be told about the symptoms of a retinal detachment and should return immediately for examination if any new floaters or photopsias occur.

STICKLER SYNDROME

In 1965, Stickler and associates described a syndrome they termed *hereditary progressive arthro-ophthalmopathy*.[42] Stickler documented the association of high myopia, total retinal detachments in the first decade of life, and premature degenerative changes of the articular cartilage. Subsequent reports have demonstrated that Stickler syndrome is inherited as an autosomal dominant trait, and it is thought to be the most common autosomal dominant connective tissue dysplasia in the American Midwest.[21]

Ocular features include high myopia (−8.00D to −18.00D) and frequent retinal detachments, often in the first decade of life. The vitreous appears optically clear with syneretic vitreous strands, vitreous membranes, and veils (Fig. 6-3). Vitreous degeneration can present as early as several months of age, or the vitreous can appear normal into the second decade of life. The retina often has perivascular pigmentary changes, but bone spicule-like pigment is not seen (Fig. 6-4). Chorioretinal degeneration and retinal breaks are prevalent, and these lead to complicated retinal detachments in up to 50% of affected eyes. Primary open-angle glaucoma or ocular hypertension occur in up to one-third of affected patients. Presenile nuclear sclerotic cataracts are often seen before age 45 and up to 20% of patients have peripheral cortical comma-shaped cataracts (Fig. 6-5) that may remain stationary throughout life.[40,46]

Systemic manifestations include orthopedic and orofacial abnormalities. Premature degenerative changes of the weight-

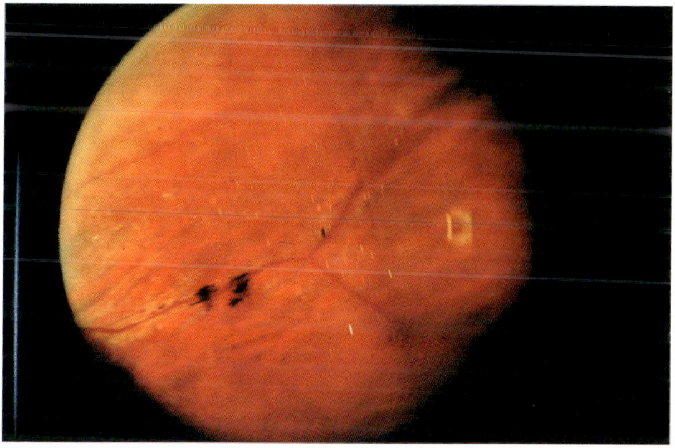

FIGURE 6-3. Syneretic vitreous veils and perivascular pigmentation in a patient with Stickler syndrome.

bearing joints are one of the most constant features of Stickler syndrome. Almost all patients complain of joint problems and exhibit generalized epiphyseal dysplasia. Radiographs reveal distortion of the distal radial carpal angle and generalized dysplastic changes of the distal femur, the proximal tibia, the distal

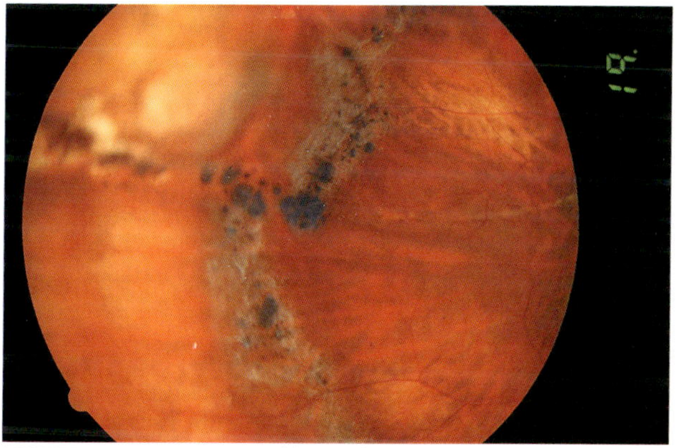

FIGURE 6-4. Severe pigmented lattice degeneration and perivascular pigmentation typical of Stickler syndrome.

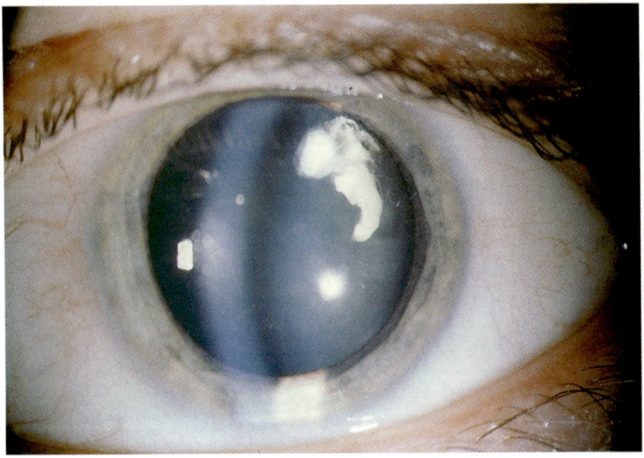

FIGURE 6-5. Peripheral cortical "wedge" cataract common in patients with Stickler syndrome.

radius, and the distal tibia (Figs. 6-6, 6-7). Orofacial anomalies such as submucous clefting of the palate, bifid uvula, and other abnormalities of the palate are noted in up to 75% of patients. Clinically, many patients appear to have midfacial flattening, but facial bone development is normal.[46] Other associations include sensorineural hearing loss and the *Pierre–Robin anomaly*. Mitral valve prolapse is also found in up to 46% of patients with Stickler syndrome.[40]

The genetic defect in many Stickler pedigrees has been shown to be individual mutations in the procollagen II gene.[1,6,27] Most of these mutations result in the premature termination of translation of the procollagen chain. Genetic heterogeneity exists because several other Stickler families have been excluded by linkage analysis at the collagen II locus.[17,26] Collagen type II is the primary fibrillar collagen of secondary vitreous and cartilage, and it is not surprising that abnormalities in the structure or function of collagen II are involved in the pathogenesis of Stickler syndrome.

Management of Stickler syndrome includes early evaluation of those at risk, long-term monitoring of those affected, timely intervention, and genetic counseling.[38] Children suspected to be affected with Stickler syndrome should have routine cycloplegic refractions, and myopic corrective lenses should be prescribed

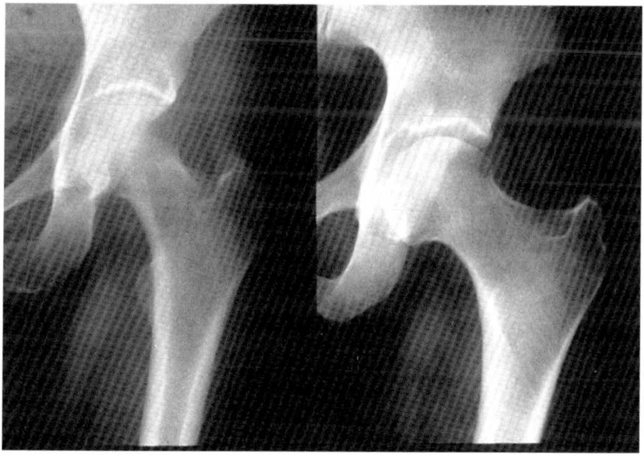

FIGURE 6-6. *Left*: normal pelvis. *Right*: anterior posterior radiograph of pelvis revealing stunting of the growth of the femoral epiphysis as well as stunting of the growth of the greater trochanter. Note irregularity of the joint surface. (Courtesy of March of Dimes Birth Defects Foundation, from Birth Defects Original Article Series, 1982;18:542.)

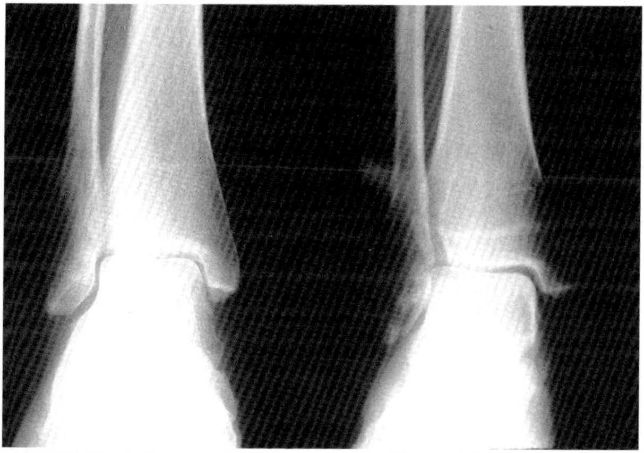

FIGURE 6-7. *Left*: normal ankle. *Right*: Stickler's syndrome anterior posterior radiograph of the ankle shows some stunting of the growth of the distal tibia with an abnormal slant to the distal tibia and shortening of the tip of the medial malleolus. (Courtesy of March of Dimes Birth Defects Foundation from Birth Defects Original Article Series, 1982;18: 542.)

when necessary to prevent ametropic amblyopia. Careful indented ophthalmoscopy looking for retinal breaks should be performed at least semiannually with treatment of new tears. Cataract extraction is often necessary when the nuclear sclerotic changes become visually significant. In cases of marked reduction of visual acuity, retinoscopy is often required to detect clear nuclear changes of the lens that can appear minimal by slit lamp examination. Retinal detachments are often difficult to manage because they can be associated with multiple posterior breaks, giant retinal tears, and cataracts. Otolaryngological consultation should be obtained to manage associated clefting and hearing abnormalities, and orthopedic evaluation should be sought to manage arthralgias and degenerative joint changes.

WAGNER'S DISEASE AND EROSIVE VITREORETINOPATHY

Wagner's disease[19,45] and erosive vitreoretinopathy[5] are two extremely rare vitreoretinal disorders that should not be confused with the common Stickler syndrome. These disorders are both linked to a similar region on chomosome 5q13–14 known to encode two proteins (link protein and versican)[4] that are involved in hyaluronan binding in the vitreous.[34] The disorders are probably allelic at the same gene, with different mutations accounting for the marked disparity in retinal detachment rates between the disorders. It is possible that these two rare disorders are only present in relatives of the two separate families.

Unlike Stickler syndrome, neither Wagner's disease nor erosive vitreoretinopathy has any of the systemic manifestations seen in Stickler syndrome. Both disorders have marked vitreous syneresis (described as optically clear), mild to moderate myopia (−3.00 to −5.00), and early cataract formation. Both disorders are characterized by a characteristic progressive retinal pigment epithelium (RPE) and choroidal atrophy (described as erosion of the RPE) that progresses to bone spicule-like pigment formation, marked constriction of visual fields, and eventual loss of central visual fields with a choroideremia-type appearance.

More than 50% of patients with erosive vitreoretinopathy have severe rhegmatogenous retinal detachments, often from giant retinal tears and multiple posterior breaks. These detachments are very difficult to repair and should be referred to very experienced vitreous surgeons. Fortunately, patients with

Wagner disease rarely demonstrate rhegmatogenous detachments,[28] although vitreous traction is described in 15% of patients.[19]

Patients have early complaints of reduced night vision, but central vision is generally normal until reduced by cataract formation at age 30 to 40. Lens changes consist of dotlike opacities on the posterior and anterior lens cortex. Vision is generally restored to normal by cataract surgery in patients, but progressive visual field loss occurs secondary to the choroidal and retinal atrophy. Patients with erosive vitreoretinopathy also lose significant vision from retinal detachments and secondary complications of retinal detachment repair.

Psychophysical tests reveal concentric constriction of the visual field in both disorders. Electroretinography reveals reduced b-wave amplitudes that may progress to an extinguished ERG.

Management of both disorders consists of genetic counseling and cataract extraction when the lens changes become visually significant. Patients with erosive vitreoretinopathy should be screened in infancy and annually for peripheral retinal pathology, with timely surgical intervention instituted for retinal breaks and detachments. No intervention is known to prevent the pigmentary degeneration of the retina in either condition.

GOLDMANN–FAVRE SYNDROME

Goldmann–Favre vitreotapetoretinal degeneration is an exceedingly rare condition consisting of progressive loss of vision due to retinoschisis, progressive cataract, and pigmentary chorioretinal degeneration with bone spicule-like formation. It is inherited in an autosomal recessive fashion. It is quite rare and shows no sex predilection.

Most patients present between the ages of 10 and 20 because of night blindness and poor vision.[41] Slit lamp examination reveals extensive liquefaction of the vitreous with multiple strands of condensed vitreous. Fundus changes include pale optic discs, sheathing of arteries and veins, and peripheral bone spicule-like pigmentary changes (Fig. 6-8). Extensive peripheral retinoschisis begins between the the equator and the ora serrata and may progressively involve the central retina. Generally, the central macula has microcystic changes and a "beaten copper" appearance. Fluorescein angiography can differentiate these

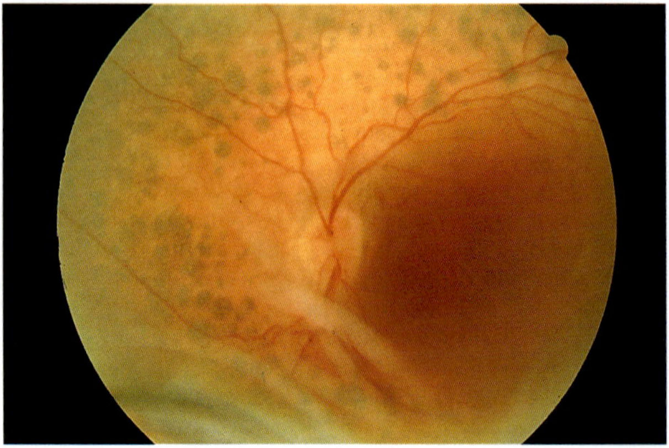

FIGURE 6-8. Vitreous strands, attenuation of retinal vessels, and peripheral pigmentary changes in a patient with Goldmann–Favre syndrome. The electroretinogram was nonrecordable.

changes from cystoid macular edema because there is no late staining of the cystic spaces in Goldmann–Favre syndrome. The macular changes may be isolated from or be continuous with the peripheral area of schisis.[38] Presenile posterior subcapsular cataracts develop in most cases.

Patients with Goldmann–Favre syndrome have nondetectable or strikingly abnormal electroretinographic responses.[14] In young patients with electroretinography (ERG) responses that are still recordable, scotopic a-waves have reduced amplitudes. The photopic and scotopic amplitudes may be essentially identical. Dark adaptation is also abnormal very early in the disease, with elevated rod thresholds or, in some cases, a monophasic cone-mediated threshold. Visual field testing reveals dense ring scotomas similar to typical retinitis pigmentosa.

Central visual loss is generally related to the macular retinoschisis and occurs early in the disease. The visual acuity is often reduced to 20/200 in childhood. The retinoschisis is presumed to be a splitting of the nerve fiber layer, and holes in both the outer and inner layer may occur.

No systemic manifestations are associated with Goldmann–Favre syndrome. Laser treatment and immunosuppressive therapy have been reported to be beneficial in some patients.

X-LINKED JUVENILE RETINOSCHISIS

Juvenile X-linked retinoschisis (also known as congenital hereditary retinoschisis, congenital vitreous veil, cystic disease of the retina in children, and sex-linked juvenile retinoschisis) was first described in 1898 by Haas.[20] Although relatively rare worldwide, juvenile X-linked retinoschisis is the most common X chromosome disorder in Finland and is the most frequent cause of bilateral impairment of vision in boys in large parts of Finland.[16] It is transmitted as an X-linked recessive trait, occurring almost exclusively in males, and is invariably bilateral. No abnormalities are found in female carriers. The disease has been mapped to the short arm of the X chromosome,[32] and individual mutations in the XLRS1 gene are identifiable in most cases of X-linked retinoschisis.[36] The protein encoded by the XLRS1 gene is thought to be involved in cell–cell interaction in the neurosensory retina.

The most constant ocular finding is a cystoid, stellate maculopathy or foveal schisis, which is present in almost every case and may be the only feature in approximately half of cases (Fig. 6-9). In older patients it often develops into an atrophic

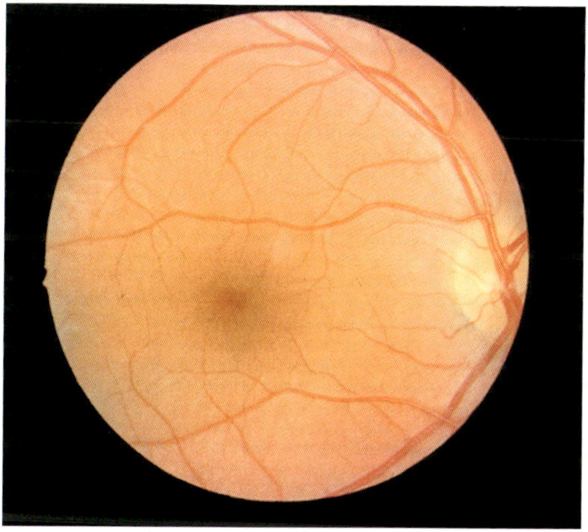

FIGURE 6-9. Cystoid stellate maculopathy or foveal schisis is present in almost every case of X-linked juvenile retinoschisis.

pigmented scar.[31] Clinically, the stellate maculopathy can mimic cystoid macular edema, but it can be differentiated by the lack of late leakage on fluorescein angiography.[38] Although bilateral inferotemporal retinoschisis has been considered the classical presentation of this disorder, only 40% of patients have peripheral retinoschisis in addition to the macular findings. The retinoschisis is a splitting of the nerve fiber layer with ballooning of the inner layer into the vitreous. The inner layer is quite thin and often contains large holes whereas the outer layer may contain small holes.[11] Unsupported retinal vessels in the inner layer may give rise to recurrent vitreous hemorrhage. Fibrous condensations of vitreous cortex (vitreous veils) often overlie the areas of peripheral retinoschisis, and vitreous bands form that extend to retinal vessels. Posterior vitreous detachment with vitreous collapse may occur and is often associated with regression of retinoschisis in the areas of vitreous detachment.[30]

X-linked juvenile retinoschisis has no known systemic manifestations. The macular changes often progress rapidly during the first 5 years of life but then progress very slowly until the sixth or seventh decade. The visual acuity is usually around 20/60 at age 20 and gradually diminishes to 20/200 by age 60.[16] Only rarely is good visual acuity maintained after the age of 60. Progression can vary from eye to eye in an affected individual or among related affected family members. Visual loss is generally related to macular involvement, although retinal detachment or vitreous hemorrhage may cause sudden visual loss.

Electroretinography in patients with juvenile X-linked retinoschisis typically reveals near normal a-waves with a selective reduction of the b-wave.[33] Oscillatory potentials can also be abnormal with decreased cone responses and almost obliterated rod responses. These ERG changes are not always present, and some patients with known mutations in the XLRS1 gene have been demonstrated to have normal electroretinography findings. Visual field testing reveals absolute scotomas in areas of peripheral retinoschisis.

Two lines of evidence suggest that an abnormality of the *Mueller cells* causes both the macular and peripheral retinal changes in juvenile X-linked retinoschisis. First, the b-wave of the ERG results from a Mueller cell response to changes in extracellular potassium levels. Second, periodic acid–Schiff staining of intraretinal filaments, presumably formed by defective Mueller cells, has been demonstrated histopathologically.[11]

Juvenile X-linked retinoschisis progresses slowly, and prophylactic treatment of schisis (even with holes in schisis cavities) is not recommended. Management includes treatment of secondary retinal detachments and vitreous hemorrhages when they occur. The goal of therapy in the treatment of combined retinal detachment and congenital retinoschisis is closure of the outer layer and full-thickness retinal breaks, which can generally be accomplished by a scleral buckling procedure.[38] No specific attempt is made to close inner layer breaks. If vitreous hemorrhage occurs, laser photocoagulation can be used to close the proximal portion of the bleeding vessel. The presence of genetic markers close to the juvenile retinoschisis gene and known mutations in the gene itself makes carrier detection and prenatal screening possible in some families.[24]

FAMILIAL EXUDATIVE VITREORETINOPATHY

Familial exudative vitreoretinopathy (FEVR) was first described by Criswick and Schepens in 1969.[12] They described heterotopia of the macula with temporal traction, posterior vitreous detachments with organized vitreous membranes, peripheral neovascularization, retinal traction with retinal breaks, and retinal detachments. The changes resemble retinopathy of prematurity, but affected patients have no history of premature birth or antenatal oxygen administration. Familial exudative vitreoretinopathy is inherited in an X-linked, autosomal recessive or autosomal dominant fashion and exhibits great variability of expression. Some patients have blinding bilateral retinal detachments in the first few years of life, whereas others have only a small area of avascular retina in the temporal periphery with no symptoms or complications throughout life.

The most constant ocular finding is an abrupt termination of retinal vessels along a scalloped edge at the equator (Fig. 6-10). The avascular area can be quite extensive or confined to only several clock hours. Often an elevated fibrovascular scar in the temporal periphery is present, very similar to the cicatricial stage of retinopathy of prematurity.[18] Peripheral neovascularization is present adjacent to this area, and the capillary bed posterior to the avascular zone is often dilated and more prominent. Maturation and organization of the fibrovascular scar produce the striking signs of retinal traction ("dragged disc" and macula

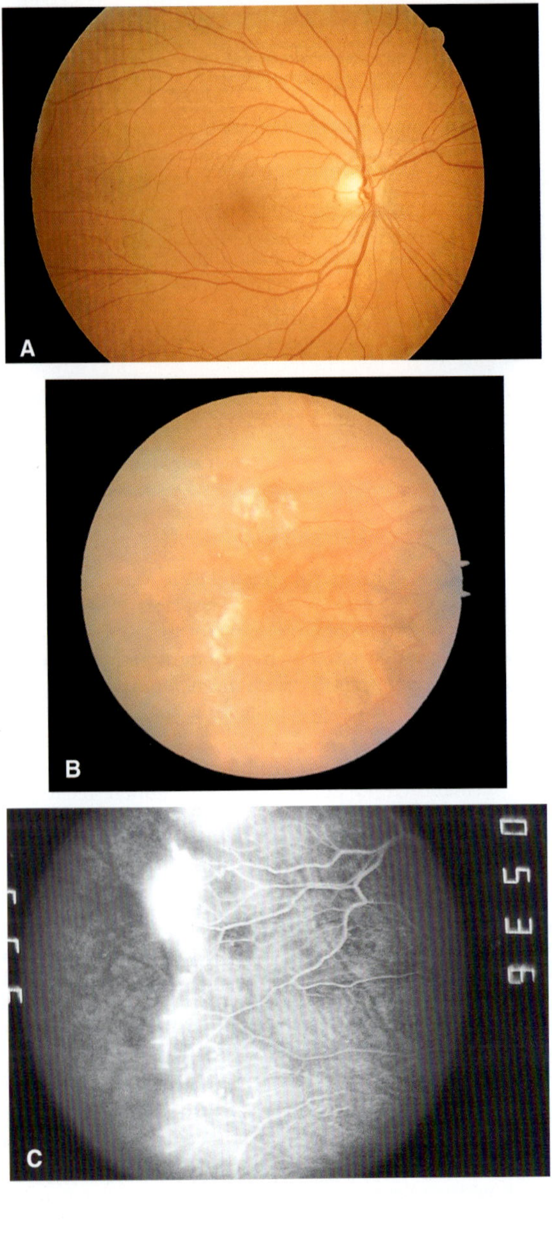
A
B
C

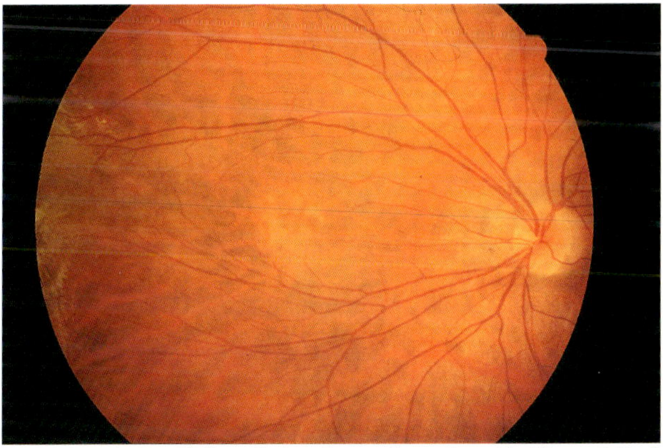

FIGURE 6-11. Familial exudative vitreoretinopathy with "dragged disc" appearance and tractional retinal detachment.

heterotopia) (Fig. 6-11). Subretinal exudates occur in only 10% to 15% of affected eyes. Retinal detachments are predominantly tractional in the first decade of life and rhegmatogenous in the second decade. The overall incidence of retinal detachment varies from 4% to 30%.[29] An ectopic macula is present in up to one-half of patients and causes a positive angle kappa. Vitreous abnormalities include posterior vitreous detachments with vitreous bands transmitting traction to the retina and thickened vitreous membranes over avascular retina.[39] Mild cases can lack vitreous abnormalities, and more than 50% of affected patients have entirely normal vitreous examinations.[44]

Fundus fluorescein angiography or angioscopy is often necessary to identify the avascular retinal areas in minimally affected patients. Retinal vessels present at the scalloped edge often leak and pool as the angiogram progresses. Defective platelet aggregation was reported in one FEVR family,[10] but subsequent reports have not substantiated this association.

FIGURE 6-10A–C. Great variability of expression in familial exudative vitreoretinopathy makes diagnosis difficult in minimally affected family members. Posterior pole of an obligate carrier reveals only "straightening" of retinal vessels (**A**). Examination of the temporal periphery reveals cessation of retinal vessels in a scalloped edge (**B**) easily demonstrated by angiography or angioscopy (**C**).

Pathophysiologically, the primary abnormality is probably abnormal maturation of the retinal vasculature and not an inherent defect in vitreous formation or function. The earliest findings in familial exudative vitreoretinopathy appear to be nonperfusion of the peripheral temporal retina with stretched retinal blood vessels and shunting with vascular leakage.[39] Secondary vitreous changes over the nonperfused areas of retina cause tractional retinal detachments that lead to visual loss.

Management of familial exudative vitreoretinopathy should include early screening and identification of affected individuals in known families. The majority of retinal detachments occur in the first decade of life, and very little progression occurs after age 10. Patients with the largest areas of nonperfused retinas are at greatest risk. Cryotherapy to large areas of avascular retina and scleral buckling surgery for tractional retinal detachments may be required. Genetic counseling is also important because asymptomatic affected patients can have severely affected children.

HEREDITARY SNOWFLAKE VITREORETINAL DEGENERATION OF HIROSE

Hirose et al. described familial snowflake vitreoretinal degeneration in 1974.[22] The disease is named after white, snowflake-like spots that are 100 to 200 μm in diameter and appear in areas of "white without pressure" (Fig. 6-12). The "snowflakes" often do not appear until after the age of 25 years, and thus the diagnosis is difficult to exclude in younger patients. Hirose's pedigree and subsequent reports have demonstrated autosomal dominant inheritance with variable expressivity.

Ocular findings include cataracts in all patients studied over 35 years of age. Nuclear sclerosis, cortical opacities, and posterior subcapsular plaques may be seen. Younger patients have fine swirling vitreous strands and liquefaction of the gel. In older patients, vitreous strands become more prominent, and posterior vitreous detachment is common. Four ophthalmoscopically distinct stages have been described. Stage I is extensive "white with pressure" in the retinal periphery. Stage II is characterized by snowflake-like spots, extending from the equator to the ora serrata. Some of these appear to be crystalline and lie in the superficial layers of the retina. The surface of the affected retina is elevated with "crater-like areas." Stage III is

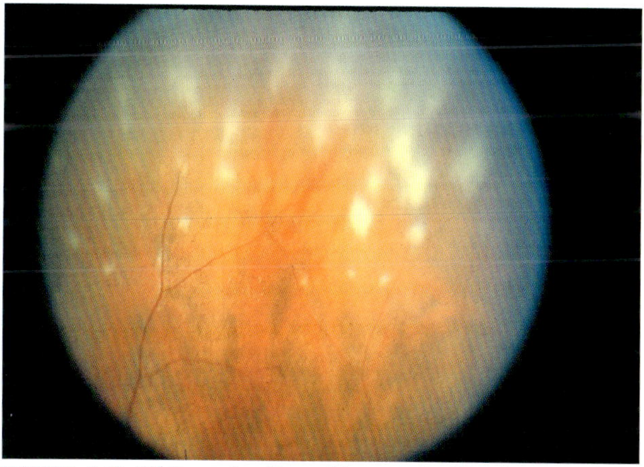

FIGURE 6-12. White and yellow-white granular-like deposits of the peripheral retina, 100–200 μm in size, characteristic of snowflake degeneration. (Courtesy of Dr. D.M. Robertson, Published courtesy of Ophthalmology 1982;89:1515.)

characterized by sheathing of retinal vessels in the area of the snowflake degeneration. The vessels become "white threads" in the periphery. Clumps of black, irregularly shaped pigment appear around the posterior margin of the snowflake degeneration. Stage IV is characterized by increased pigmentary changes and disappearance of retinal vessels. Snowflake degeneration is associated with an increased incidence of retinal detachment, and surgical repair is rarely successful.

Although patients do not complain of nyctalopia, snowflake degeneration is associated with constriction of the visual field and elevation of rod thresholds in dark adaptation tests.[23] Electroretinography demonstrates a decreased amplitude of the scotopic b-wave in almost all patients.

Management consists of cataract extraction when the lens changes become visually significant and routine peripheral retinal examinations. Because retinal detachments are common and are associated with poor outcomes, laser photocoagulation is recommended for any type of retinal break.[35] No treatment is indicated for the snowflake degenerative changes alone.

Robertson and colleagues reported 10 patients in four families with lesions similar to those of stage I and stage II snowflake generation.[37] These patients did not have associated vitreous traction and did not progress to arteriolar attenuation. Robertson stated that the snowflake lesions themselves may be an innocent peripheral retinal finding unless associated with other conditions such as lattice degeneration.

AUTOSOMAL DOMINANT VITREORETINOCHOROIDOPATHY (ADViRC) AND AUTOSOMAL DOMINANT NEOVASCULAR INFLAMMATORY VITREORETINOPATHY (ADNIV)

In 1982, Kaufman and colleagues described a unique vitreoretinal degeneration that they called autosomal dominant vitreoretinochoroidopathy (ADViRC).[25] The condition is characterized by an abnormal chorioretinal hypopigmentation and hyperpigmentation that is found between the vortex veins and the ora serrata for 360°. There is a distinct posterior boundary near the equator (Fig. 6-13). Patients have retinal arteriolar narrowing and occlusion, small punctate white opacities in the retina, and, in some cases, choroidal atrophy. Most affected family members have cystoid macular edema, diffuse retinal vascular incompetence, vitreous cells, and presenile cataracts; many have retinal neovascularization. Vitreous changes include only mild degenerative changes, vitreous cells, and early posterior vitreous

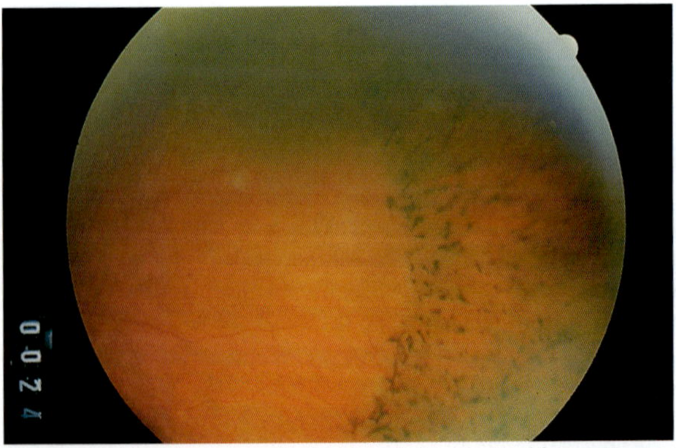

FIGURE 6-13. Distinct posterior border of chorioretinal hyperpigmentation near the equator in a patient with autosomal dominant vitreoretinochoroidopathy (ADViRC). (Courtesy of Dr. D.P. Han.)

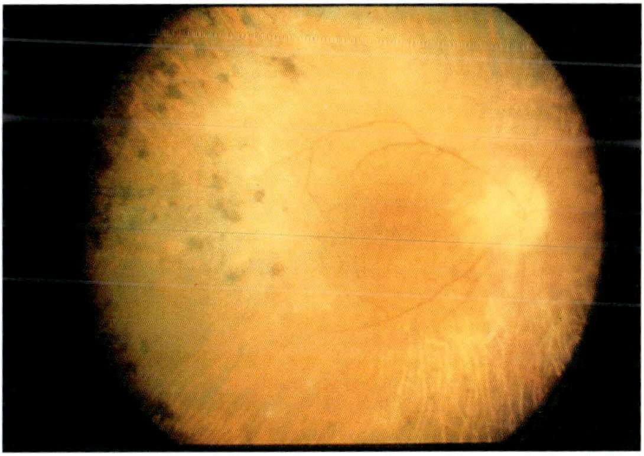

FIGURE 6-14. Peripheral hyperpigmentation with no defined distinct posterior border, arteriolar attenuation, and pale optic nerve in a patient with end-stage autosomal dominant neovascular inflammatory vitreoretinopathy (ADNIV). (Courtesy of Dr. J.C. Folk. Published courtesy of Ophthalmology 1990;97:1128.)

detachments. Patients have no systemic abnormalities and do not complain of nyctalopia. Electroretinography is normal in younger individuals and only moderately affected in older patients.[3]

Cystoid macular edema or vitreous hemorrhage can occur in children as young as age 7 years with ADViRC. The condition progresses slowly and is not associated with retinal detachments.

Bennett and colleagues described a similar entity in 1990 that they called autosomal dominant neovascular inflammatory vitreoretinopathy (ADNIV).[2] The ADNIV gene has recently been mapped to chromosome 11q13.[43] ADNIV, like ADViRC, has prominent cystoid macular edema, generalized leakage from retinal vessels, peripheral retinal neovascularization, closure of peripheral retinal vessels, pigmentary changes in the retina including both hyperpigmentation and hypopigmentation, vitreous cells and hemorrhage, and cataracts.[13] Unlike ADViRC, electroretinography shows selective loss of the b-wave in all patients. Other distinctive features of ADNIV include anterior uveitis, development of neovascular glaucoma, and tractional retinal detachments in up to 20% of patients. The pigmentary changes of ADNIV do not have the distinct posterior boundary of ADViRC (Fig. 6-14).

In contrast to ADViRC, which appears to remain stable, ADNIV is a progressive disease. Patients with ADNIV are generally asymptomatic until their midtwenties, but vitreous cells can be observed biomicroscopically and a selective loss of the b-wave can be seen with electroretinography. Later, peripheral retinal scarring and pigmentation, peripheral arteriolar closure, and neovascularization of the peripheral retina or optic disc develop. Cystoid macular edema, vitreous hemorrhage, tractional retinal detachment, and neovascular glaucoma can cause profound visual loss. Vitrectomy is often necessary to repair the retinal detachments.

References

1. Ahmad NN, Ala-Kokko L, Knowlton RG, et al. Stop codon in the procollagen II gene (COL2A1) in a family with the Stickler syndrome (arthro-ophthalmopathy). Proc Natl Acad Sci USA 1991;88:6624–6627.
2. Bennett SR, Folk JC, Kimura AE, Russell SR, Stone EM, Raphtis M. Autosomal dominant neovascular inflammatory vitreoretinopathy. Ophthalmology 1990;97:1125–1135.
3. Blair NP, Goldberg MF, Fishman GA, Salzano T. Autosomal dominant vitreoretinochoroidopathy (ADVIRC). Br J Ophthalmol 1984;68: 2–9.
4. Brown DM, Graemiger RA, Hergersberg M, et al. Genetic linkage of Wagner disease and erosive vitreoretinopathy to chromosome 5q13-14. Arch Ophthalmol 1995;113:671–675.
5. Brown DM, Kimura AE, Weingeist TA, Stone EM. Erosive vitreoretinopathy—a new clinical entity. Ophthalmology 1994;101:694–704.
6. Brown DM, Nichols BE, Weingeist TA, Sheffield VC, Kimura AE, Stone EM. Procollagen II gene mutation in Stickler syndrome. Arch Ophthalmol 1992;110:1589–1593.
7. Byer NE. A clinical definition of lattice degeneration of the retina and its variations. Mod Probl Ophthalmol 1975;15:58–67.
8. Byer NE. Lattice degeneration of the retina. Surv Ophthalmol 1979; 23:213–248.
9. Byer NE. Vitreous in lattice: discussion. Ophthalmology 1984;91: 457.
10. Chaudhuri PR, Rosenthal AR, Goulstine DB, Rowlands D, Mitchell VE. Familial exudative vitreoretinopathy associated with familial thrombocytopathy. Br J Ophthalmol 1983;67:755–758.
11. Condon GP, Brownstein S, Wang N, Kearns AF, Ewing CC. Congenital hereditary (juvenile X-linked) retinoschisis: histopathologic and ultrastructural findings in three eyes. Arch Ophthalmol 1986;104: 576–583.

12. Criswick VG, Schepens CL. Familial exudative vitreoretinopthy. Am J Ophthalmol 1969;68:578–594.
13. Fishman GA. ADNIV: discussion. Ophthalmology 1990;97:1135–1136.
14. Fishman GA, Jampol LM, Goldberg MF. Diagnostic features of the Favre–Goldmann syndrome. Br J Ophthalmol 1976;60:345–353.
15. Foos RY, Simons KB. Vitreous in lattice degeneration of retina. Ophthalmology 1984;91:452–457.
16. Forsius H, Krause U, Helve J, et al. Visual acuity in 183 cases of x-chromosomal retinoschisis. Can J Ophthalmol 1973;8:385–393.
17. Francomano CA, Rowan BG, Liberfarb RM, et al. The Stickler and Wagner syndromes. Evidence for genetic heterogeneity. Am J Hum Genet 1988;43:A83.
18. Gow J, Oliver GL. Familial exudative vitreoretinopathy—an expanded view. Arch Ophthalmol 1971;86:150–155.
19. Graemiger RA, Niemeyer G, Schneeberger SA, Messmer EP. Wagner vitreoretinal degeneration. Follow-up of the original pedigree. Ophthalmology 1995;102:1830–1839.
20. Haas J. Uber das zusammenvorkommen von veranderungen der retina und choriodea. Arch Augenheilkd 1898;37:343–348.
21. Herrmann J, France TD, Spranger JW, Opitz JW, Wiffler C. The Stickler syndrome (hereditary arthroophthalmopathy). Birth Defects 1975;11:76–103.
22. Hirose T, Lee KY, Schepens CL. Snowflake degeneration in hereditary vitreoretinal degeneration. Am J Ophthalmol 1974;77:143–153.
23. Hirose T, Wolf E, Schepens CL. Retinal functions in snowflake degeneration. Ann Ophthalmol 1980;12:1135–1146.
24. Kaplan J, Pelet A, Hentati H, et al. Contribution to carrier detection and genetic counselling in X-linked retinoschisis. J Med Genet 1991; 28(6):383–388.
25. Kaufman SJ, Goldberg MR, Orth DH, Fishman GA, Tessler H, Mizuno K. Autosomal dominant vitreoretinochoroidopathy. Arch Ophthalmol 1982;100:272–278.
26. Knowlton RG, Weaver EJ, Struyk AF, et al. Genetic linkage analysis of hereditary arthro-ophthalmopathy (Stickler syndrome) and the type II procollagen gene. Am J Hum Genet 1989;45:681–688.
27. Korkko J, Ritvaniemi P, Haataja L, et al. Mutation in Type II procollagen (COL2A1) that substitutes aspartate for glycine α 1-67 and that causes cataracts and retinal detachment: evidence for molecular heterogeneity in the Wagner syndrome and the Stickler syndrome (arthro-ophthalmopathy). Am J Hum Genet 1993;53:55–61.
28. Maumenee IH, Stoll HU, Mets MB. The Wagner syndrome versus hereditary arthroophthalmopathy. Trans Am Ophthalmol Soc 1982; 80:349–365.
29. Miyakubo H, Inohara N, Hashimoto K. Reinal involvement in familial exudative vitreoretinopathy. Opththalmologica 1982;185: 125–135.

30. Neetens A. Hereditary vitreoretinal diseases. In: Schepens CL, Neetens A (eds) The vitreous and vitreoretinal interface. New York: Springer-Verlag, 1987:241–272.
31. Odland M. Congenital retinoschisis. Acta Ophthalmol 1981;59:649–658.
32. Oudet C, Weber C, Kaplan J, et al. Characterisation of a highly polymorphic microsatellite at the DXS207 locus: confirmation of very close linkage to the retinoschisis disease gene. J Med Genet 1993; 30(4):300–303.
33. Peachey NS, Fishman GA, Derlacki DJ, Brigell MG. Psychophysical and electroretinographic findings in X-linked juvenile retionschisis. Arch Ophthalmol 1987;105:513–516.
34. Perveen R, Hart-Holden N, Dixon MJ, et al. Refined genetic and physical localization of the Wagner disease (WGN1) locus and the genes CRTL1 and CSPG2 to a 2- to 2.5-cM region of chromosome 5q14.3. Genomics 1999;57:219–226.
35. Pollack A, Uchenik D, Chemke J, Oliver M. Prophylactic laser photocoagulation in hereditary snowflake vitreoretinal degeneration. Arch Ophthalmol 1983;101:1536–1539.
36. The Retinoschisis Consortium. Functional implications of the spectrum of mutations found in 234 cases with X-linked juvenile retinoschisis. The Retinoschisis Consortium. Hum Mol Genetics 1998;7:1185–1192.
37. Robertson DM, Link TP, Rostvald JA. Snowflake degeneration of the retina. Ophthalmology 1982;12:1513–1517.
38. Robertson JE, Meyer SM. Hereditary vitreoretinal degenerations. In: Ryan SJ (ed) Retina, vol 1. St. Louis: Mosby, 1989:469–479.
39. Sebag J. The vitreous. Structure, function, and pathobiology. New York: Springer-Verlag, 1989.
40. Seery CM, Pruett RC, Liberfarb RM, Cohen BZ. Distinctive cataract in Stickler syndrome. Am J Ophthalmol 1990;110:143–148.
41. Spallone A. Differential diagnosis of hereditary vitreoretinopathy. Milano: Fogliazza Ediatore, 1989.
42. Stickler GB, Belau PG, Farrell FJ, et al. Hereditary progressive arthoophthalmopathy. Mayo Clin Proc 1965;40:433–455.
43. Stone EM, Kimura AE, Folk JC, et al. Genetic linkage of autosomal dominant neovascular inflammatory vitreoretinopathy to chromosome 11q13. Hum Mol Genet 1992;9:685–689.
44. van Nouhuys CE. Dominant exudative vitreoretinopathy and other vascular developmental disorders of the peripheral retina. Doc Ophthalmol 1982;54:1–414.
45. Wagner H. Ein bisher unbekanntes Erbleiden des Auges (degeneratio hyaloideo-retinalis hereditaria), beobachtet im Kanton Zurich. Klin Monatsbl Augenheilkd 1938;100:840–857.
46. Weingeist TA, Hermsen V, Hanson JW, Bumsted RM, Weinstein, SL, Olin WH. Ocular and systemic manifestations of Stickler's syndrome: a preliminary report. Birth Defects 1982;18:539–560.

7

Retinal Vascular Disorders

Richard M. Feist, Christopher F. Blodi, and Peter H. Spiegel

Retinal vascular disorders in children, unlike those in adults, rarely represent the sequelae of chronic systemic insults such as hyperglycemia or hypertension. Children are more likely to suffer from developmental, infectious, neoplastic, or traumatic retinal vascular disorders. As with any other cause of visual loss in childhood, prompt treatment of retinal vascular disorders can be essential to the avoidance of amblyopia. Table 7-1 lists the usual age of presentation for the entities discussed in this chapter.

SICKLE CELL DISEASE

Eight percent of the African-American population in the United States is heterozygous for the sickle trait (AS) (Table 7-2). With the exception of some Mediterranean and Indian populations, the sickle trait is very rare in Americans of Asian or European descent. Sickle hemoglobin (S Hb) varies from normal hemoglobin (A Hb) at position six of the beta-hemoglobin chain. The substitution of valine for glutamic acid at this position produces a hemoglobin that offers some protection against malaria because the *Plasmodium* organism is unable to break down Hb S. Heterozygous patients are generally asymptomatic systemically and ophthalmically. Unfortunately, Hb S polymerizes under hypoxic conditions, leading to rigid, sickle-shaped erythrocytes. Homozygous (SS) patients can develop systemic complications such as splenic autoinfarction, hemolysis, severe and chronic anemia, and blast crisis. However, only 8.8% of these patients develop proliferative sickle retinopathy and only 3% develop vitreous hemorrhage. In contrast, proliferative sickle

TABLE 7-1. Usual Age of Presentation of Various Retinal Vascular Disorders.

Disease	*Age of presentation*
Background sickle retinopathy	Late childhood
Proliferative sickle retinopathy	Adolescents and young adults
Coats' disease	Prepubertal; first or second decade of life
Von Hippel syndrome	Young adults; may present in late childhood or adolescence
Retinal cavernous hemangioma	First or second decade of life; congenital?
Sturge–Weber syndrome	Congenital
Wyburn–Mason syndrome	Congenital
Background diabetic retinopathy	50% of patients after 7 years of disease
Proliferative diabetic retinopathy	Rare before puberty; 50% of postpubertal patients after 15 years type I disease
Hypertensive retinopathy	Rare before puberty; acute changes may occur in pregnant adolescents (greater risk of eclampsia in this age group)
Terson's syndrome	May occur following an intracranial hemorrhage; may occur at any age
Shaken baby syndrome	Infants and toddlers
Purtscher's retinopathy	May occur at any age
Eales disease	Young adults
Hypomelanosis of Ito	Congenital
Incontinentia pigmenti	Infancy
Goodpasture syndrome	Any age
Allergic granulomatosis	Any age after infancy
Takayasu's arteritis	Adolescence
Norrie's disease	Congenital
Fascioscapulohumeral dystrophy	Young adults
Anemic retinopathy	May occur at any age
Leukemic retinopathy	May occur at any age
Hyperviscosity syndromes	May occur at any age
Kawasaki's disease	First or second decade of life
Carotid cavernous fistula	May occur following trauma at any age
Vein occlusions	Rare in children
Congenital vascular loops	Congenital

TABLE 7-2. Incidence of Various Hemoglobinopathies in the U.S. Black Population.

AS, 8%
AC, 2%–3%
SS, 0.2%
SC, 0.1%
SThal, 0.003%

AS, sickle cell heterozygous; AC, heterozygous for hemoglobulin A and C; SS, sickle cell homozygous; SC, heterozygous for sickle hemoglobin and hemoglobin C; SThal, sickle hemoglobin and thalassemia heterozygous.

Source: Goldberg MF. Sickle cell retinopathy. In: Tasman W, Jeager EA (eds) Duane's clinical ophthalmology, vol 3, chapter 17. Philadelphia: Lippincott, 1990, with permission.[16]

retinopathy develops in up to 72% of those patients heterozygous for sickle hemoglobin and hemoglobin C (Hb SC) and in 33% of patients heterozygous for sickle hemoglobin and thalassemia (SThal).

The underlying etiology of *sickle retinopathy* is sickling of erythrocytes in response to hypoxia in the peripheral retinal circulation. The low incidence of proliferative retinopathy in homozygous hemoglobin S patients has been postulated to be the result of a protective effect of lowered blood viscosity that results from the relatively low hematocrit. The relative frequency of various hemoglobinopathies in the African-American population is listed in Table 7-2.[16]

Fundus findings in background sickle cell retinopathy include *salmon patch hemorrhages* (Fig. 7-1), which are full-thickness intraretinal hemorrhages (often with some subinternal limiting membrane blood) that occur distal to arteriolar occlusions. As these hemorrhages reabsorb over time, these areas may develop into *iridescent spots* or into *black sunbursts* (Fig. 7-2). The former are thought to be schisis cavities containing hemosiderin whereas the latter result from hypertrophy, hyperplasia, and migration of the retinal pigment epithelium.

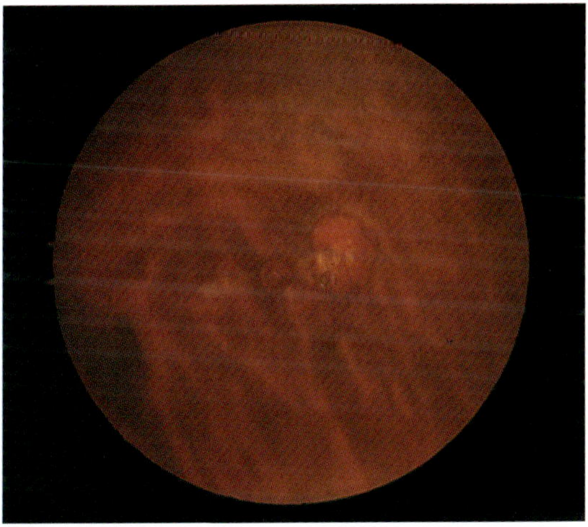

FIGURE 7-1. This "salmon patch" represents an intraretinal hemorrhage that extends from the internal limiting membrane and may involve the entire thickness of the retina. These hemorrhages typically have a bright red appearance.

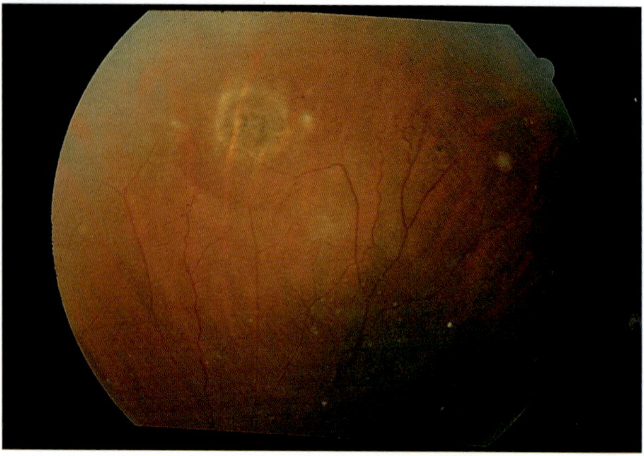

FIGURE 7-2. Black sunbursts represent hypertrophy, hyperplasia, and migration of the retinal pigment epithelium following resolution of a salmon patch hemorrhage.

Cotton wool spots may occur in the posterior pole, and the thinning of the retina that follows their resolution may be seen as a "macular depression." The *sickle disc sign* refers to comma-shaped capillaries on the disc that are caused by chronic sludging of blood. A similar finding can occasionally be seen in conjunctival capillaries. Iris atrophy may also be observed in patients with sickle cell retinopathy (Fig. 7-3).[48] Additional fundus changes include *angioid streaks* and tortuosity and dilation of the retinal venules. Retinal arteriolar occlusions have been reported in both a 5.5-year-old and a 9-year-old with SS hemoglobinopathy.[1,7] A 31-year-old with hemoglobin SC with a spontaneous central retinal artery occlusion was recently reported.[12] These cases of posterior disease stand in contrast to the more common picture of peripheral vascular occlusion.

Proliferative sickle retinopathy typically occurs in young and middle-aged adults but may occur in the second decade of life, usually following puberty. Patients with proliferative sickle retinopathy develop peripheral vascular occlusions followed by arteriovenous anastamoses and, eventually, peripheral neovascularization. The peripheral neovascular tufts typically have a shape similar to the aquatic plant *Gorgonia flabellum* and were consequently termed *sea fans* by Welch and Goldberg (Fig. 7-4).[48] Patients with these findings are at risk for vitreous

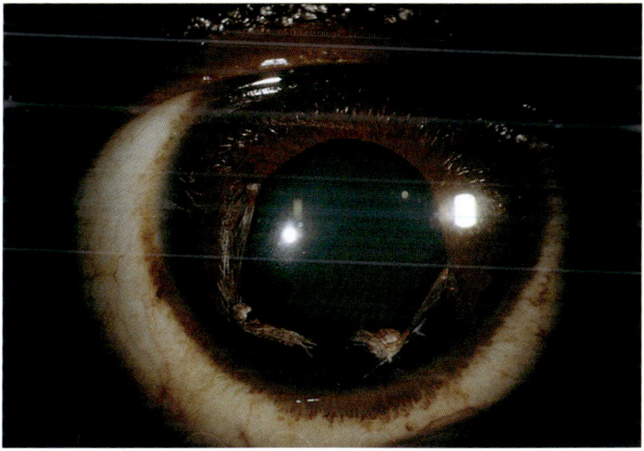

FIGURE 7-3. Iris atrophy in a patient with sickle cell disease.

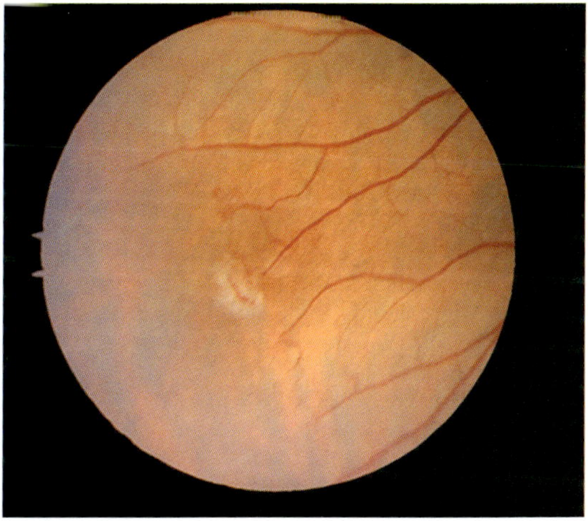

FIGURE 7-4. Peripheral neovascular tufts in the shape of a sea fan are found at the anterior edge of perfused retina in proliferative sickle retinopathy.

hemorrhage as well as tractional and rhegmatogenous retinal detachment.

Penman et al., reporting on the Jamaican sickle cohort, found that proliferative sickle retinopathy was more likely to occur in those with vascular morphological abnormalities (abrupt terminations, vascular buds) at the border of nonperfused retina compared to patients with more normal-appearing peripheral vascular beds.[32]

Scatter laser photocoagulation is recommended for patients with more than 60° of proliferative sickle retinopathy. If scatter treatment alone is insufficient to induce nonperfusion in the proliferative tufts, then supplemental feeder vessel treatment may be required. Feeder vessel treatment should not be considered as primary treatment because of an increased risk of rhegmatogenous retinal detachment following argon photocoagulation.[10] Patients with less than 60° of peripheral neovascularization are at a lower risk for both vitreous hemorrhage and retinal detachment, and there is insufficient evidence to make any treatment recommendation for these patients.[10]

In patients with cloudy media from vitreous hemorrhage, or small pupils, transscleral cryotherapy or transscleral diode laser photocoagulation may be employed.[38]

COATS' DISEASE

Coats' disease is an idiopathic, typically nonhereditary condition in which telangiectatic and aneurysmal retinal vessels are associated with massive subretinal exudate. The classic, adolescent form of the disease may occur at as early as 4 months of age with two-thirds of cases occurring before 10 years of age; 80% of cases are unilateral, and there is a 3:1 male predilection.[17]

Clinical diagnosis of Coats' disease is often made following the incidental findings of strabismus or of a white pupillary reflex. On fundus examination, yellowish to greenish subretinal exudate or intraretinal or intravitreal hemorrhage may be seen. Exudates and hemorrhage may be minimal but also may be massive, resulting in large areas of retinal detachment and obscuration of fundus details (Fig. 7-5). Although exudates and hemorrhages are usually located posteriorly, the underlying defect is a localized area of telangiectasias and aneurysms of the retinal vessels. These vascular changes may occur adjacent to exudates or may be more peripherally located. In some cases,

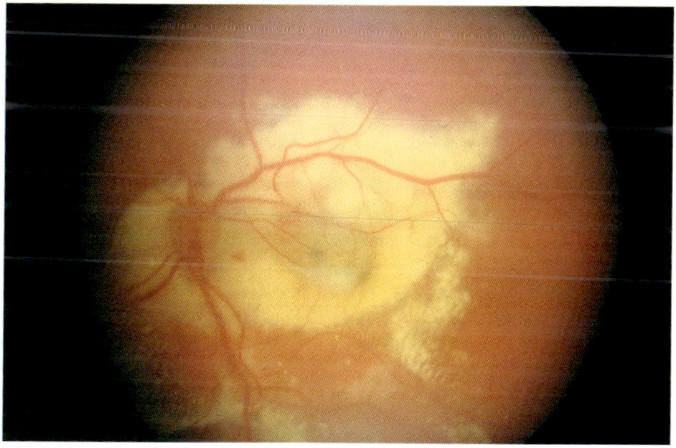

FIGURE 7-5. Although the retinal vascular telangiectasias of Coats' disease are located peripherally, the subretinal exudate typically occurs in the posterior pole, reducing vision dramatically in some cases.

fluorescein angiography is necessary to identify the location and extent of vascular changes. Angiography demonstrates early and persistent leakage from the areas of vascular abnormality as well as surrounding areas of capillary nonperfusion.

Coats' disease is a progressive disorder and when untreated may lead to permanent loss of central vision. Treatment consists of transcleral cryoablation of anterior areas of telangiectasis and laser photocoagulation of posterior areas. Multiple treatments may be necessary for ablation of areas of telangiectasia. Eyes with extensive retinal detachment may be treated with modern vitreoretinal techniques, including vitrectomy, drainage of subretinal fluid, placement of expandable gas, cryotherapy, and photocoagulation.[22,41] Shields et al. developed a staging classification of Coats' disease that may be useful in determining prognosis and in guiding treatment decisions (Table 7-3).[41] Of 124 affected eyes treated as necessary and followed for at least 6 months, 20% achieved a visual acuity of 20/100 or better; 24% had acuities from count fingers to 20/200; 40% had hand motions vision or no light perception; and 16% required enuculation. Poor visual outcomes were caused by complications such as subfoveal fluid and fibrosis, foveal exudation, and macular edema. Enucleation was usually reserved for those with

TABLE 7-3. Staging Classification of Coats' Disease.

Stage 1.	Retinal telangiectasia only
Stage 2.	Telangiectasia and exudation
	A. Extrafoveal exudation
	B. Foveal exudation
Stage 3.	Exudative retinal detachment
	A. Subtotal detachment
	1. Extrafoveal
	2. Foveal
	B. Total retinal detachment
Stage 4.	Total retinal detachment and glaucoma
Stage 5.	Advanced end-stage disease

Source: Shields JA, Shields CL, Honavar SG, et al. Classification and Management of Coats disease: the 2000 Proctor lecture. Am J Ophthalmol 2001;131:572–583, with permission.[41]

total retinal detachment and glaucoma (stage 4).[41] Pauleikhoff and Wessing reported complete resolution of subretinal exudates in 67.3% of cases with no retinal detachment and in 33% of cases with retinal detachment.[31a] Final visual acuity in their series was between 20/30 and 20/200 in 39.4% of cases and better than 20/30 in 15.3%.[3]

PHAKOMATOSES (NEUROCUTANEOUS DISEASES)

The phakomatoses are a group of disorders that affect multiple organs, typically the eyes, the skin, and the central nervous system. The phakomatoses that are associated with retinal or choroidal vascular lesions are *Von Hippel syndrome*, *Sturge–Weber syndrome*, and *Wyburn–Mason syndrome*.

Von Hippel syndrome is an autosomal dominantly inherited disorder in which retinal capillary hemangiomas occur. The gene that is mutated in this disease has been mapped to chromosome 3p25–3p26.[2] Penetrance in this syndrome is approximately 80%. In approximately one-half of cases, multiple hemangiomas may occur. These hemangiomas may remain asymptomatic or may cause reduced visual acuity due to subretinal exudate. Approximately one-half of patients have an associated infratentorial hemangioblastoma of the cerebellum, brainstem, or spinal cord, in which case the disorder is called Von Hippel–Lindau syndrome. Patients with Von Hippel–Lindau syndrome are at increased risk of renal cell carcinoma, pheochromocytoma, and cysts of the pancreas, epididymis, kidney, liver, lung, adrenal gland, bone, omentum, or mesocolon. Symptomatic hemangiomas can be treated with laser photocoagulation using long-duration burns or with cryotherapy. Multiple treatment sessions may be required.

Retinal cavernous hemangioma is characterized by dark, grapelike clusters of intraretinal aneurysms. Their clinical appearance is distinct from retinal capillary hemangioma. On fluorescein angiography, separation of the serum and cellular components of blood may be seen. These vascular hamartomas are symptomatic in approximately 10% of cases and may cause subretinal, intraretinal, and vitreous hemorrhage. Treatment is indicated only in symptomatic cases, and the value of treatment in these cases is still unproven. Choroidal hemangiomas may occur in a localized or a diffuse form. Sturge–Weber syndrome is a noninherited clinical condition characterized by a facial nevus flammeus (hemangioma of skin with capillary and cavernous channels) with ipsilateral intracranial hemangioma. In 40% of patients with Sturge–Weber syndrome, an associated diffuse, ipsilateral choroidal hemangioma may be found. Secondary hyperopia may occur with diffuse choroidal hemangioma as well as overlying retinal detachment in one-half of cases. Treatment of retinal detachment in these cases is by placement of light photocoagulation scars over the entire tumor in an attempt to strengthen the adhesion between the retina and the underlying pigment epithelium. In patients with diffuse choroidal hemangioma associated with Sturge–Weber syndrome, the median age at onset of ocular symptoms is 9 years. Patients with isolated, localized choroidal hemangiomas have a median age of onset of 39 years.

Wyburn–Mason syndrome is characterized by the association of abnormal retinal arteriovenous anastomoses with similar lesions in the ipsilateral midbrain. This condition is nonhereditary and is only rarely associated with subretinal exudation. The degree of arteriovenous anastomosis in the involved retina is variable and may be minor or involve the entire retinal circulation. Vision is dependent on the relative sparing of the macular circulation. Neurological sequelae are similarly variable. Only rarely is photocoagulation indicated for subretinal exudate or iris neovascularization.[40]

DIABETIC RETINOPATHY

The major retinal complications of diabetes are retinal neovascularization (proliferative diabetic retinopathy), diabetic macular edema, and capillary nonperfusion. These conditions are all related to the duration of chronic hyperglycemia and are quite rare before puberty. Following puberty, the incidence of *diabetic retinopathy* in type I diabetes begins to rise sharply such that 50% of patients have proliferative disease after 15 years. A similar acceleration of activity of diabetic retinopathy occurs with pregnancy. Pregnant women without advanced proliferative diabetic retinopathy are unlikely to develop exuberant proliferation and severe visual loss, but pregnant women with active proliferative disease are at significant risk. Women with background disease are at risk for both proliferative disease and diabetic macular edema. Follow-up examination of diabetics should be at least twice yearly during puberty and every 1 to 2 months during pregnancy.[4]

HYPERTENSIVE RETINOPATHY

Fundus findings of *hypertensive retinopathy* consist of widening of the arteriolar reflex associated with diffuse arteriolar narrowing, nicking (focal narrowing) of the veins distal to arteriovenous crossings, intraretinal hemorrhages, and disc edema. These changes result from arteriolosclerosis following chronic hypertension and are not usually seen in children. The acute fundus changes of hypertension are more common in the adolescent age group, specifically in the clinical setting of preeclampsia. *Preeclampsia* is a hypertensive disorder of pregnancy that occurs in the absence of other etiologies. It usually begins following the 12th week of gestation and is more common in the primigravida and in the adolescent. In preeclampsia, as in other acute hypertensive episodes, the primary fundus findings are focal constriction of retinal arterioles, cotton wool spots, choroidal infarctions with secondary serous retinal detachments (usually in the macula), and optic disc edema not associated with elevated intracranial pressure (Fig. 7-6). Prompt obstetrical evaluation and treatment are essential for pregnant patients with these fundus findings.[36,43]

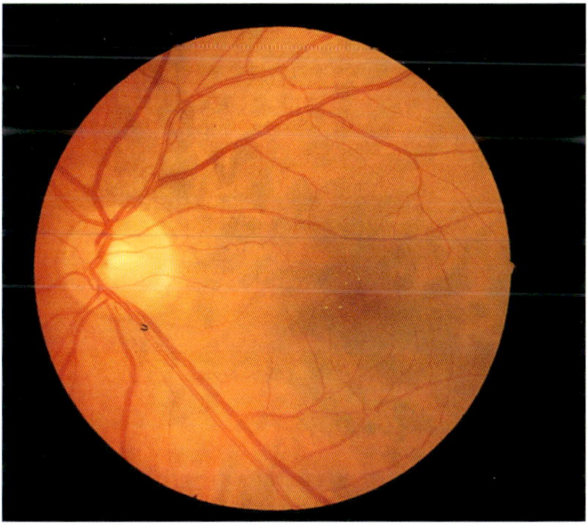

FIGURE 7-6. Choroidal infarction caused by preeclampsia typically produces a serous macular detachment.

TERSON'S SYNDROME

Intraocular hemorrhage is a known complication of subarachnoid hemorrhage and occurs in approximately 20% of these patients (Fig. 7-7). *Terson's syndrome* refers to cases in which vit-

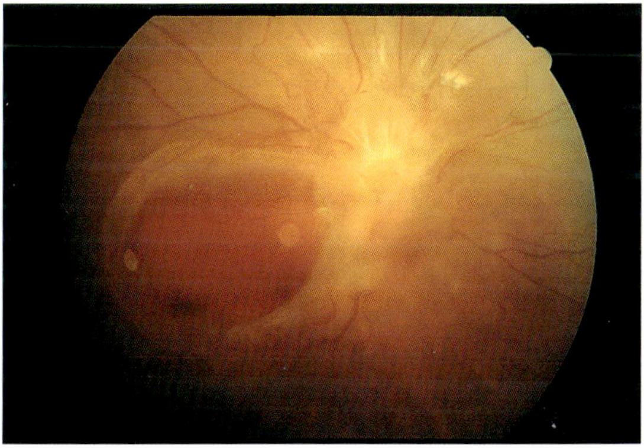

FIGURE 7-7. Terson's syndrome is often associated with subinternal limiting membrane hemorrhages.

reous hemorrhage accompanies subarachnoid hemorrhage. It is probably more appropriate to consider intraocular hemorrhage in this setting as a spectrum ranging from mild intraretinal hemorrhage to massive vitreous hemorrhage. This finding is highly significant because mortality from subarachnoid hemorrhage increases from 19.7% to 53.6% when associated with intraocular hemorrhage. Terson believed that a sudden increase in venous pressure following an abrupt elevation of intracranial pressure caused the intraocular hemorrhage. It is interesting that similar findings may occur following traumatic subdural hemorrhage.[39]

SHAKEN BABY SYNDROME

Blunt trauma of the head is the leading cause of death in child abuse. Blunt trauma in this setting may lead to ocular findings ranging from the anterior segment to the retina and optic nerve. When violent shaking of a small child occurs (*shaken baby syndrome (SBS)*, the typical fundus finding is a diffuse, often massive, intraretinal and vitreous hemorrhage. The intraretinal hemorrhages are typically located in the nerve fiber layer and may be unilateral or bilateral. This fundus appearance may closely resemble Terson's syndrome. However, the mechanism of injury in shaken baby syndrome differs from that in Terson's syndrome, and the latter designation should not be used to describe the intraocular hemorrhages in SBS.[28] A typical perimacular fold of the retina may also be seen in SBS and in few other entities.

Dense vitreous hemorrhages are associated with poor visual outcome because of both ocular disease and concomitant damage to the visual pathways.[25] The presence of a midline shift of brain structures on neuroimaging, and of nonreactive pupils, were both strongly predictive of mortality in one study.[26]

Historical details provided by caregivers are often inconsistent with the functional level of the child. Any time a diagnosis of child abuse is suspected, a report should be made to the proper authorities so that investigation can be undertaken.[49]

PURTSCHER'S RETINOPATHY

Sudden elevation of the venous pressure following chest compression can cause diffuse cotton wool spots and nerve fiber layer hemorrhages throughout the fundus. Suggested etiologies for these findings include aberrant coagulation and physical injury due to direct transmission of the elevated venous pressure. Fluorescein angiography shows leakage corresponding to areas of cotton wool spots and staining of small arterioles. *Purtscher's retinopathy* may be seen following motor vehicle accidents or cardiopulmonary resuscitation and in child abuse cases, especially those involving sexual abuse.

EALES DISEASE

Eales disease is an idiopathic peripheral retinal vasculitis with the peak onset of symptoms between the ages of 20 and 30 years. Eales disease is rare in the United States but is a significant cause of uveitis in the Middle East and India. Historically, Eales disease has been described as a peripheral periphlebitis, but more recent studies have suggested an equal amount of arteriolar sheathing. Nonperfusion of the peripheral retina is a hallmark of the disease and most often involves the temporal retina. Retinal neovascularization occurs in up to 80% of patients and often leads to vitreous hemorrhage. Although serious complications such as rubeosis iridis with neovascular glaucoma or macular nonperfusion may occur, the visual prognosis of Eales disease is usually quite good, with two-thirds of patients maintaining vision of 20/40 or better.[15]

INCONTINENTIA PIGMENTI

Incontinentia pigmenti is characterized by abnormalities in ectodermal structures such as the eyes, skin, teeth, and central nervous system. Affected patients usually present in infancy with a vesicular eruption of the skin that evolves into a whorling pattern of abnormal pigmentation (Fig. 7-8A). These whorls become less visible with increasing age and may be nearly invisible by the third decade of life. Patches of alopecia may be seen as well.

Ophthalmic findings include strabismus, nystagmus, blue sclera, cataract, and microphthalmia. Fundus findings may include optic nerve atrophy or papillitis, retinal hemorrhages or neovascularization, retinal edema, and chorioretinitis (Fig. 7-8B).[47] Holmstrom and Thoren found serious and vision-threatening ocular disease in 45% of their 30 patients.[19] Retinal

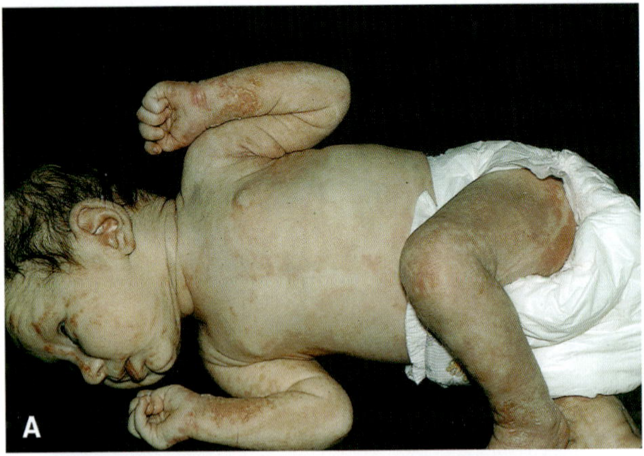

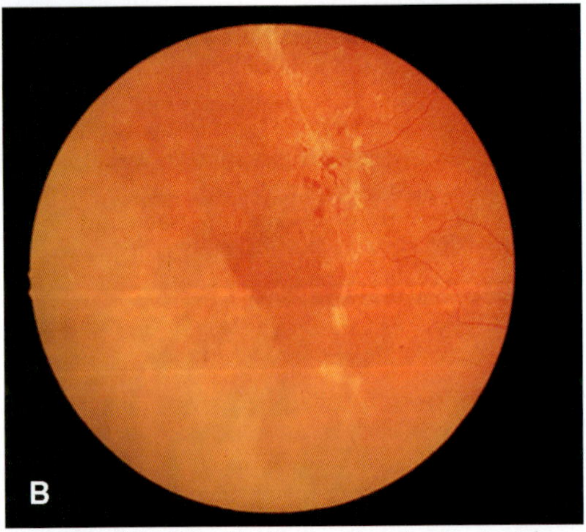

FIGURE 7-8A,B. **(A)** Blister-like lesions that develop in infancy, then evolve into whorls of brown pigment, are characteristic of incontinentia pigmenti. (Courtesy of Mary S. Stone, M.D.) **(B)** Peripheral retinal neovascularization may be seen in incontinentia pigmenti and may be associated with vitreous hemorrhages in some cases.

disease is the greatest threat to vision. The natural history of ocular disease in IP is poorly defined. However, a screening schedule for retinal examinations has been proposed and includes examinations shortly after birth and then monthly for 3 to 4 months. This schedule is followed by examinations at 3-month intervals for an additional year, then by semiannual examinations until age 3.[19,29]

The condition is most commonly inherited as an X-linked dominant that is lethal in males (Bloch–Sulzberger syndrome). One gene has been localized to the long arm of the X chromosome (Xq28).[19] Thus, almost all affected patients are female. Some pedigrees have been reported in which affected males have transmitted the disease to daughters, but no male-to-male transmission has been documented.[23]

HYPOMELANOSIS OF ITO

Hypomelanosis of Ito is a rare syndrome characterized by bizarre, patterned, hypopigmented streaks along the lines of Blashko. Hypomelanosis of Ito is also distinguishable from incontinentia pigmenti in that the skin lesions are not preceded by the inflammatory vesicles that are seen in the latter disease. Ophthalmic findings can include nystagmus, strabismus, heterochromia irides, iris coloboma, microphthalmia, myopia, corneal pannus, choroidal atophy, retinal hypopigmentation, and retinal detachment.[35] Half these patients have systemic findings that may include central nervous system dysfunction (delayed development or seizure) and musculoskeletal anomalies.[37]

GOODPASTURE SYNDROME

Goodpasture syndrome is a chronic, relapsing autoimmune disease characterized by episodic bouts of hemoptysis, dyspnea, and glomerular nephritis caused by immunoglobulin G deposition in the basement membrane of lung alveoli and renal glomeruli. An episcleritis may develop in some patients resembling that seen with rheumatoid arthritis. Patients may also develop choroidal infarctions with secondary serous retinal detachment or macular edema.[21] A 40-year-old patient with Goodpasture's syndrome developed bilateral peripapillary subretinal neovascular membranes that were successfully treated with laser ablation.[34]

ALLERGIC GRANULOMATOSIS (CHURG–STRAUSS DISEASE)

Churg–Straus disease is a systemic allergic disease that is characterized by a granulomatous and eosinophil-rich inflammation involving the respiratory tract, with necrotizing vasculitis. The primary complications of Churg–Strauss disease of interest to the ophthalmologist are orbital inflammatory pseudotumor and ischemic vasculitis.[44] Branch and central retinal artery occlusion, and ischemic optic neuropathy, have been reported.[44] Diagnosis is aided by the presence of blood eosinophilia and perinuclear antineutrophil cytoplasmic antibodies.[8]

TAKAYASU'S ARTERITIS

The inflammatory condition called *Takayasu's arteritis* primarily affects the aorta and its branches in children and young women. It is rare in the United States and Europe but common in Japan and other parts of the Orient. Synonyms for this disease include "pulseless disease" and "aortitis syndrome." Histologically, the disease is characterized by a granulomatous panarteritis. Systemic findings may include fatigue, weight loss, low-grade fever, diminished pulses, orthostatic syncope, intermittent claudication, and seizures. The reported mortality rates vary from 10% to 75%, depending in part on the length of follow-up. Death usually results from a cerebrovascular accident or complications of congestive heart failure. Ophthalmic findings result from ischemia. Mild ischemia is associated with retinal vasodilation and formation of microaneurysms. Severe ischemia leads to arteriovenous shunting, capillary dropout, cotton wool spots, anterior segment ischemia, neovascular glaucoma, vitreous hemorrhage, retinal detachment, and optic atrophy.[6,13,45] Treatment with prednisone or other glucocorticoids may alleviate symptoms and induce a remission in many patients but has yet to be proven to increase life expectancy.[13,45] Neovascularization may be treated with photocoagulation. In cases with carotid artery narrowing, endarterectomy should be considered to improve blood pressure to the eye.[6]

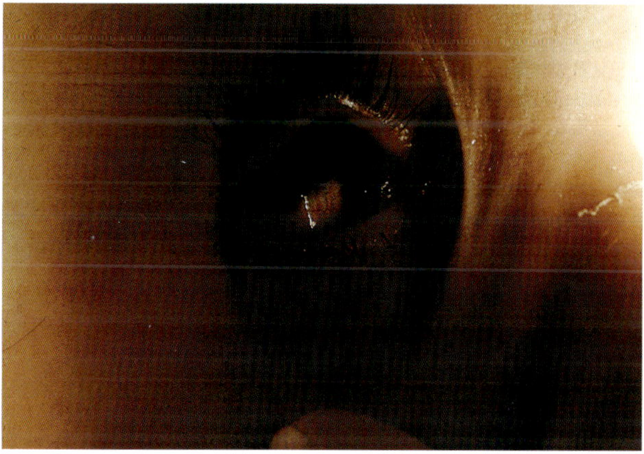

FIGURE 7-9. Microphthalmos is the most common clinical appearance of the eye in Norrie's disease.

NORRIE'S DISEASE

Norrie's disease, a rare, X-linked disorder, is also known as Andersen–Warburg syndrome. Clinical findings include mental retardation in two-thirds of cases and deafness that typically occurs between childhood and middle age. Ophthalmic findings include retinal detachments, usually with microphthalmos and blindness from birth (Fig. 7-9). In the fundus, there is formation of pseudotumors by dysplastic retinal tissue. Clinical findings can range from a clear anterior segment with retinal pseudotumors resembling retinopathy of prematurity to complete disorganization of all intraocular contents.[18,46] Dozens of mutations in the Norrie disease gene, resulting in abnormalities of the protein, *norrin*, have been identified as causative. This protein is normally expressed in the brain, retina, and choroid.[31]

FASCIOSCAPULOHUMERAL DYSTROPHY

The autosomal dominant form of muscular dystrophy called *fascioscapulohumeral dystrophy* predominantly affects the muscles of the shoulders and may be associated with sensorineural hearing loss and peripheral retinal telangiectasis similar to those of Coats' disease. Similar retinal telangiectasis has also been described in a patient with scapuloperoneal muscular dystrophy, a rare myopathy of the muscles of the proximal shoulder and anterior thigh. Sporadic, autosomal dominant and X-linked cases of scapuloperoneal dystrophy have been described.[9,42]

ANEMIA

Patients with *anemia* may have a variety of fundus findings including retinal hemorrhages, cotton wool spots, hard exudates, venous dilation and tortuosity, and disc edema (Fig. 7-10). The retinal hemorrhages associated with anemia may vary from flame shaped, to white centered, to subinternal limiting membrane. Fundus findings in anemia are most often seen with moderate to severe anemia of acute onset; children have these findings less commonly than adults. Associated thrombocytopenia may play an etiological role in anemic retinopathy. Vision may be normal but can also be profoundly affected when macular hemorrhage or optic nerve ischemia occur.[20]

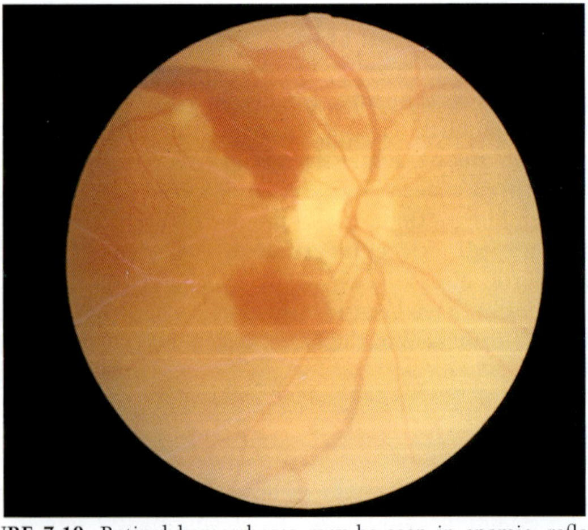

FIGURE 7-10. Retinal hemorrhages may be seen in anemia, reflecting a combination of poor endothelial oxygenation and deficient platelet function.

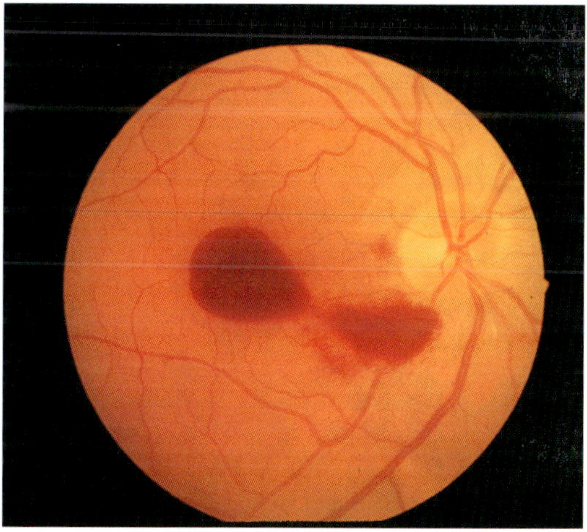

FIGURE 7-11. Retinal hemorrhages may occur in leukemia, often in those cases that involve blast crisis and anemia.

LEUKEMIA

The retinal findings of *leukemia* resemble those of patients with severe anemia and include retinal hemorrhages, venous dilation and tortuosity, and hard exudates (Fig. 7-11). Additional findings may include microaneurysmal changes in peripheral retinal vessels, capillary nonperfusion, neovascularization of the retina or optic nerve, and direct leukemic infiltration of the choroid, optic nerve, retina, or vitreous. Fundus findings in leukemia are most often associated with acute leukemic episodes or with relapses and may be related to coexisting anemia or hyperviscosity. If a leukemic patient develops optic disc swelling, increased intracranial pressure should be ruled out and prompt treatment begun with some combination of irradiation, steroids, and chemotherapy to prevent permanent, profound visual loss.[20,33]

HYPERVISCOSITY SYNDROMES

Several disorders may result in hyperviscosity of the blood, including *Waldenstrom's macroglobulinemia*, *polycythemia*, and *multiple myeloma*. Waldenstrom's macroglobulinemia

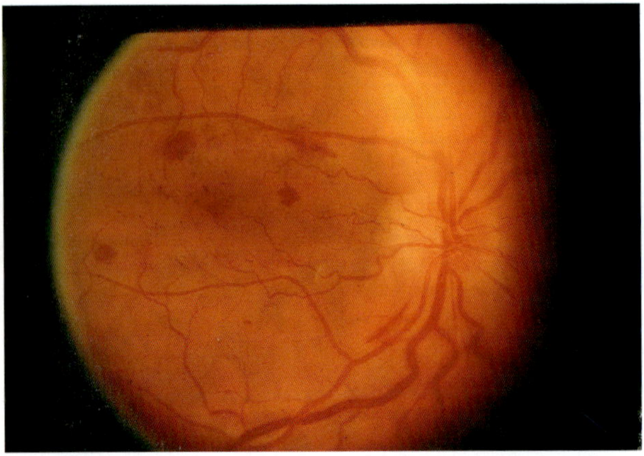

FIGURE 7-12. Multiple myeloma may lead to a hyperviscosity syndrome with intraretinal hemorrhages and, in some cases, to retinal vascular occlusions.

is characterized by production of monoclonal IgM protein with hyperviscosity. Systemic findings may include fatigue, headaches, and epistaxis. Fundus findings are similar to those of anemia or leukemia and involve retinal hemorrhages, venous tortuosity and dilation, and optic disc edema (Fig. 7-12). Multiple myeloma is a plasma cell neoplasm and results in osteoporosis, a tendency to fractures, and amyloid deposits throughout the body. Fundus findings may be suggestive of hyperviscosity. Polycythemia is an overproduction of erythrocytes and may be a primary bone marrow disorder or a response to a hypoxic environment such as high altitude. Fundus findings typical of hyperviscosity may be observed in many of these patients.[11,24]

KAWASAKI'S DISEASE

Kawasaki's disease, also known as mucocutaneous lymph node syndrome, is an idiopathic, acute, febrile illness of children. The disease is characterized by fever of 5 or more days duration, petechial rash of the palms and soles, nonpurulent cervical lymph node swelling, bilateral conjunctival injection, and transient anterior uveitis during the acute phase of the disease. Retinal arterial obstruction may occur secondary to arteritis in these patients. Careful medical follow-up of these patients is necessary because approximately 3% of patients with this disorder die of coronary arteritis. Mortality can be reduced by appropriate and early intervention.[14]

CAROTID CAVERNOUS FISTULA

Carotid-cavernous fistulas in children are almost always the result of trauma. Rupture of the internal carotid artery inside the cavernous sinus produces a high-pressure arteriovenous shunt. Reversal of flow in vessels that ordinarily drain into the cavernous sinus results in "arterialization" with engorgement of the veins of the orbit, conjunctiva, and lids on the affected side (Fig. 7-13). Exophthalmos, glaucoma, and an orbital bruit may also become evident. Cranial nerves III through VI may become affected in their intracavernous course. Fundus changes can include disc edema, retinal hemorrhages, and central retinal vein occlusion.

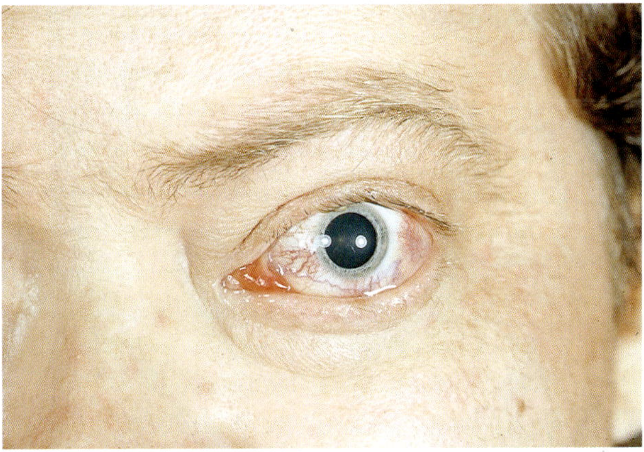

FIGURE 7-13. Arterialization of the conjunctival circulation in patients with carotid cavernous fistulas may lead to a mistaken diagnosis of "pink eye."

VEIN OCCLUSIONS

Branch retinal *vein occlusion* in adults is typically associated with chronic systemic hypertension and occurs at arteriovenous crossings. This type of branch retinal vein occlusion is exceedingly rare in children. Branch retinal vein occlusions may occur in children in association with hyperviscosity syndromes, sickle hemoglobinopathies, and retinal venous loops. Central retinal vein occlusion in children is even less common than branch retinal vein occlusion and probably has a similar etiology.[30]

CONGENITAL VASCULAR LOOPS

Dilated vascular loops may be located on or near the optic disc. These loops are arterial in approximately 80% of cases and involve the inferior retinal circulation in approximately two-thirds of cases (Fig. 7-14). Cilioretinal arteries are an associated finding in the majority of eyes. Complications are infrequent but include occlusion of an arterial loop with resultant branch retinal arterial occlusion, occlusion of a venous loop with result-

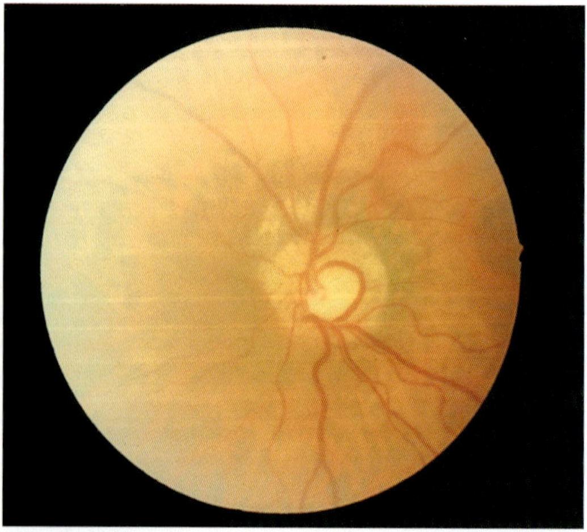

FIGURE 7-14. Although retinal vascular loops at the optic disc are typically arterial, venous loops may be seen in 20% of these cases.

ant branch retinal venous occlusion, vitreous hemorrhage from traction on a loop, amaurosis fugax, and hyphema.[5]

Acknowledgments. The preparation of this chapter was supported in part by an unrestricted grant from Research to Prevent Blindness, Inc.

References

1. Al-abdulla NA, Haddock TA, Kerrison JB, et al. Sickle cell disease presenting with extensive perimacular arteriolar occlusions in a nine-year-old boy. Am J Ophthalmol 2001;131:275–276.
2. Alper SL, Lodish HF. Impact of molecular biology of nephrology. In: Wilson (eds) Harrison's principles of internal medicine, 12th edn. New York: McGraw-Hill, 1991:1132.
3. Asdourian G. Vascular anomalies of the retina. In: Peyman GA, Sanders DR, Goldberg MF (eds) Principles and practices of ophthalmology. Philadelphia: Saunders, 1980:1299.
4. Benson WE, Tasman W, Duane TD. Diabetes mellitus and the eye. In: Tasman W, Jaeger EA (eds) Clinical ophthalmology, vol 3. Philadelphia: Lippincott, 1990.
5. Brown G, Tasman W. Congenital anomalies of the optic disc. New York: Grune & Stratton, 1983.
6. Chun YS, Park S, Park IK, et al. The clinical and ocular manifestations of Takyasu arteritis. Retina 2001;21(2):132–140.
7. Clarke WN, Vomiero G, Leonard BC. Bilateral simultaneous retinal arteriolar obstruction in a child wih hemoglobin SS sickle cell disease. JAAPOS 2001;5:126–128.
8. Cury D, Breakey AS, Payne BF. Allergic granulomatous angiitis associated with uveoscleritis and papilledema. Arch Ophthalmol 1956; 55:261.
9. Dickey JB, Daily MJ. Retinal telangiectasis in scapuloperoneal muscular dystrophy. Am J Ophthalmol 1991;112:348–349.
10. Farber MD, Jampol LM, Fox P, et al. A randomized clinical trial of scatter photocoagulation of proliferative sickle cell retinopathy. Arch Ophthalmol 1991;109(3):363–367.
11. Feman SS, Stein RS. Waldenstrom's macroglobulinemia, a hyperviscosity manifestation of venous stasis retinopathy. Int Ophthalmol 1981;4(1-2):107–112.
12. Fine LC, Petrovic V, Irvine AR, et al. Spontaneous central retinal artery occlusion in hemoglobin SC disease. Am J Ophthalmol 2000; 130:680–681.
13. Font RF, Naumann G. Ocular histopathology in pulseless disease. Arch Ophthalmol 1969;82:784.
14. Font RL, Mehta RS, Streusand SB, O'Boyle TE, Kretzer FL. Bilateral retinal ischemia in Kawasaki disease. Ophthalmology 1983;90:569.

15. Gieser SC, Murphy RP. Eales disease. In: Ryan SJ (ed) Retina, vol 2. St. Louis: Mosby, 1989:538.
16. Goldberg MF. Sickle cell retinopathy. In: Tasman W, Jeager EA (eds) Duane's clinical ophthalmology, vol. 3. Philadelphia: Lippincott, 1990.
17. Haller JA. Coats' disease. In: Ryan SJ (ed) Retina, vol 2. St. Louis: Mosby, 1989:491.
18. Holmes LB. Norrie's disease: an X-linked syndrome of retinal malformation, mental retardation, and deafness. N Engl J Med 1971;284:367.
19. Holmstrom G, Thoren K. Ocular manifestations of incontinentia pigmenti. Acta Ophthalmol Scand 2000;78:348–353.
20. Holt JM, Gordon-Smith EC. Retinal abnormalities in diseases of blood. Br J Ophthalmol 1969;53:145.
21. Jampol LM, Lahav M, Albert DM, Craft J. Ocular clinical findings and basement membrane changes in Goodpasture's syndrome. Am J Ophthalmol 1975;79:452.
22. Kreusel K, Krause L, Broskamp G, et al. Pars plana vitrectomy and endophotocoagulation for paracentral Coats' disease. Retina 2001;21:270–271.
23. Kurczynski TW, Bun JS, Johnson WE. Studies of a family with incontinentia pigmenti variously expressed in both sexes. J Med Genet 1982;19:447.
24. Luxenbourg MN, Mausolf FA. Retinal circulation in the hyperviscosity syndrome. Am J Ophthalmol 1970;70:588.
25. Matthews GP, Das A. Dense vitreous hemorrhages predict poor visual and neurological prognosis in infants with shaken baby syndrome. J Pediatr Ophthalmol Strabismus 1996;33:260–265.
26. McCabe CF, Donahue SP. Prognostic indicators for vision and mortality in shaken baby syndrome. Arch Ophthalmol 2000;118:373–377.
27. Miller NR. Walsh and Hoyt's clinical neuro-ophthalmology, 4th edn, vol 4. Baltimore: Williams & Wilkins, 1988:2165.
28. Mills MD. Terson syndrome. Ophthalmology 1998;105:2161–2162.
29. Nguyen JK, Brady-McCreery KM. Laser photocoagulation in preproliferative retinopathy of incontinentia pigmenti. JAAPOS 2001;5:258–259.
30. Orth DH, Patz A. Retinal branch vein occlusion. Surv Ophthalmol 1978;22:357.
31. Ott S, Patel RJ, Appukuttan B, et al. A novel mutation in the Norrie disease gene. JAAPOS 2000;4:125–126.
31a. Pauleikhoff D, Wessing A. Long-term results of the treatment of Coats' disease. Fortschr Ophthalmol 1989;86(5):451–455.
32. Penman AD, Talbot JF, Chaung EL, et al. New classification of peripheral vascular changes in sickle cell disease. Br J Ophthalmol 1994;78:681–689.
33. Ridgway EW, Jaffe N, Walton DS. Leukemic ophthalmopathy in children. Cancer (Phila) 1976;38:1744.

34. Rowe PA, Mansfield DC, Dutton GN. Ophthalmic features of fourteen cases of Goodpasture's syndrome. Nephron 1994;68:52–56.
35. Ruggieri M, Pavone L. Hypomelanosis of Ito: clinical syndrome or kust phenotype. J Child Neurol 2000;15:635–644.
36. Scheie HG. Evaluation of ophthalmoscopic changes of hypertension and arteriolosclerosis. Arch Ophthalmol 1953;49:117.
37. Schwartz MF Jr, Esterly NB, Fretzin DF, Pergament E, Rozenfeld IH. Hypomelanosis of Ito (incontentia pigmentia achromans), a neurocutaneous syndrome. J Pediatr 1977;90:236.
38. Seiberth V. Trans-scleral diode laser photocoagulation in proliferative sickle cell retinopathy. Ophthalmology 1999;106:1828–1829.
39. Shaw HE Jr, Landers MB III. Vitreous hemorrhage after intracranial hemorrhage. Am J Ophthalmol 1975;80:207.
40. Shields JA, Shields CL. The phakomatoses (the systemic hamartoses. In: Nelson LB, Calhoun JH, Harley RD (eds) Pediatric ophthalmology, 3rd edn. Philadelphia: Saunders, 1991:427.
41. Shields JA, Shields CL, Honavar SG, et al. Classification and management of Coats disease: the 2000 Proctor lecture. Am J Ophthalmol 2001;131:572–583.
42. Small RG. Coats' disease and muscular dystrophy. Trans Am Acad Ophthalmol Otolaryngol 1968;72:225.
43. Sunness JS. The pregnant woman's eye. Surv Ophthalmol 1988;32: 219.
44. Takanashi T, Uchida S, Arita M, et al. Orbital inflammatory pseudotumor and ischemic vasculitis in Churg–Strauss syndrome. Ophthalmology 2001;108:1129–1133.
45. Tanaka T, Shimizu K. Retinal arteriovenous shunts in Takayasu's disease. Ophthalmology 1987;94:1380.
46. Warburg M. Norrie's disease and falciform detachment of the retina. In: Goldberg MF (ed) Genetic diseases in ophthalmology. Boston: Little, Brown, 1974:430.
47. Watzke RC, Stevens TS, Carney RG Jr. Retinal vascular changes of incontinentia pigmenti. Arch Ophthalmol 1976;94:743.
48. Welch RB, Goldberg MF. Sickle cell hemoglobin and its relation to fundus abnormality. Arch Ophthalmol 1966;75:353.
49. Williams DF, Mieler WF, Williams GA. Posterior segment manifestations of ocular trauma. Retina 1990;10:S35.

8

Nonvascular Hamartomas

Chittaranjan V. Reddy and Arlene V. Drack

This chapter discusses some of the nonvascular hamartomas and choristomas of the retina, retinal pigment epithelium (RPE), and choroid that may be seen in the pediatric population. Although many of the lesions discussed in this chapter are present in childhood, they are frequently discovered later in life during routine examination or when late visual symptoms develop.

CHOROIDAL NEVUS

Choroidal nevi are tumors consisting of benign uveal melanocytes that are derived embryologically from the neural crest. Choroidal nevi are believed to be developmental tumors; they are rarely seen at birth or during infancy but increase in frequency around puberty.[8] The pathogenesis of choroidal nevi is poorly understood, but they are similar to nevi involving other parts of the uveal tract. Clinically evident choroidal nevi are estimated to occur in 1% to 2% of the general population, but they are found in 6.5% of autopsied eyes.[11] There is no known sexual predilection, but whites have these lesions more commonly than blacks.

Ophthalmoscopically, choroidal nevi usually appear as brown to slate gray lesions with fairly distinct margins (Fig. 8-1). However, lesions may be amelanotic or show variable pigmentation.Choroidal nevi vary from 0.5 to 10 mm in diameter, but they are usually approximately one disc area in size. Choroidal nevi are usually flat but may be elevated 1 to 3 mm. Most choroidal nevi are located posterior to the equator. In contrast, choroidal freckles, also frequently seen, are fairly indis-

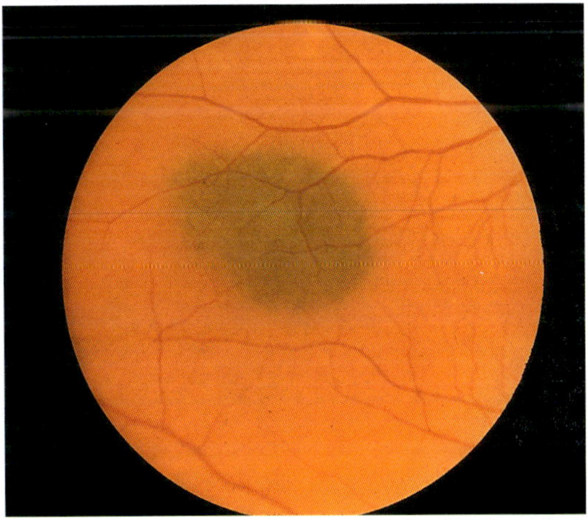

FIGURE 8-1. Choroidal nevus. Note the well-defined border of the lesion.

tinct, flat lesions. Choroidal freckles simply represent localized increased choroidal pigmentation.

Over several years, the clinical appearance of a choroidal nevus may change secondary to degeneration within the tumor or in the overlying tissue. Changes include the appearance of drusen, RPE atrophy, and pigment migration into the retina that can appear as bone spicules at the edge of the lesion. Clumps and patches of orange pigmentation can also be seen overlying the nevus (Fig. 8-2). Orange pseudohypopyon with metamorphopsia, which resolved without treatment, has been reported.[16a] Serous detachment of the retina, RPE detachments, and choroidal neovascular membranes (CNVM) can occur in association with choroidal nevi. Laser photocoagulation has been helpful in some cases.[5] The visual prognosis is dependent on the secondary changes and on the location of the choroidal nevus. Macular lesions have the worst prognosis. For most nevi, the visual prognosis is quite good.

Choroidal nevi may undergo malignant transformation into melanomas. Over a 10-year period, approximately 1 in 500 patients with choroidal nevi develop choroidal melanoma.[6] Thus, most patients with choroidal nevi do not develop melanoma. It is not clear what percentage of melanomas arise de novo and what percentage arise from preexisting choroidal

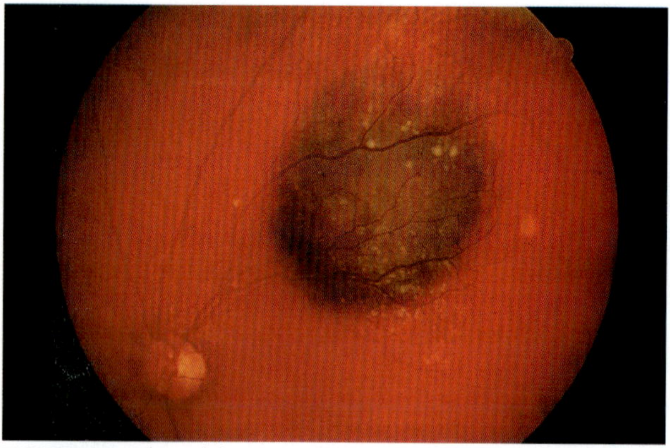

FIGURE 8-2. Choroidal nevus with pigmentary changes and overlying drusen suggesting chronicity.

nevi. Features that are associated with an increased risk of malignant transformation include largest diameter greater than 3 mm, elevation greater than 1 to 2 mm, and overlying orange pigmentary changes.[1] Suspicious lesions require examination and photography every 6 to 12 months to look for evidence of growth.

The diagnosis of a choroidal nevus is usually based on the ophthalmoscopic appearance. Echography is of little help in differentiating nevi from small melanomas. Histologically, nevi are comprised of four benign cell types (occurring in decreasing frequency): polyhedral cells, spindle cells, fusiform or dendritic cells, and balloon cells. Individual nevus cells may be pigmented or nonpigmented.

The mnemonic TFSOM (To Find Small Ocular Melanoma) has been suggested by Shields and Shields[22a] to help differentiate between nevi and malignancies. Thickness >2mm, Fluid subretinally, Symptoms, Orange pigment, and Margin touching the disc are all risk factors. Tumors with no factors have a 3% chance for growth at 5 years, those with one factor have a 38% chance and those with two or more factors have a 50% chance and often require treatment as they are actually small melanomas.[22a]

MELANOCYTOMA (MAGNOCELLULAR NEVUS)

The term melanocytoma refers to a dark brown or black variant of a choroidal nevus composed histopathologically of highly pigmented, plump, round to oval nevus cells. Melanocytomas can be seen anywhere in the uveal tract, but most are seen near the optic nerve head (Fig. 8-3). Although most are well circumscribed, diffuse forms of the lesion exist. It is difficult to determine the exact incidence of this unusual tumor because some may be confused with typical choroidal nevi. Melanocytomas are probably present at birth, but the diagnosis is usually made at a later age. Although there is no significant sexual predilection, there is a strong racial predisposition to melanocytomas. Approximately one-third to one-half of melanocytomas occur in blacks, in strong contrast to malignant melanomas, of which less than 1% occur in blacks. When melanocytomas occur in whites, they are usually seen in those of Hispanic or Italian descent.[12]

A melanocytoma of the optic nerve head is usually an incidental finding. If the lesion is fairly large, the patient may complain of slight blurring of vision. Additionally, an afferent pupillary defect and visual field abnormalities may be seen. In approximately half the cases, a typical choroidal nevus is con-

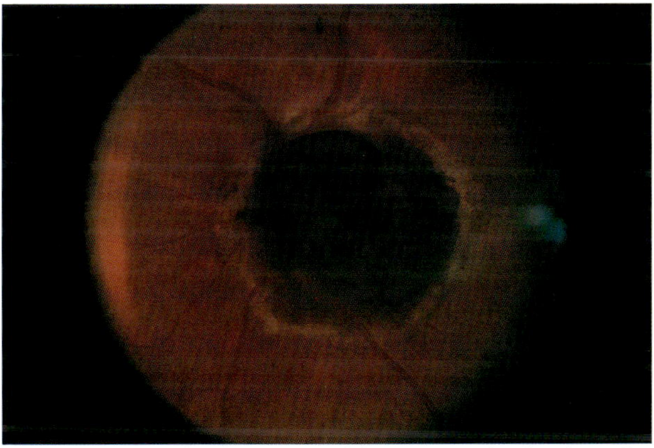

FIGURE 8-3. Typical melanocytoma of the optic nerve head with an adjacent choroidal nevus. (Courtesy of Dr. F.C. Blodi.)

tiguous with the melanocytoma at the optic nerve head. Extrapapillary melanocytomas are quite similar to other uveal nevi but tend to be much more pigmented.

In about 15% of cases, a subtle growth of the tumor at the optic nerve head is seen. Some larger melanocytomas may also undergo necrosis and liberate pigmentary debris into the vitreous cavity. Retinal vascular occlusion at the optic nerve head can occur with melanocytomas. In extremely rare cases, malignant transformation to melanomas has been described.[2,21]

Diagnosis is usually made by ophthalmoscopy alone. Fundus photography, fluorescein angiography, and visual field testing may be helpful for comparison on follow-up visits. Echography is not necessary in most cases.

CONGENITAL HYPERTROPHY OF THE RETINAL PIGMENT EPITHELIUM

Congenital hypertrophy of the retinal pigment epithelium (CHRPE) is fairly commonly seen on routine ophthalmoscopy and usually does not cause any symptoms. There are two recognized clinical forms: solitary lesions and multifocal grouped pigmentation of the RPE, also known as *bear tracks*. The lesions seen in these two variants are similar histologically and probably have a similar pathogenesis. The lesions are typically hyperpigmented although amelanotic lesions are seen as well.

CHRPE has no racial predilection, in contrast to choroidal nevi, choroidal melanomas, and melanocytomas, which may be related to the fact that the other tumors are derived from uveal melanocytes rather than the RPE. The diagnosis of CHRPE lesions is typically made on the basis of the clinical appearance of the lesion. Visual field testing has demonstrated defects in older individuals that are secondary to degeneration of the overlying photoreceptors. Therefore, lesions in the macula may cause visual loss with time.

Solitary CHRPE lesions are usually hyperpigmented with a sharply demarcated border that may be smooth or scalloped (Fig. 8-4). The lesions are usually flat, vary from 1 to 6 mm in diameter, and are more commonly found in the temporal fundus. CHRPE lesions may show central lacunae or peripheral depigmentation (Fig. 8-5). Overlying retinal vessels may be attenuated, but there is typically no invasion into the retina. Some solitary CHRPE lesions may be completely nonpigmented.

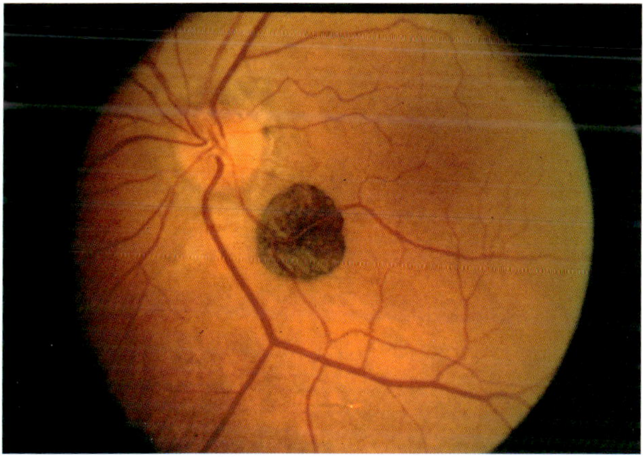

FIGURE 8-4. Congenital hypertrophy of the retinal pigment epithelium (CHRPE). Note the fairly distinct border of the lesion.

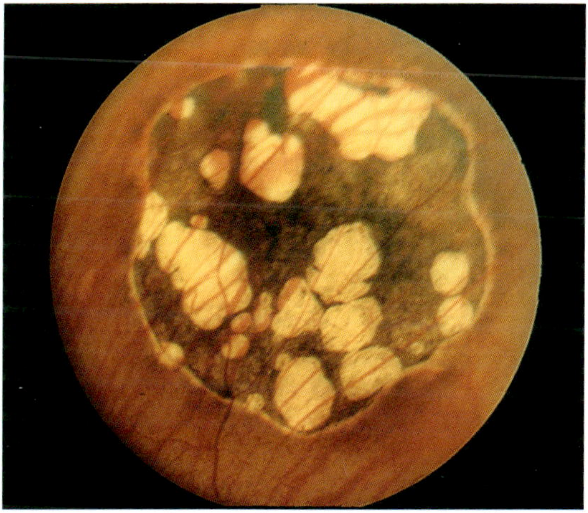

FIGURE 8-5. CHRPE lesion with several hypopigmented lacunae and a surrounding halo.

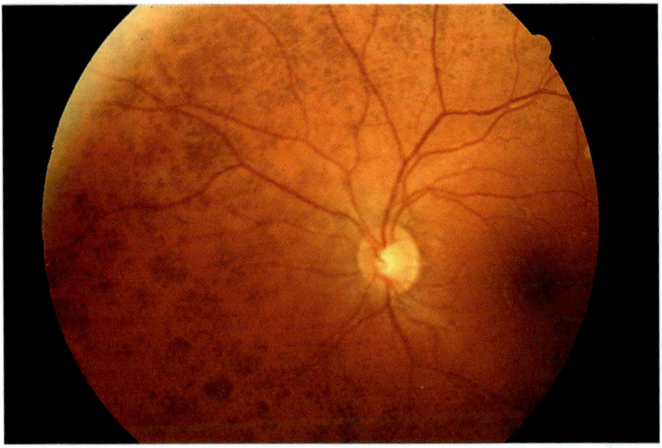

FIGURE 8-6. Multifocal CHRPE or "bear tracks."

There may be one to three lesions per eye, but bilateral involvement occurs only in 1% to 2% of cases.[18] Although growth of these lesions may occur, there is no known potential for malignant transformation.

The multifocal variant of CHRPE, similar to the solitary form, does not usually cause symptoms. Ophthalmoscopically, multifocal CHRPE lesions are usually grouped in one sector of the fundus (Fig. 8-6). Several small, variably sized lesions are arranged such that they resemble animal footprints (*bear tracks*). They do not typically have the lacunae or halos of depigmentation that are noted in the solitary form of CHRPE. Occasionally lesions may be amelanotic and are sometimes referred to as *polar bear tracks*.

CHRPE AND INHERITED GASTROINTESTINAL POLYPOSIS

CHRPE lesions have been associated with familial adenomatous polyposis, Gardner's syndrome, and Turcot's syndrome.[16,24] These autosomal dominant syndromes are associated with a very high risk of developing adenocarcinoma of the colon by age 50 years. Polyps may develop in early childhood. These patients may also have skeletal hamartomas and various other soft tissue tumors. The identification of typical CHRPE lesions may provide very useful diagnostic information to potentially affected offspring whose intestinal manifestations develop at a later age. Mutations of the APC gene are causative in some patients.[20a]

The presence of four or more CHRPE lesions not restricted to one sector of the fundus or bilateral involvement should make one suspicious of a familial polyposis syndrome. In addition, the CHRPE lesions seen in these patients have a characteristic appearance (Fig. 8-7). They tend to be oval in shape, oriented horizontally, and typically have a hypopigmented area that gives them a fishtail or comet-like appearance. There is no known histopathological difference between the CHRPE lesions associated with familial polyposis and those that are not.

Histopathologically, CHRPE lesions consist of focal areas of taller retinal pigment epithelial cells densely packed with pigment granules that are also larger than those found in the normal surrounding RPE. Within the lesions, areas of decreased density of the pigment granules have been noted and probably

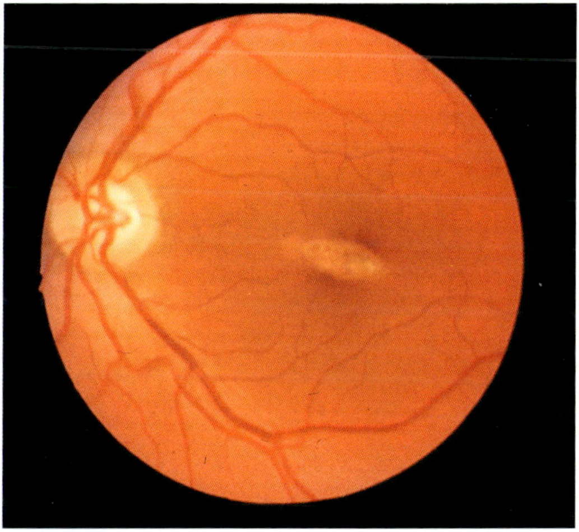

FIGURE 8-7. Macular CHRPE lesion in a patient with intestinal polyposis. Note the horizontal orientation of the "fishtail" lesion. (Courtesy of Dr. T.A. Weingeist. Previously published in Ophthalmology 1991;98: 113, used with permission.)

correspond to the depigmented lacunae seen clinically. The overlying Bruch's membrane may be thickened, and the photoreceptors are usually very sparse or absent.

CONGENITAL HYPERPLASIA OF THE RETINAL PIGMENT EPITHELIUM

Congenital hyperplasia of the retinal pigment epithelium (RPE) (Figs. 8-8, 8-9) is far less common than CHRPE. Asymptomatic children and adults have been diagnosed with this condition following ophthalmoscopic examination. Unlike typical CHRPE lesions, these hamartomas are composed of hyperplastic RPE cells that extend anteriorly into the overlying retina. Histopathologically, these lesions are probably characterized by sheets of increased numbers of fairly normal sized RPE cells.[4] There has been no demonstrated malignant transformation of these lesions.

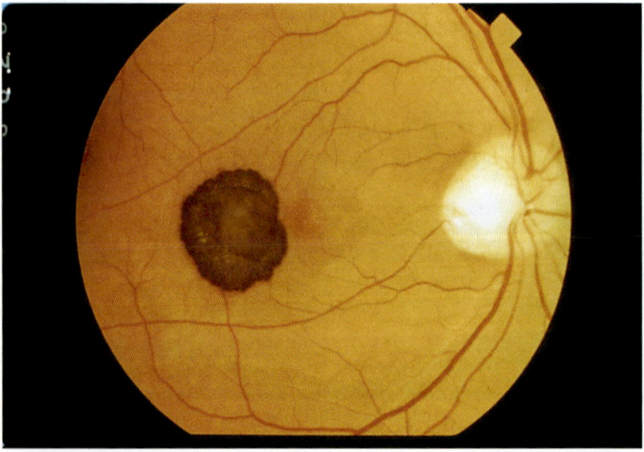

FIGURE 8-8. Congenital hyperplasia of the retinal pigment epithelium (RPE). (Courtesy of Dr. S. Pautler.)

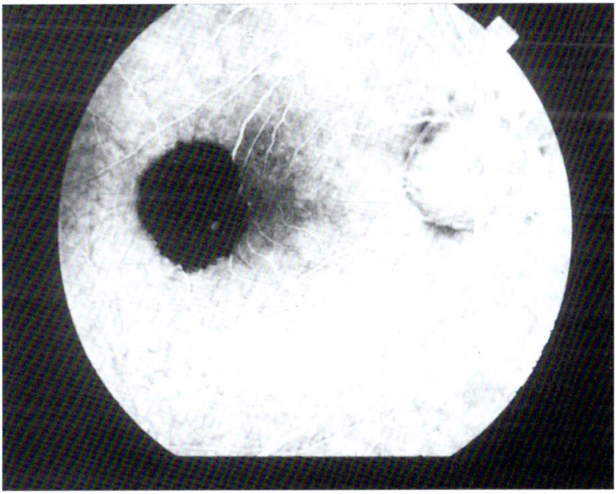

FIGURE 8-9. Fluorescein angiogram of the lesion in Figure 34-8. Note extension of the tumor into the overlying retina with retinal vascular changes.

COMBINED HAMARTOMA OF THE RETINAL PIGMENT EPITHELIUM AND RETINA

The clinical entity of a combined hamartoma of the retinal pigment epithelium and sensory retina was first clearly defined by Gass.[7] These tumors are quite rare. Clinically, the lesions may be found at any age including early childhood and infancy. The previous clinical history is often noncontributory, and the patient's visual complaints are dependent on the location of the tumors.

Ophthalmoscopically, the tumors may be located in a juxtapapillary (Figs. 8-10, 8-11) or peripheral distribution. Patients with juxtapapillary tumors are more commonly seen in young adulthood because of decreased or distorted vision. The tumors tend to be poorly-defined, elevated, variably pigmented, and involve part of the optic nerve and the adjacent retina. Tortuosity of the large retinal vessels emanating from the optic nerve head, a prominent feature, may be worsened by contraction of the fibroglial tissue. Additionally, the tumors may have a

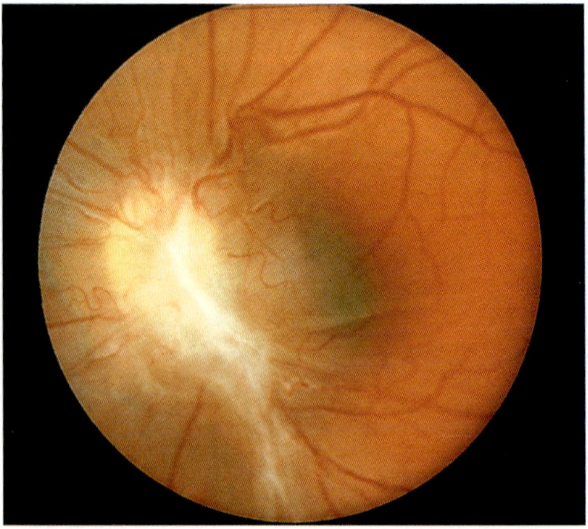

FIGURE 8-10. Juxtapapillary combined hamartoma of the RPE and retina.

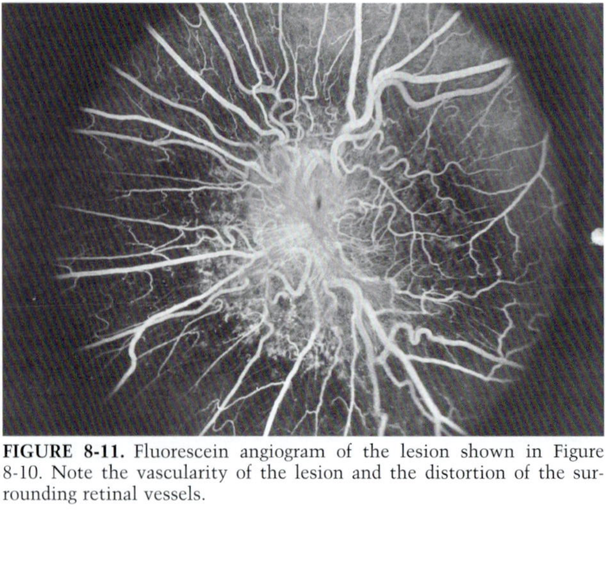

FIGURE 8-11. Fluorescein angiogram of the lesion shown in Figure 8-10. Note the vascularity of the lesion and the distortion of the surrounding retinal vessels.

prominent capillary network that can lead to macular exudation. Retinoschisis, intraretinal and subretinal lipid deposition, and retinal hole formation have been described.[20] Rarely, retinal hemorrhage, vitreous hemorrhage, or choroidal neovascular membranes occur. When located peripherally, dragging of the retinal vessels is a prominent feature. Regardless of location, the tumors have a variable composition of glial tissue and RPE.

The visual prognosis is dependent on the location of the tumor. Most peripheral lesions are asymptomatic and tend to be associated with good vision. Visual acuity in juxtapapillary lesions is dependent on the extent of macular distortion or optic nerve involvement. Overall, approximately 40% of patients maintain vision of 20/40 or better and approximately 30% of patients have vision that is 20/200 or worse.[19] Vitrectomy to relieve traction caused by epiretinal membrane formation usually does not improve vision.[15]

The diagnosis of combined hamartomas is based on the clinical appearance of the lesions. Fluorescein angiography may provide useful information regarding the vascular abnormalities associated with the tumor. Echography is of little value.

The pathogenesis of these lesions is not fully understood, but they may be developmental or arise secondary to inflammation. Evidence to support the notion that these are developmental tumors comes from cases in which the combined hamartomas are associated with neurofibromatosis, congenital anomalies of the optic disc, incontinentia pigmenti, X-linked retinoschisis, and facial hemangiomas.[10] Histopathologically, disorganization of retinal architecture is noted. Sheets of proliferating RPE are seen along with increased numbers of blood vessels. Fibroglial tissue on the inner surface of the retina and vitreous condensations are a prominent feature in some cases.

CHOROIDAL OSTEOMA

Choroidal osteomas are benign tumors of the choroid consisting of mature bone that are usually found in a juxtapapillary or a macular location (Fig. 8-12). They are typically discovered in women in their teens and twenties. Occasionally, they may be seen in men and adults older than 30.The symptoms at the time of diagnosis are dependent on the location of the osteoma as well as the presence or absence of an associated serous or hemorrhagic detachment of the retina. The lesions may be bilateral in

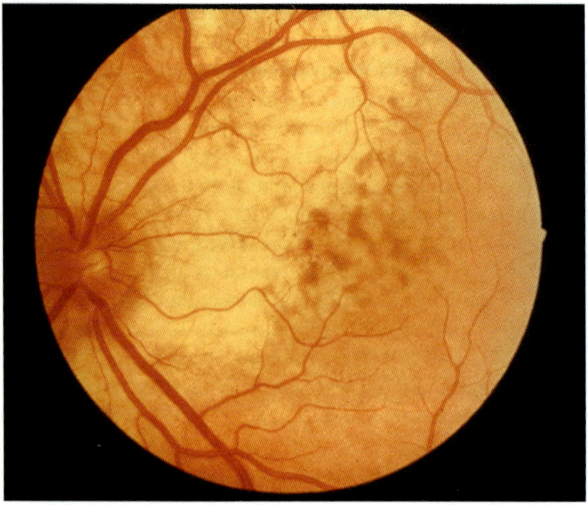

FIGURE 8-12. Juxtapapillary choroidal osteoma extending into the macula. Note the pigmentary changes in the macula.

20% to 25% of cases. There is no known predilection for race. The exact incidence of choroidal osteoma is not known.

Ophthalmoscopically, a choroidal osteoma typically appears as a slightly elevated, yellow to orange subretinal lesion. At the time of diagnosis, mottling of the overlying retinal pigment epithelium is frequently present. Multicentric lesions may occur, but solitary lesions are the norm. A pathognomonic feature of choroidal osteoma is the appearance of small vascular tufts that emerge on the anterior surface of the tumor. These tufts are particularly evident with fluorescein angiography and represent feeder vessels exiting from the spaces between the cancellous bone that make up the tumor. These blood vessels do not cause exudation or hemorrhage.[9] The presence of subretinal fluid or hemorrhage are signs of choroidal neovascular membrane development. Laser photocoagulation should be considered if the choroidal neovascular membrane appears to be vision threatening. Several treatment sessions may be required to eradicate the new blood vessels.

The visual prognosis of a choroidal osteoma is dependent on its location. Subfoveal lesions tend to have the worst prognosis, with gradual visual loss secondary to progressive degeneration of the overlying retina or serous detachment. Most patients with juxtapapillary osteomas tend to have a better prognosis.

Diagnosis of choroidal osteomas is best made by ophthalmoscopic examination and fluorescein angiography. Echography may be useful in differentiating choroidal osteomas from similar lesions. A-scan ultrasound typically shows a sharp high-intensity echo spike from the anterior surface of the tumor, along with high internal reflectivity (Fig. 8-13). A CT scan may show the characteristic appearance of a radioopaque lesion at the level of the choroid.

The exact pathogenesis of choroidal osteomas is unknown. Intraocular calcification has been noted in association with trauma, inflammation, congenital malformations, and long-standing retinal detachment, as well as abnormalities of calcium and phosphorus metabolism. Choroidal osteomas have similarly been described following a history of trauma or intraocular inflammation but most are seen in the absence of any associated ophthalmic problems. Female hormones probably play a role in the pathogenesis of choroidal osteomas given its preponderance in women. Familial occurrence of choroidal osteomas has also been reported.[17]

Two conditions that may be confused with typical choroidal osteomas are *sclerochoroidal calcification* and the *nevus sebaceous of Jadassohn*. Sclerochoroidal calcifications are typically seen along the superotemporal arcade and are more frequently multifocal. In older patients, they may occur in the absence of any abnormalities of calcium or phosphorus metabolism and probably represent calcification at the site of insertion of the superior oblique muscle.[23] The linear nevus sebaceous syndrome (of Jadassohn) consists of midline facial skin lesions, seizures, mental retardation, and ophthalmologic abnormalities. The ophthalmic abnormalities include conjunctival lipodermoids, colobomata of the lids, iris, choroid, and disc, angiomas of the orbit, osseous choristomas of the choroid (similar to typical choroidal osteomas), and subretinal neovascularization.[13]

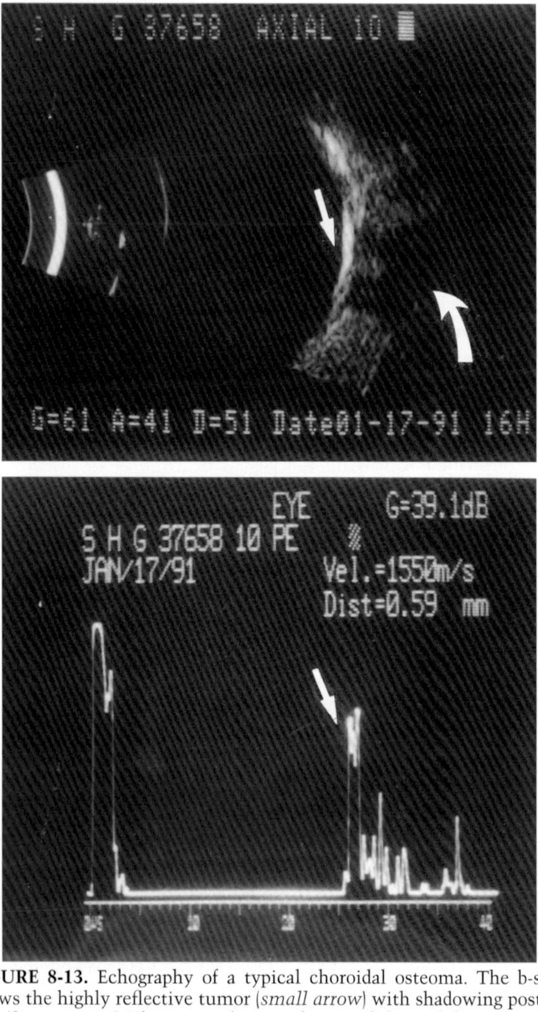

FIGURE 8-13. Echography of a typical choroidal osteoma. The b-scan shows the highly reflective tumor (*small arrow*) with shadowing posteriorly (*large arrows*). The a-scan shows a sharp peak (*arrow*) that represents the anterior surface of the tumor with decreasing echoes posteriorly. (Courtesy of Dr. K. Ossonig.)

TUBEROUS SCLEROSIS

Tuberous sclerosis, first described by Bourneville in 1880, consists of the triad of adenoma sebaceum, seizures, and variable mental retardation. There are many other cutaneous, CNS, and systemic features, discussed elsewhere in this volume.

The most characteristic fundus lesion seen in tuberous sclerosis is an *astrocytic hamartoma* of the optic nerve head or the retina; these are estimated to occur in approximately 50% of the patients with tuberous sclerosis. Astrocytic hamartomas are not a pathognomonic feature of tuberous sclerosis, as they may occur in neurofibromatosis as well. Moreover, it is unclear what percentage of astrocytic hamartomas is associated with tuberous sclerosis. Most patients with astrocytic hamartomas are asymptomatic, but gradual visual loss may be related to tumors at the optic nerve head or in the macula. These tumors can occur in the pediatric population.

Ophthalmoscopically, one or more elevated, white, fairly well circumscribed lesions arising from the inner retinal surface or the optic nerve are seen (Fig. 8-14). In younger patients, the lesions may be smaller, less opaque, and have poorly defined

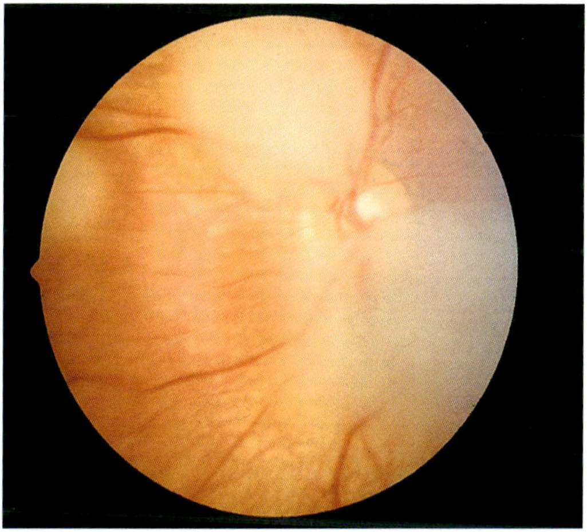

FIGURE 8-14. Typical "gelatinous" retinal astrocytoma in a patient with tuberous sclerosis. (Courtesy of Dr. F. Judisch.)

margins; these may be mistakenly diagnosed as retinoblastoma. Another striking feature of astrocytic hamartomas is the characteristic nodular calcification that may give a mulberry appearance that has also been likened to fish eggs or tapioca (Fig. 8-15). The calcification seen in retinoblastoma is usually dull and chalky white as opposed to the more glistening yellow, nodular calcification that is seen with astrocytic hamartomas. Dilated, tortuous retinal feeder vessels are a more common feature of retinoblastomas than of astrocytic hamartomas.[22]

Diagnosis of astrocytic hamartomas is usually made on the basis of the ophthalmoscopic appearance and associated findings of tuberous sclerosis. Fluorescein angiography reveals varying degrees of vascularity within and on the surface of the tumor. There is an invariable leakage of dye from the tumor vessels late in the angiogram, which may pool within the cystic areas of the tumor. Echography is helpful for larger tumors but is of little value with smaller tumors.

Histopathologically, the tumors are composed of well-differentiated, spindle-shaped fibrous astrocytes with round or oval nuclei and abundant eosinophilic cytoplasm. Some authors have stressed the importance of the vascular component of these lesions, which may suggest a link between these typically glial

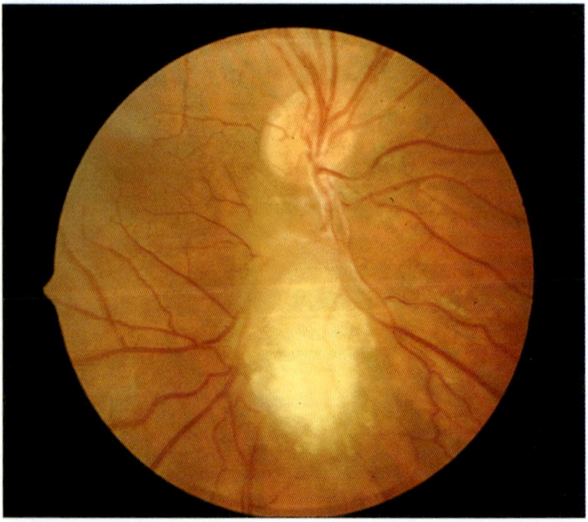

FIGURE 8-15. Retinal astrocytoma with calcifications appearing like "tapioca."

tumors and the retinal capillary hemangiomas seen in von Hippel–Lindau syndrome.[3] The calcification seen clinically has been verified histopathologically. The most common retinal finding in tuberous sclerosis is usually reported to be a flat, hypopigmented macule which appears similar to ash leaf spots on the skin, however a large British study found this punched-out lesion in only 39% of patients, compared to a flat translucent hamartoma in 70%. "Mulberry" lesions were found in 55%.[18a] Mutations of the TSC1 and TSC2 genes cause tuberous sclerosis.[11a]

NEUROFIBROMATOSIS

Neurofibromatosis is a syndrome with skin, neurological, and ophthalmic manifestations and is discussed more fully elsewhere in this volume. The most common ocular features are the iris Lisch nodules (probably nevi), neurofibromas of the eyelids, large corneal nerves, and optic nerve gliomas and meningiomas.

The most frequent retinal lesion seen with neurofibromatosis is an astrocytic hamartoma, although these occur less frequently than in patients with tuberous sclerosis. The astrocytic hamartomas seen in both phakomatoses are identical clinically and histologically. Additional retinal findings include myelinated nerve fibers. Multifocal congenital hypertrophy of the RPE (*bear tracks*) probably occurs more frequently in association with neurofibromatosis than in the general population.[14] Additionally combined hamartomas of the RPE and retina have been described in patients with neurofibromatosis, lending support to the idea that the combined hamartomas may be developmental in origin.[10]

Choroidal lesions similar to iris Lisch nodules have been described. Histopathologically, these hamartomas are probably nevi. Malignant melanomas are also more common in patients with neurofibromatosis and may be related to the greater number of nevi.[25] Additionally, some patients have thickened long ciliary nerves (neurilemoma) or may have diffuse thickening of the uveal tract (neurofibroma), which is probably caused by proliferation of neurons and Schwann cells of the ciliary nerves. Choroidal neurofibromas and neurilemomas occur more frequently in neurofibromatosis than in the general population, with the former tumor occurring in approximately 35% to 50% of patients.

Acknowledgments. Revision of this chapter was supported in part by the Georgia Lions Children's Eyecare Center.

References

1. Augsburger JJ, Schroeder RP, Terito CL, Gamel JW, Shields JA. Clinical parameters predictive of enlargement of choroidal melanocytic lesions. Br J Ophthalmol 1989;74:911–917.
2. Baker–Griffith AE, McDonald PR, Green WR. Malignant melanoma arising in a choroidal magnocellular nevus. Can J Ophthalmol 1976; 11:140–146.
3. Barsky WB, Wolter JR. The retinal lesions of tuberous schlerosis: angiomatous hamartoma? J Pediatr Ophthalmol 1971;8:261–265.
4. Duke JR, Maumenee AE. An unusual tumor of the retinal pigment epithelium in an eye with early open angle glaucoma. Am J Ophthalmol 1959;47:311–317.
5. Folk JC, Weingeist TA, Coonan P. The treatment of serous macular detachment secondary to choroidal melanomas and nevi. Ophthalmology 1989;96:547–551.
6. Ganley JP, Comstock GW. Benign nevi and malignant melanomas of the choroid. Am J Ophthalmol 1973;76:19–25.
7. Gass JDM. An unusual tumor of the pigment epithelium and retina simulating choroidal melanoma and retinoblastoma. Trans Am Ophthalmol Soc 1973;71:171–183.
8. Gass JDM. Problems in the differential diagnosis of choroidal nevi and malignant melanomas: the XXXIII Edward Jackson Memorial Lecture. Am J Ophthalmol 1977;83:299–323.
9. Gass JDM. New observations concerning choroidal osteomas. Int Ophthalmol 1979;1:71–84.
10. Gass JDM. Discussion of: Schachat AP, Shields JA, Fine SL, et al. Combined hamartomas of the retina and retinal pigment epithelium. Ophthalmology 1984;91:1615.
11. Hale PN, Allen PA, Straatsma BR. Benign melanomas (nevi) of the choroid and ciliary body. Arch Ophthalmol 1965;74:532–538.

11a. Hodges A, et al. Pathologic mutations in TSC1 and TSC2. Hum Molec Genet 2001;10(25):2899–2905.

12. Joffe L, Shields JA, Osher R, Gass JDM. Clinical follow-up studies of melanocytomas of the optic disc. Ophthalmology 1979;86:1067–1078.
13. Lambert HM, Sipperley JO, Shore JW, Dieckert JP, Evans R, Lowd DK. Linear nevus sebaceous syndrome. Ophthalmology 1987;94: 278–282.
14. Lewis RA, Riccardi VM. Von Recklinghausen neurofibromatosis. Incidence of iris hamartoma. Ophthalmology 1981;88:348–354.
15. McDonald HR, Abrams GW, Burke JM, Neuwirth J. Clinicopathologic results of vitreous surgery for epiretinal membranes in

patients with combined retinal and retinal pigment epithelial hamartomas. Am J Ophthalmol 1976;100.227–231.
16. Munden PM, Sobol WM, Weingeist TA. Ocular findings in Turcot Syndrome (glioma-polyposis).Ophthalmology 1991;98:111–114.
16a. Naseripour M et al. Pseudohypopyon of orange pigment overlying a stable choroidal nevus. Am J Ophthalmol 2001;132(3):416–417.
17. Noble KG. Bilateral choroidal osteoma in three siblings. Am J Ophthalmol 1990;109:656–660.
18. Purcell JJ, Shields JA. Hypertrophy with hyperpigmentation of the retinal pigment epithelium. Arch Ophthalmol 1975;93:1122–1126.
18a. Rowley SA et al. Ophthalmic manifestations of tuberous sclerosis: a population based study. BJO 2001;85(4):420–423.
19. Schachat AP, Shields JA, Fine SL, et al., and The Macula Society Research Committee. Combined hamartomas of the retina and retinal pigment epithelium. Ophthalmology 1984;91:1609–1614.
20. Schachat AP, Glaser BM. Retinal hamartoma, acquired retinoschisis, and retinal hole. Am J Ophthalmol 1985;99:604–605.
20a. Scott RJ, et al. Familial Adenomatous Polyposis: more evidence for disease diversity and genetic heterogeneity. Gut 2001;48(4):508–514.
21. Shields JA, Shields CL, Eagle RG, Lieb WE, Stern S. Malignant melanoma associated with melanocytoma of the optic disc. Ophthalmology 1990;97:225–230.
22. Shields JA, Shields CL. Intraocular tumors. Philadelphia: Saunders, 1992:432.
22a. Shields C, Shields J. Clinical features of small choroidal melanoma. Curr Opin Ophthalmol 2002;13(3):135–141.
23. Sivalingam A, Shields CL, Shields JA, et al. Idiopathic sclerochoroidal calcification. Ophthalmology 1991;98:720–724.
24. Traboulsi EI, Krush AJ, Gardner EJ, et al. Prevalence and importance of pigmented ocular fundus lesions in Gardner's syndrome. N Engl J Med 1987;316:661–667.
25. Wiznia RA, Freedman JE, Mancini AD, Shields JA. Malignant melanoma of the choroid in neurofibromatosis. Am J Ophthalmol 1978;86:684–687.

9

Retinoblastoma and Other Malignant Intraocular Tumors

A. Linn Murphree and Laurie E. Christensen

RETINOBLASTOMA

Early Detection and Treatment

Much of the vision loss that we as pediatric ophthalmologists accept as normal with retinoblastoma can be prevented or reversed with aggressive screening, early diagnosis, and treatment. In fact, we are convinced that in the coming decades detecting early disease by lowering the average age at initial diagnosis will prove to be a much more efficient and cost-effective way to manage retinoblastoma than developing exotic new drugs or gene therapy for advanced disease. For retinopathy of prematurity (ROP), we readily accept that early detection and treatment can prevent vision loss. The problem there, however, seems a bit more manageable; the children at risk for ROP all belong to a small and easily identifiable group based on low birth weight.

In the absence of a family history of retinoblastoma, the problems of screening for retinoblastoma would, on first glance, appear to be a logistical nightmare. Changing practice patterns to include instillation of a mydriatic drop as a routine part of well-child care can be a simple, easy-to-perform, effective adjunct to the red-reflex exam already used by pediatricians. Unfortunately, achieving that change in practice patterns, even for something as simple as a single instillation of a drop in each eye (a 10-second, 15-cent, intervention), will require overcoming major conceptual hurdles.

The first hurdle is the rarity issue. The argument goes like this: "Retinoblastoma is so rare, that I (the pediatrician) will see only 2 to 3 cases in my 30 years of practice. Are you telling me I must screen 25,000 to 35,000 infants to find those 2 to 3 cases early?" The response to that argument is simple. Well-child care is all about screening and prevention.

Most pediatricians already screen for retinoblastoma. Currently they either perform, or know that they need to perform, the pupillary red-reflex exam. As a result, the proposed change in practice patterns to include pupil dilation as part of well-child care does not add a single step to the physical examination that is already a part of the well-child visit. The current practice of performing the pupillary red-reflex exam with an undilated pupil is like listening for a heart murmur without a stethoscope; it is hardly worth the trouble.

It is true that retinoblastoma is rare, affecting at most only 1 in 12,000 infants. However, if the incidence of retinoblastoma is combined with congenital cataracts, the other major treatable congenital developmental anomaly of the eye, intraocular pathology that can be treated successfully before the end of the third month of life would be found in 1 of every 750 infants screened. To put these numbers in perspective, the incidence of congenital heart disease is about 1 in 500 live births; congenital dislocation of the hip affects 1 in 1,000 infants. A major reason neonatal well-child examinations exist is to screen for both these developmental disorders because early diagnosis and treatment is essential for the well-being of the child. During the 1- or 2-month well-child visit, pediatricians accurately listen for faint heart murmurs and competently manipulate the hip joint for evidence of a congenital dislocation. They do not, as yet, adequately screen for treatable intraocular pathology.

The second hurdle to achieving practice pattern changes that encourage dilation of the pupil in the primary care office relates to their personal past experience screening for intraocular pathology with an undilated pupil. Most pediatricians received little medical school training in ophthalmology and feel unprepared to screen for intraocular pathology. They all, however, know that the red-reflex examination is the best way to screen for retinoblastoma. They are generally now uncomfortable, however, with the routine results they get from the undilated red-reflex screen. The pupil is so small, often 2 mm or less, that the data from the test are inconclusive. The rationale for checking the "eyes normal" box is that because the disease is rare, the chances of being right are very high. Unfortunately, the chances of overlooking the presence of a large intraocular tumor are also high.

The third hurdle to the concept of pupil dilation in the primary care office is the misperceived burden that a single instillation of a mydriatic drop would impose on the doctor, office staff, and office routine. Poorly or misremembered information from medical school mixed with past personal experience contributes to this problem. Examples of misremembered information include (1) dilating the pupils causes glaucoma; (2) dilating the pupil takes three instillations of drops 5 min apart and then a wait of 30 min; (3) holding down a child to put in dilating drops requires three or four office staff members and totally disrupts the office routine; (4) dilating the pupils requires more work from the pediatrician that will not be separately reimbursed; and (5) dilating the pupils will obscure critical information that could be gathered from the pupil exam before dilation.

Each of the five misremembered "facts" about pupil dilation commonly used by those opposed to the use of dilation as a part of the 1- or 2-month well-baby examination is pure myth.

1. Pupillary dilation causes glaucoma in older adults with narrow anterior chambers, not in infants. Iatrogenic glaucoma has not been a concern or a finding in the hundreds of thousands of tiny infants dilated for ROP screening in the last decade.

2. A single instillation of a single agent, 1% tropicamide, gives 5 to 6 mm of dilation at 20 min, more than adequate for red-reflex screening

3. Three or four people might be required to hold down a 3- or 4-year-old to put in eye drops, but the subjects of our interest are newborn infants no more than 1 to 2 months old. When they are placed supine to be weighed, the nurse makes a "lake" of 2 to 3 drops of tropicamide over the inner edge of the lid fissure. If the "lake" wets the lashes to the lateral edge of the fissure and excess runs down the temple toward the ear, the drop is "in." There is no need or benefit of holding the lids open. If the drop does not get "in" immediately, gentle manipulation of the upper lid with the thumb on the brow will accomplish the trick. Holding the infant down is not necessary.

4. Dilating the pupil as part of the well-baby examination requires no extra effort on the part of the pediatrician. In fact,

pediatricians who have been doing this routinely in their practice for more than 8 years report that except that they now get a wonderfully informative red-reflex examination on virtually every baby, they are not consciously aware of the mechanics of the dilation process. They always performed the red-reflex examination. The only difference is that now they get useful information.[2]

5. Drops are not instilled during the first examination of the child by the pediatrician, which usually occurs before discharge from the hospital. Significant anisocoria or papillary pathology would be noted on that exam.

Finally, failure to recognize the signs of retinoblastoma early can often be blamed on poor communication between parents and pediatrician. Several factors contribute to this problem: (1) parents see the leukocoria and pediatricians generally do not (because of the small pupil); (2) pediatricians find it hard to believe that the parents or other lay family members can see signs of disease that they (the trained professionals) cannot; and (3) parents accept reassurance from the pediatrician because they question their own observations of the abnormal white "glow" that is present only some times. When an irritated authority figure suggests that they might be imagining things and that they are overreacting, the parents often question the validity of their own observations and quietly acquiesce to the opinion of the professional.

Clinical Presentation

Any white or yellow lesion in the posterior segment of the eye in a child under 5 years of age should raise the possibility of retinoblastoma. This disease is highly curable in its early stages but can be fatal if the diagnosis is missed or delayed. When the fundus of a young child cannot be seen clearly for whatever reason, a CT scan or ocular ultrasound is essential to rule out the presence of intraocular calcium before surgically entering the eye.

Retinoblastoma rarely, if ever, causes pain and discomfort unless secondary glaucoma is present. Evidence that the child does not see well is nonexistent in unilateral disease where one eye is normal. Even in bilateral disease, it is rare for the macula in both eyes to be destroyed by the tumor, although in advanced disease this can happen.

Clinical signs of retinoblastoma relate to the tumor location, size, and color (Table 9-1). In the majority of cases, the diagnosis of retinoblastoma is straightforward. In a large majority of children with this disease, a parent or family member first notes the presence of a white pupillary reflection or reflex (leukocoria). A posterior pole tumor as small as 3 to 5 mm in diameter has the capacity to create leukocoria.

The term that parents use for the leukocoria observation is rarely the textbook-cited "cat's eye." Usually it is a "g" word, such as "gleam, glow, glare, or glint" (Fig. 9-1). Parents are often unsure of their observation because they see it only intermittently. It is most obvious near the end of the day when the light is low and the pupil dilates naturally. It is common for parents to seek brighter light for a better look. A combination of the child's near pupillary reflex (from the parent's face near the child) and the brighter light almost always defeats that effort, leaving the parent questioning their earlier observation.

In other infants, loss of binocularity and central vision in one eye because of a tumor in the macula is the reason that strabismus may be the first sign of the tumor. In the genetically predisposed individual in whom the tumor appears in the first few months of life, there seems to be a predilection for the posterior pole, most likely because of the number of dividing retinoblasts in the macula at this stage of retinal development. In any case, a macular tumor is likely to be in position to reflect incident light, and create leucocoria (see Fig. 9-1). It is rare for a retinoblastoma to be initially discovered during a dilated fundus exam done for an unrelated reason. However, we have found

TABLE 9-1. Differential Diagnosis of Leukocoria.
1. Retinoblastoma
2. Persistent hyperplastic primary vitreous (PHPV)
3. Cataract
4. Retinopathy of prematurity
5. Toxocariasis
6. Coloboma of choroid
7. Uveitis
8. Coats' disease
9. Vitreous hemorrhage
10. Retinal dysplasia
11. Tumors other than retinoblastoma
12. Retinal detachment
13. Corneal opacity
14. Myelinated nerve fibers

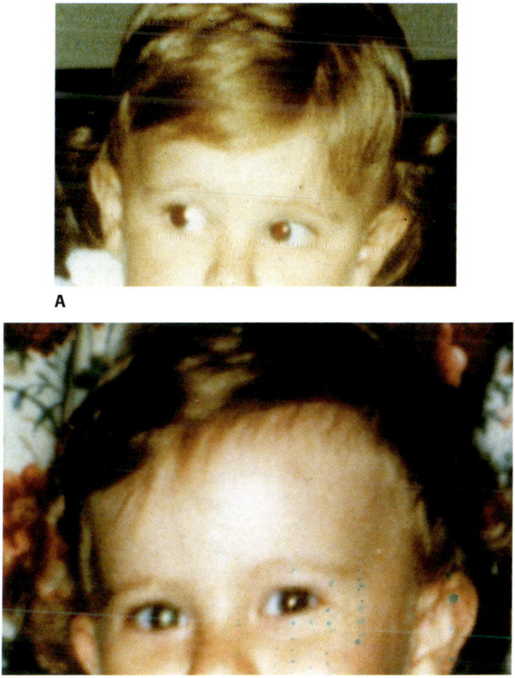

A

B

FIGURE 9-1A,B. Snapshots obtained from family of an 18-month-old child with unilateral retinoblastoma OS. **(A)** At 15 months of age, red reflexes are evident bilaterally. **(B)** At 17 months of age, leukocoria is obvious in the left eye. Old photographs can be helpful in dating the onset of leukocoria or strabismus.

three unsuspected retinoblastomas during routine screening for retinopathy of prematurity in at-risk infants.

Unfortunately, unless there is bilateral retinoblastoma in a parent, appropriate screening for retinoblastoma is rarely a part of well-child care. This unfortunate situation accounts for the average age of diagnosis of 12 months for sporadic new bilateral disease. The suspected diagnosis of retinoblastoma is confirmed when ophthalmoscopy reveals one or more nodular masses that appear creamy white. Tumors larger than 3 mm will have intralesional vascularization (Fig. 9-2). Atypical cases of

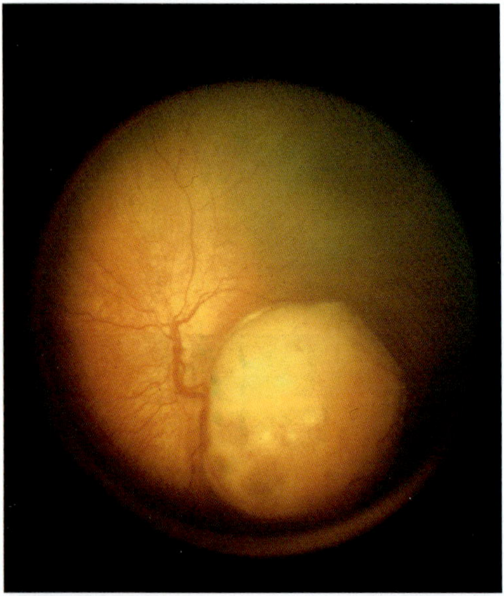

FIGURE 9-2. Fundus photograph of typical endophytic retinoblastoma: right eye of an 18-month-old child who presented with a 2-month history of an "unusual glint or reflex" in the right pupil. There is no tumor in the left eye, and the family history is entirely negative for evidence of retinoblastoma or other childhood cancers. This tumor has the smooth, regular margins that are characteristic of endophytic retinoblastoma. Calcium inclusions can sometimes be seen in these tumors, and they are present in this case. The "lacunae" or clear spaces within the tumor mass are areas of glial differentiation. The creamy, yellow-white, yogurt-like appearance indicates viable retinoblastoma. The initial diagnosis made well into the second year of life, the unifocal, uniocular nature of the tumor, and the absence of a family history are strongly suggestive of sporadic, nonhereditary retinoblastoma. However, these clinical findings do not allow one to be absolutely certain about the genetic status of this child because 15% of genetically predisposed individuals develop retinoblastoma in only one eye.

retinoblastoma are of concern because they can be confused with other disorders. Traumatic hyphema, vitreous hemorrhage, or glaucoma can obscure an underlying retinoblastoma. Such misdiagnoses can lead to an inappropriate surgical intervention. Opening an eye containing an unsuspected retinoblastoma dramatically increases the risk of tumor spread outside the eye.

When the tumor presents as just described, the diagnosis is relatively straightforward. Unfortunately, events in the natural growth cycle of this tumor can create presenting symptoms that mimic other conditions (Figs. 9-3, 9-4, 9-5, 9-6). One of the most commonly misdiagnosed clinical signs of intraocular retinoblastoma is an orbital cellulitis-like picture caused by massive necrosis of the intraocular tumor[21,42,60] with subsequent transscleral diffusion of a chemical inflammatogenic molecule(s). Because the necrosis can frequently be accompanied by bleeding, a vitreous hemorrhage associated with a partial or complete hyphema may also be the presenting sign of a retinoblastoma.[37,53] A fundus examination should be part of any workup of a preseptal or orbital cellulitis.

When the fundus of a child cannot be seen adequately for whatever reason, an imaging study (either ultrasound or CT scan) is essential (Fig. 9-6); this is especially important before undertaking a vitrectomy to evacuate the blood. An eye massively filled with retinoblastoma may lead to angle-closure glau-

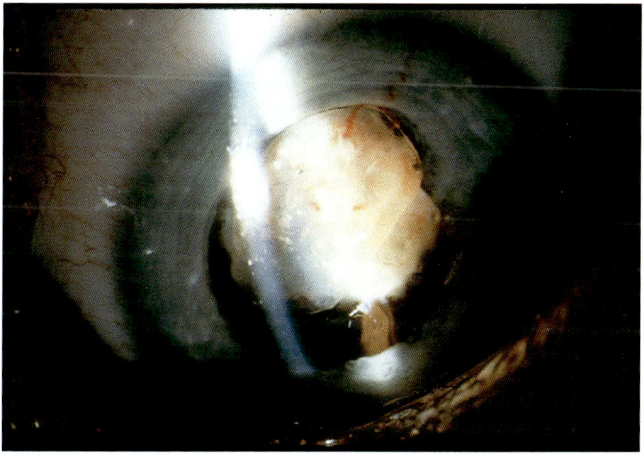

FIGURE 9-3. Eye of a 3-year-old child who presented with an intraocular mass OD. There was concern about the possibility of an intraocular ocular malignancy. The cornea in the right eye was 1 mm smaller than in the left eye. Slit lamp exam showed a vascularized membrane with anterior synechia. Ultrasound showed a stalk going from the back of the lens to the nerve head, and a diagnosis of persistent hyperplastic primary vitreous (PHPV) was made. However, one can appreciate that this could be confused with retinoblastoma.

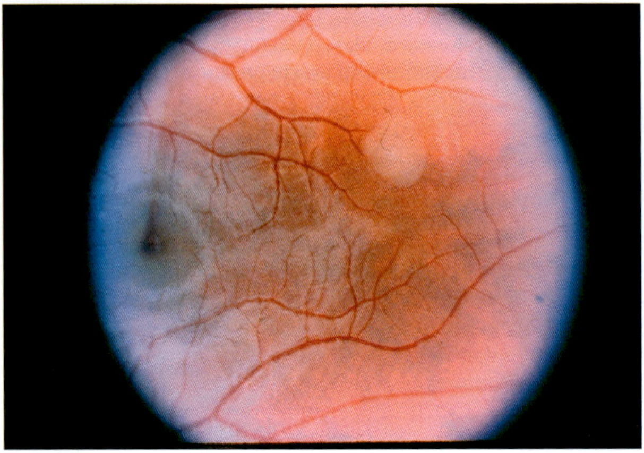

FIGURE 9-4. Fundus photograph of a 5-year-old child with tuberous sclerosis. This whitish elevated lesion, slightly smaller than one disc in diameter, looks very much like retinoblastoma. This is the early form of the astrocytic hamartoma associated with tuberous sclerosis. Eventually such lesions take on the typical mulberry appearance characteristic of tuberous sclerosis. At this point, however, it could be confused with an active or regressed retinoblastoma.

coma by pushing the lens–iris diaphragm forward and occluding the anterior chamber angle. A surgical procedure for glaucoma should not be undertaken in a child without either a clear view of the posterior pole or an imaging study that rules out the presence of an intraocular mass. In most cases, the presence of a retinoblastoma in an eye does not cause pain. If, however, there is associated hemorrhage or angle-closure glaucoma, then pain may be a presenting symptom.

Epidemiology

Retinoblastoma is a rare disease but is disproportionately important because its misdiagnosis is one of the few errors in the practice of ophthalmology that can lead to the death of a child. The prevalence of retinoblastoma in the developed world seems to be about 11 cases per 1 million children under 5 years of age. A less useful but more commonly used measure is the incidence rate. The incidence is expressed as a ratio of the number of cases

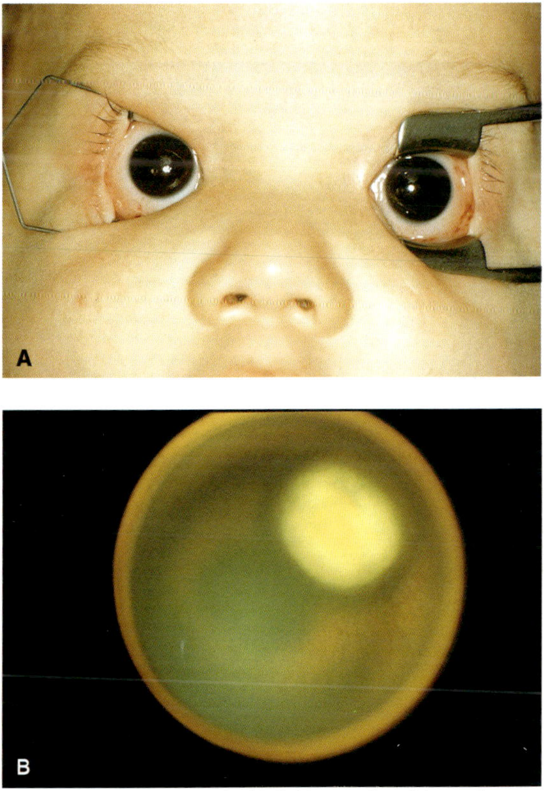

FIGURE 9-5A,B. This 4-month-old child was referred for evaluation of a mass in the right eye, which was noted to be smaller than the left at birth. A right esotropia developed at 2 months of age. **(A)** Clinical appearance of the child at 4 months of age with the smaller right eye. **(B)** Fundus examination revealed a white mass centered over the optic nerve with a pigmented ring around the base. About 40 fine radial vessels entered the mass around the perimeter. The left eye was normal. Initially the mass did not demonstrate calcification, and the clinical impression was that the mass represented some type of developmental anomaly. Retinoblastoma was not considered a strong possibility because that tumor does not arise from the optic nerve. Repeat examination 5 weeks later showed that the mass had doubled in size. Repeat CT scan confirmed the increased size but still showed no evidence of calcification. The right eye was subsequently enucleated for diagnostic reasons. Histopathology revealed a total retinal detachment with retinal dysplasia. The mass appeared to be a choristomatous malformation of the optic nerve consisting of an abnormal localization of meningothelial cells around the central retinal vessels.

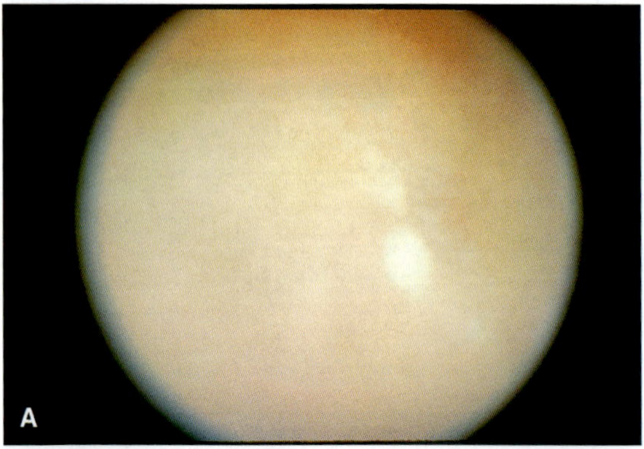

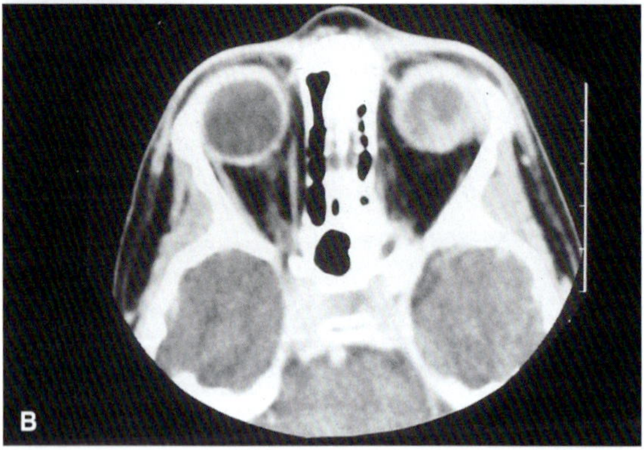

FIGURE 9-6A,B. A 7-year-old boy presented with pain and redness of the left eye of 1 week duration. **(A)** Physical examination revealed hand motions vision, a mild anterior chamber reaction, and an intense vitreous reaction. The other eye was normal. Because of the child's age and the presence of anterior and posterior chamber inflammation, toxocara and toxoplasmosis were high on the list of differential diagnoses. **(B)** Ultrasound and CT demonstrated a posterior pole mass but no evidence of calcification. Because of the presence of the mass (even without calcification), a diagnosis of retinoblastoma was under consideration.

newly diagnosed in any given year to the number of live births recorded in that year. Obviously not all new cases of retinoblastoma are diagnosed in the first year of life, but the ratio is a useful one. The incidence rate most commonly cited is 1 case of retinoblastoma per 15,000 to 18,000 live births.[11,33,45,62]

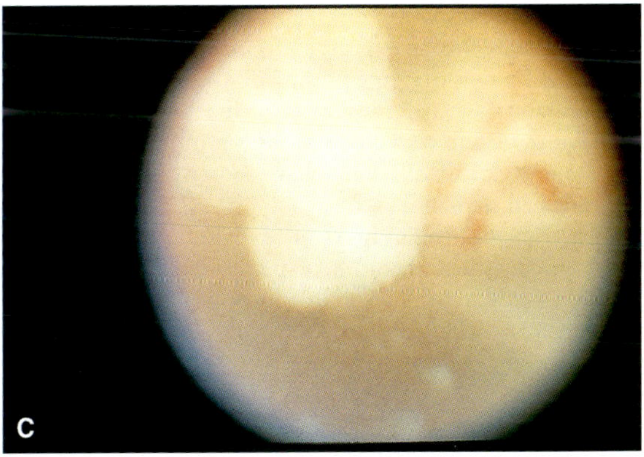

FIGURE 9-6C. (C) The child was treated with a short 3-day course of oral corticosteroids, and the vitreous cleared, revealing a classic retinoblastoma. A repeat CT scan showed calcification for the first time. All the presenting findings in this child were "out of character" for retinoblastoma. A correct diagnosis would not have been made without a high index of suspicion.

The estimate, from several decades ago, of 1 in 15,000 to 1 in 18,000 either is an underestimate or the perceived total number of new cases today is an overestimate. An overestimate could result when the family of a child with retinoblastoma seeks treatment advice in several ocular oncology centers and is counted several times. According to the 2000 census figures, there were 4,340,000 live births in the United States and Canada during that year. If the number of new cases of retinoblastoma generally agreed upon (300 in the United States and 50 in Canada) are, in fact, diagnosed annually, then the incidence figure for retinoblastoma in North America is 1 in 12,400 live births. The incidence rate more commonly cited of 1 in 15,000 require that only 289 cases of retinoblastoma be newly diagnosed in the United States and Canada. There is a great need for a national registry to answer questions such as this. The newly organized *Children's Oncology Group* (COG), formed from a merger of the Children's Cancer Group (CCG) and the Pediatric Oncology Group (POG), is interested in establishing a national retinoblastoma registry.

Worldwide there is evidence that unilateral retinoblastoma may be much more common in some underdeveloped countries, particularly in Mexico and Central America, in the countries of central Africa, and on the Indian subcontinent. There is evidence in one study reported from Mexico that a high incidence of endemic human papilloma viral (HPV) infection may be associated with the larger than expected number of cases of retinoblastoma.[43a] It is known that one of the HPV proteins can bind with and inactivate the Rb-1 protein pRb. Inactivating the protein could have the same effect as a mutation in the gene manufacturing the protein: insufficient active protein is available to the cell to halt cell division.

In Los Angeles, the number of Rb patients with Latino surnames is higher than would be expected based on population. We will be studying this issue in collaboration with the author of the report on the HPV as a possible causal factor for the increased number of unilateral cases of retinoblastoma.

Etiology

The protein product of the gene (Rb-1) associated with retinoblastoma is known to be an indispensable component of the normal cell machinery for regulation of its own growth. The normal role of this growth suppressor gene product can be thought of as a stoplight to the traffic of cell growth. For the cell to divide, it must change the light to green (which it accomplishes by attaching a phosphate group and temporarily inactivating the suppressor protein). After completion of one cell division, the traffic light again turns to red (the phosphate group is removed, reactivating the growth suppressor protein). We now know that loss or inactivation of the product of the retinoblastoma gene, RB-1, is required for transformation of a retinoblast into a malignant cell.[39] This protein may be missing or defective as a result of either an inactivating mutation or deletion of both maternal and paternal alleles of the Rb gene in chromosomal region 13q14. Knudson predicted that two mutational events were required for the appearance of retinoblastoma, but there was no evidence at that time that the mutational events were allelic (present in both the maternal and paternal copies of the gene).[32] It was not until Cavenee and colleagues demonstrated the presence of recessive cancer genes through reduction to homozygosity that the allelic nature of the retinoblastoma mutations was clearly delineated.[9]

The nongenetic form of retinoblastoma (unifocal, unilateral disease) can result when two independent, inactivating mutations happen by chance to occur together in a single retinal cell. Another possible etiology, as already discussed, is the presence of a viral protein that inactives the Rb-1 gene product. In both scenerios, the germline is uninvolved and thus genetic transmission of a predisposition to Rb is impossible. Approximately 60% of all retinoblastoma cases are of the unilateral, nonhereditary type. A basic hypothesis of Knudson's classic publication was that two independent mutational events would take a longer time to occur than a single one, which would explain the observation that children with unilateral, nonheritable retinoblastomas are older on the average than those with an inherited predisposition.[30,31,32]

In the other 40% of patients, an inactivating mutation or deletion in one of the two alleles of the RB-1 gene (we refer to this event as the "predisposing mutation") is either inherited from one parent who is known to be affected (10%), or occurs spontaneously in the sperm or egg (90% of spontaneous new mutations are paternal in origin) at or near the time of conception. This event accounts for the common clinical finding of a negative family history of retinoblastoma following the birth of a child with bilateral retinoblastoma. Regardless of whether the predisposing mutation was inherited from a parent or occurred de novo in a sperm or egg, all the cells of the developing child carry the predisposing mutation and have only one normal copy of the Rb gene.

The presence of a single predisposing, inactivating mutation is not, however, sufficient to cause the tumor. A second inactivating mutation is required for tumor formation and occurs in one or more individual retinal cells in each eye, usually as a result of an error at mitosis. Because the frequency of such an event is approximately 1 per million developing retinal cells, and there are several million cells at risk in each eye, several discrete, independently arising retinoblastomas would be expected to occur in each eye of genetically predisposed "gene carriers," and this is exactly what is observed.

As the second (tumorigenic) mutation occurs by chance alone, the number of tumors in each eye assumes a normal distribution, and about 15% of patients who "carry the gene" develop tumors in only one eye. Such individuals are at risk for transmitting the disease to their children even though they have only unilateral disease. If the tumorigenic mutation does not occur in either eye, the individual is a nonexpressing "gene carrier."

In approximately 3% of retinoblastoma cases, a karyotypically visible deletion of chromosomal region 13q14 is present. The clinical appearance or phenotype of these patients relates to the extent of the deletion (Fig. 9-7).

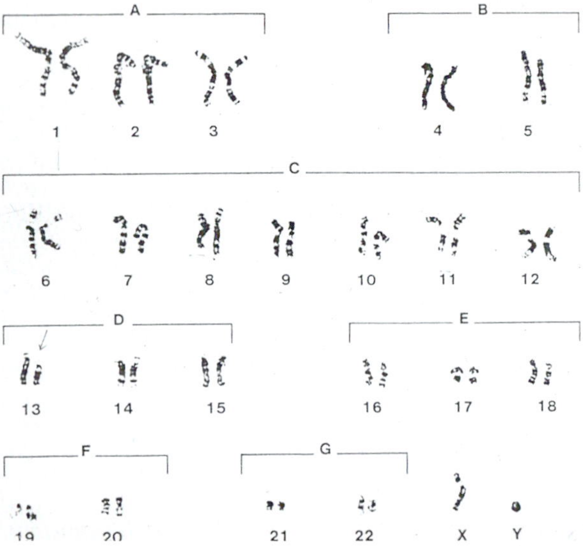

A

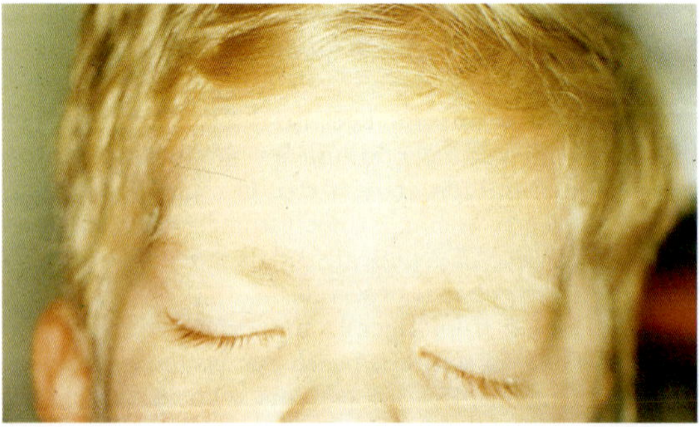

B

FIGURE 9-7A,B. This 2-year-old child was diagnosed with bilateral retinoblastoma at 4 months of age. **(A)** Chromosomal analysis demonstrated a significant deletion of one of the two chromosome 13s, including region 13q14, the site of the retinoblastoma gene. **(B)** The facial photograph shows the features of the 13 q-syndrome: low-set ears and facial dysmorphism. The child was developmentally delayed. At 25 months of age, a preauricular mass was noted on the left side of the child's face. Excisional biopsy confirmed a primitive neuroectodermal tumor. This second malignant neoplasm occurred within the field of the previous external beam radiotherapy.

Staging of Retinoblastoma

The terminology in this area is treacherous. "Staging" is generally used in oncology to define how extensively a tumor has become disseminated throughout the body. Because spread of retinoblastoma outside the eye is rare in the developed world, the use of the word staging should be reserved for the child with known metastatic disease. In ocular oncology, because we are almost always contending with tumor confined to the eye when retinoblastoma is first diagnosed, the term grouping is more appropriate.

The currently available Reese–Ellsworth grouping of retinoblastoma is outdated and needs revision. The Reese–Ellsworth (R-E) classification was originally developed in the late 1960s and early 1970s as a guide to predicting visual prognosis in eyes treated primarily with external beam radiotherapy.[47] Both tumor size and location were assigned major roles in the R-E grouping. More than 10 years ago, most ocular oncology centers treating this disease began using chemotherapy as primary therapy.

With primary chemotherapy, tumor size and location is less important than the presence of intraocular dissemination of the tumor in predicting ultimate outcome. The beta version of a new classification for intraocular retinoblastoma is currently being evaluated in a number of major centers internationally. Publication is expected soon.

Clinical Presentation

Natural History

The natural history of retinoblastoma is to fill the eye, then continue local expansion into the periocular tissues (Fig. 9-8), and finally the brain. Bloodborne metastases may occur before, during, or after local extension and spread the tumor to distant sites, primarily bone and bone marrow. The disease is uniformly fatal if left untreated. Occasionally, an apparent retinoblastoma (retinoma) may display evidence of involution and appear as a treated scar (Fig. 9-9).

Early retinoblastoma lesions are barely perceptible, round elevations in the retina, and are sometimes found only by detecting the circular retinal reflex formed by their shape. Multiple lesions appear at various times in genetically predisposed

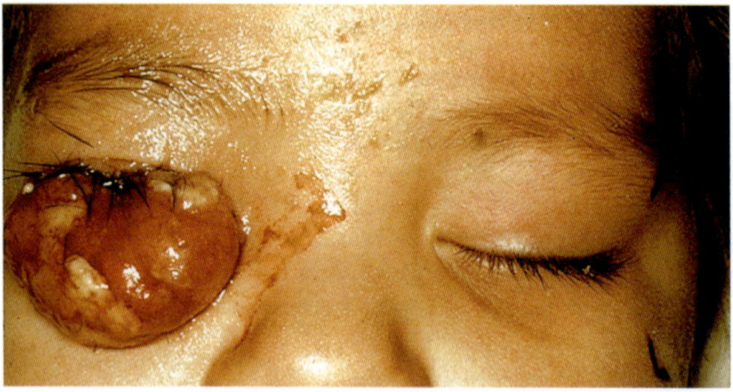

A

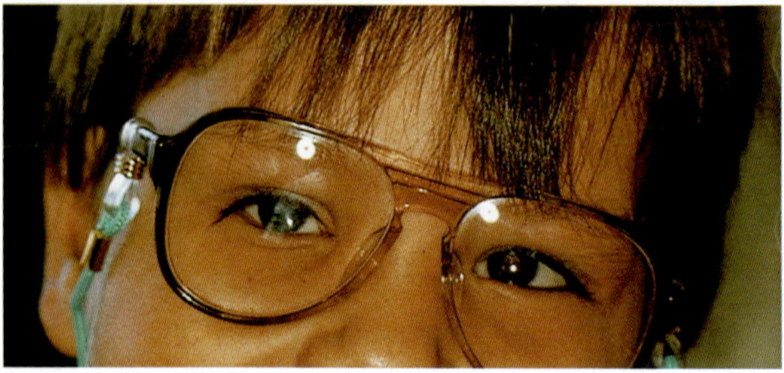

B

FIGURE 9-8A,B. Extraocular retinoblastoma in the United States is rare. However, in Third World countries it may be the most common presenting sign of the disease. **(A)** 3.5-year-old child from Mexico presented with extraocular disease in the right eye and intraocular disease in the left. On CT scan, there was no evidence of intracranial disease. He was treated with chemotherapy for the extraocular disease, which responded dramatically. External beam radiotherapy was given for the intraocular disease in the left eye with approximately 60% of the dose delivered across the midline to the right orbit. Subsequently, the right eye became shrunken and phthisical. The eye was then removed. Fortunately, the disease had extended only anteriorly and had not invaded the optic nerve or the retrobulbar space. **(B)** Patient is wearing his ocular prosthesis and safety glasses. Five years later he was free of retinoblastoma recurrence but had developed an osteosarcoma of the left arm.

patients (Fig. 9-10). The earliest lesions do not appear to have tumor vascularization. These very small lesions may be virtually transparent, but as they enlarge they become more opaque. Once a retinoblastoma has reached one disc diameter in size, it usually has the characteristic appearance of frozen yogurt. Untreated tumors are fairly uniform. This opacity distinguishes them from treated and inactive tumors that are "gauzy" or partially transparent (type II regression).

As tumors enlarge, clonal overgrowth frequently leads to an asymmetrical spread away from the original tumor base; this can be particularly evident in tumors of the posterior pole, which frequently "overhang" the disk or macula. During the course of treatment, it is often a pleasant surprise to see the macula or disc appear from beneath the retreating tumor mass.

As tumors grow and their demand for a blood supply increases, the nearest retinal vessels are recruited as tumor "feeder" vessels. As the flow increases, the size and tortuosity of these vessels increase. During tumor therapy, a decrease in the size and tortuosity of these vessels is a positive sign that the treatment is at least partially successful.

With endophytic growth (growth into the vitreous as a single mass), two things eventually happen. As the base expands and as more incompetent tumor vessels form, fluid accumulates beneath the retina and a serous retinal detachment appears around the base of the tumor. As the fluid increases, it tends to move dependently. With large tumors, it is not uncommon to see a total serous retinal detachment.[59] In the presence of a tumor-associated detachment, it is common for the tumor to "seed" the subretinal space. Where these small clumps of malignant cells attach to the retinal pigment epithelium (RPE) or the underside of the detached retina, new tumors may appear in the distribution of the retinal detachment even if the fluid resolves with treatment. Visibly detectable tumor nodules on the underside of the detached retina at the time of diagnosis make the salvage of the eye unlikely.

With continued expansion of an *endophytic tumor*, the pseudocapsule surrounding the tumor eventually breaks down, allowing the loosely adherent tumor cells access to the vitreous cavity. Initially, their growth is stunted by lack of oxygen and nutrients in this new environment. Eventually, however, they coalesce into spheres consisting of an inner core of necrotic tumor cells and an outer shell composed of only two viable cell layers. The thickness of the vitreous "seeds" is determined by

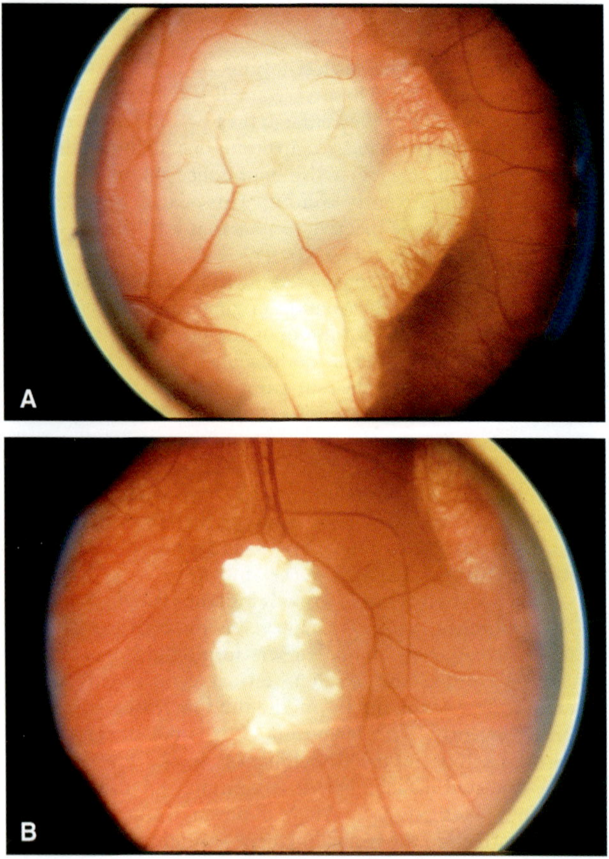

FIGURE 9-9A–D. A 7-year-old child was evaluated in an emergency room following minor head trauma. The ER physician noted poor acuity in the left eye and also noted an afferent pupillary defect on the left. Subsequent ophthalmologic evaluation revealed multifocal inactive retinoblastoma in the left fundus. The child had no previous diagnosis or treatment of retinoblastoma lesions. **(A)** Appearance of the larger lesion at age 7 years. This lesion shows a type II regression pattern (gray, semitransparent). Adjacent to it is a rather large section of RPE depigmentation. **(B)** Image of a second lesion demonstrating a type I regression pattern in which the residual mass is composed entirely of calcium, giving the tumor a cottage cheese-like appearance. **(C,D)** Photographs of the same two lesions 3 years later show an absence of growth and the maturing of the regression patterns. The typical pattern of regression and the associated depigmentation of the RPE supports the diagnosis of retinoma or retinocytoma. (Courtesy of Dr. I. Hsu, Portland, OR.)

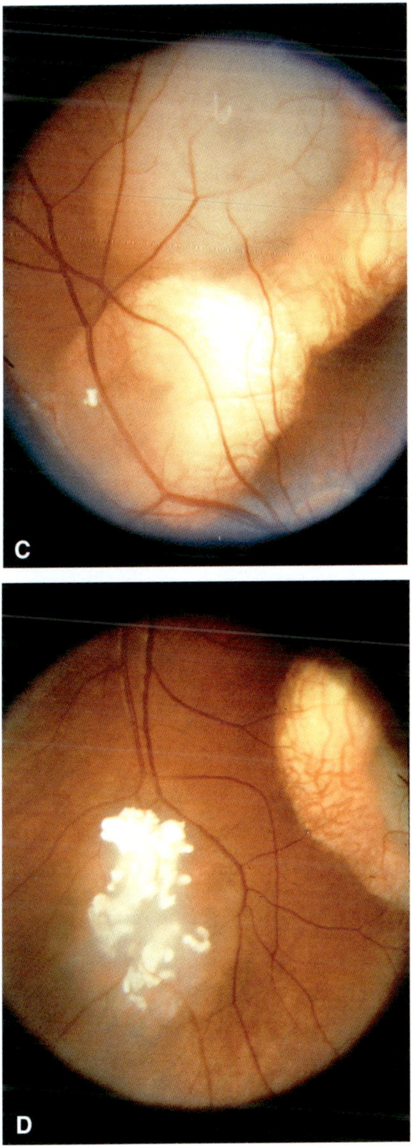

FIGURE 9-9A–D. (continued)

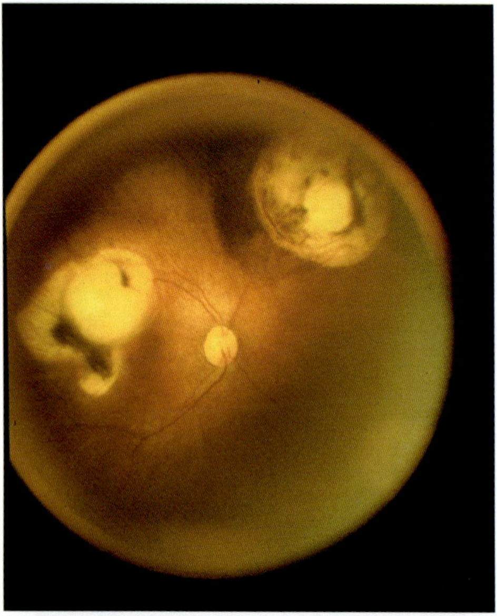

FIGURE 9-10. Fundus photograph of a child with multifocal, bilateral retinoblastoma. With the exception of one reported case, tumor has not been documented to spread from one eye to the other; these tumors have all arisen independently of each other. The findings in this child would be statistically impossible unless he is genetically predisposed to develop the tumor. Without genetic predisposition, each of these tumors could only have arisen as a result of two chance DNA events in the same retinal cell. Each of those events occurs spontaneously with a frequency approaching once per 1 million retinoblasts. The frequency of even one tumor arising in the absence of genetic predisposition is the product of the individual frequencies or once per 1,000,000,000,000 retinoblasts. In contrast, if this child is genetically predisposed, he carries one of the two DNA events necessary for tumor formation in every cell. Only one additional "once per million" event must occur for a tumor to arise. Because children have approximately 3 million retinoblasts at birth, a second tumorigenic event would be expected to occur in an average of three retinal cells in each eye. Three tumors is about the average number seen in each eye in patients with genetically predisposed retinoblastoma.

the oxygen diffusion gradient in the vitreous. The use of the term seeds to describe these structures is most appropriate because these are relatively dormant carriers ready to "seed" tumor wherever they can reattach and recruit a blood supply (Fig. 9-11). An eye with diffuse extensive vitreous seeding is almost impossible to treat successfully.

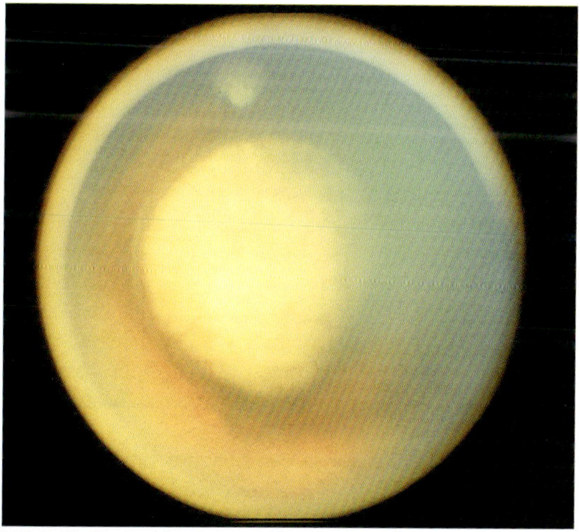

FIGURE 9-11. Retinoblastoma can break through its smooth surface and spread tumor cells into the vitreous. Not infrequently, the early stages of vitreous "seeding" is a localized event, occurring just over the surface of an individual tumor. In this figure, the localized vitreous seeding is arising from a "nipple" or candy kiss-like structure on the surface of a previously smooth tumor mass. This geographic feature is likely the result of the rapid overgrowth of a clone of daughter cells, all arising from one tumor cell, which happened to undergo a mutation that further releases restraints on growth rate. These spontaneous mutations within tumors that confer growth advantages are frequently the result of chromosome rearrangement during tumor cell mitosis and are collectively known as "progression of malignancy." As clones of these cells overgrow their cousins, the nature of the entire malignancy rapidly changes character toward a more aggressive and life-threatening tumor.

Diffuse infiltrating retinoblastoma is a rare subtype of the disease that may be diagnosed in older children (average age, 6.1 years). There is no definite mass and the condition is frequently misdiagnosed as a posterior uveitis. Pseudohypopyon is common.[5]

WORKUP

The only essential laboratory study in the systemic workup of a newly diagnosed retinoblastoma is an imaging study to demonstrate the presence of calcium in the eye, either a CT scan with contrast or echography or both. Magnet resonance imaging (MRI) is helpful if the retinoblastoma is suspected to be present outside the eye, either in the optic nerve or in the orbit. It is unnecessary to order bone scans, extensive blood studies (including liver function studies), a lumbar puncture, or a bone marrow aspiration and biopsy in the typical case of intraocular retinoblastoma in which the classic fundus picture is present and calcification is clearly demonstrable with an imaging study (Fig. 9-12).

Because retinoblastoma most commonly metastasizes to bone and bone marrow, any unusual bone lesion should be suspected to be caused by metastatic retinoblastoma or, if the patient is genetically predisposed, by a second malignant neoplasm (most commonly osteogenic sarcoma) (Fig. 9-13).[59] One of our patients with bilateral retinoblastoma was treated in another hospital for several months for a nonhealing bone abscess in the mandible. Eventually, this lesion was shown to be an osteogenic sarcoma.

An inflammatory reponse can obscure the classic features of retinoblastoma. Figure 9-6 shows findings in a 7-year-old patient whose clinical diagnosis of toxocara granuloma was made at grand rounds in a major teaching center. An intraocular mass was present without clear evidence of calcium on CT scan. After 3 days of high-dose systemic steroids, the vitreous cleared dramatically and revealed a typical endophytic retinoblastoma. Repeat echography showed clear evidence of calcification in the mass, and a correct diagnosis of retinoblastoma was made.

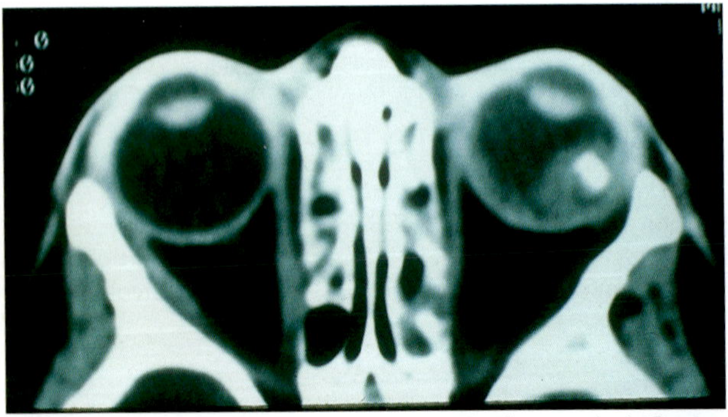

FIGURE 9-12. Precontrast CT demonstrates a bright spot of calcification within the tumor mass in the left eye. Pre- and postcontrast scans both show calcification, but contrast may be very useful in demonstrating extraocular involvement. MRI scans do not define calcification but may prove to be useful in demonstrating optic nerve involvement.

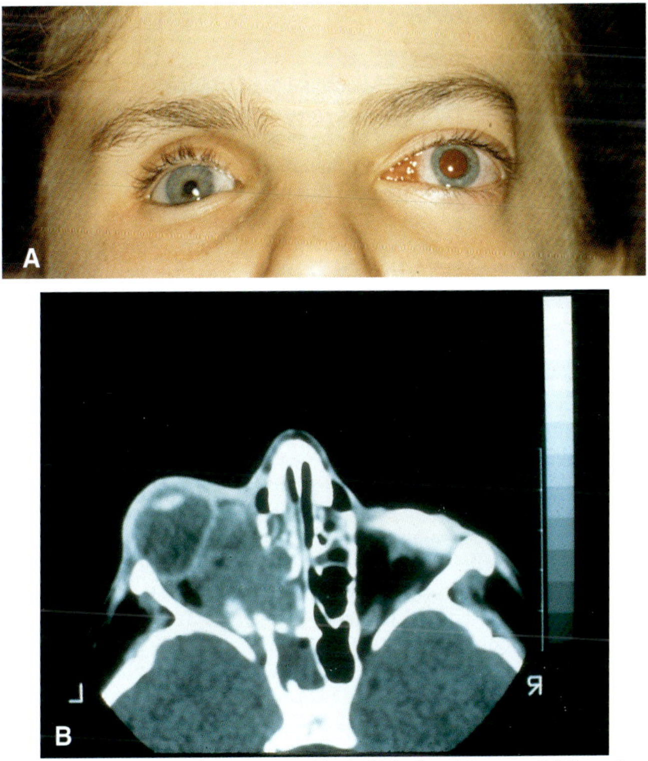

FIGURE 9-13A,B. This 12-year-old child had a history of bilateral retinoblastoma diagnosed at age 2 years. The right eye was removed at the time of diagnosis, and the left eye was treated with external beam radiotherapy and cryotherapy. There was no history of ocular tumor recurrence. At age 11, the child began complaining of a "fullness" behind her left eye. An ophthalmologist examined her three times during the subsequent 8 months and noted no active retinoblastoma. She then developed orbital aching, headaches, nausea, vomiting, and a 15-pound weight loss. Multiple pediatricians evaluated her and thought she was suffering from a "chronic viral syndrome." She then developed proptosis and the inability to move her left eye. (**A**) Patient's clinical appearance at this time. The left eye was proptotic and there was conjunctival congestion and chemosis. In this photograph she is attempting to look up but cannot. The right orbit contains a prosthesis. (**B**) CT appearance at the same time. A large mass is present in the ethmoid sinus and left orbit inside the radiated field. Biopsy confirmed the clinical diagnosis of osteosarcoma. This child had symptoms for 8 months before diagnosis. The delay was primarily caused by the failure of her physicians to consider the possibility of a second malignant neoplasm and to order an imaging study of the left orbit. Similar cases have prompted the development of a medi-alert card.

Genetic Counseling

Genetic counseling is becoming a more integrated part of the management of retinoblastoma. Genetic counseling requires a team approach. The need for fresh tumor tissue for adequate genetic counseling is one of the best arguments for the treatment of all retinoblastoma, including the primary enucleation of unilateral sporadic retinoblastoma, at a major ocular oncology center. Experienced genetic counselors will have all the necessary information about which blood and tumor specimens are needed and to which labs they should be sent. Turnaround time is improving in most of the laboratories; results may now be available in 8 to 12 weeks. Costs associated with these DNA tests have not decreased, but more insurance companies are now paying these charges.

The genetics of retinoblastoma is well understood, and our tools for affordable, reliable, gene-based genetic counseling are improving. The "retinoblastoma" gene was cloned almost simultaneously in Boston[14] and Los Angeles.[15] Most people have two normal copies of the Rb gene in each cell. Individuals genetically predisposed to retinoblastoma have only one normal copy. The second copy is defective and does not produce an active protein. If the single good copy is mutated or otherwise becomes defective, then the cell is completely released from the growth restraint imposed by this system. The loss of both copies of the growth-suppressing gene is required for retinoblastoma to develop. The loss of both copies of this gene also occurs in some cases of other malignancies, including breast, lung, and prostate.[63] In these tumors, the two Rb mutations are not involved in tumor initiation but are part of the cascade of events known as progression of malignancy. Gene products that target and bind the Rb gene protein, such as the SV40 large T antigen, the E6 antigen of human papilloma virus, and the E1A antigen of adenovirus, can also cause malignant transformation of cells.[16] Homologues of these genes (human oncogenes) are present in normal cells. Because the Rb gene product binds to oncogene products, the Rb gene seems to function as an anti-oncogene.

Histopathological Risk Factors for Metastatic Disease

Unlike choroidal melanoma, the most differentiated retinoblastomas appear to have the same metastatic potential as the least differentiated ones. However, histological examination of the enucleated specimen is important for another reason. If there is tumor in the optic nerve past the lamina cribrosa, or massive invasion of the choroid, or both, then prophylactic chemotherapy is recommended. However, if the nerve is free of tumor past the lamina cribrosa, and if there is no evidence of spread through the choroid into the sclera, then additional treatment is not necessary. Efforts should be made to obtain as long a piece of optic nerve as possible. Clinical follow-up is especially important in patients with a genetic predisposition.

Treatment of Intraocular Retinoblastoma

The treatment of intraocular retinoblastoma has evolved significantly in the last decade and since the first edition of this textbook. The primary use of traditional teletherapy (external beam radiotherapy) in the treatment of intraocular tumor is rare. Enucleation of eyes with advanced intraocular retinoblastoma in unilaterally affected patients is appropriate and common. Retinoblastoma in patients with bilateral disease or only moderately advanced unilateral disease diagnosed today are treated with a protocol of systemic chemotherapy (generally carboplatin, etoposide, and vincristine) given intravenously every 3 to 4 weeks followed by consolidation (the use of a different dose of the same drug, a different drug, or different treatment modality) with the focal surgical techniques of direct tumor photocoagulation or cryotherapy or both.[40]

One of the authors (ALM) first suggested the use of the term chemoreduction for what we were beginning to do in the treatment of retinoblastoma in the Franschescetti Lecture at the International Symposium on Retinoblastoma in Switzerland in 1992. At the time, he thought it might be a convenient shorthand way to describe the use of primary systemic chemotherapy to reduce the volume of the tumor followed by local surgical modalities (laser or cryo) to consolidate the initial massive, but incomplete, tumor cell kill by the chemotherapy.

We no longer use that term, because it implies that in treating retinoblastoma we are using an approach unique to this tumor. That is not the case. In fact, every effective treatment regimen for solid tumors that includes primary systemic chemotherapy requires consolidation to accomplish complete tumor destruction. Systemic chemotherapy alone, in virtually no solid tumor, will sterilize the tumor. A better terminology would be "primary systemic chemotherapy followed by local consolidation."

During the slightly more than one decade that primary systemic chemotherapy has been employed as the preferred treatment for intraocular retinoblastoma, there is an increasing body of evidence that supports care of these patients is best delivered in ocular oncology centers. There is no such animal as a "simple enucleation for retinoblastoma." Harvesting of fresh tumor is an essential part of the management of unilateral retinoblastoma under 2 years of age. Genetic counseling can only be done adequately if tumor DNA and peripheral white cell DNA are available for comparison. Once the eye with retinoblastoma is in formalin, the ability to carry out adequate genetic counseling has probably been lost.

Ideally, ophthalmologists with oncology training should be treating retinoblastoma. Because it is a rare tumor, even most pediatric oncologists do not have much experience treating this tumor. They know the drugs—carboplatin, etoposide, and vincristine—but require close collaboration with an experienced ocular oncologist for treatment planning.

Because the pediatric ophthalmologist may be aware that chemotherapy is being used in the treatment of this tumor, lack of experience by both ophthalmologist and oncologist can lead to grossly inappropriate therapy. For example, there is rarely, if ever, an indication to treat advanced unilateral retinoblastoma with systemic chemotherapy for the intraocular disease. Parents with a child newly diagnosed with retinoblastoma will have searched the Internet. They are aware of the chemotherapy option and often push for attempts to salvage the eye through the use of systemic chemotherapy. This approach is, in most cases, not advised.

Another not uncommon mistake made by pediatric ophthalmologists during surveillance exam under anesthesia (EUAs) on the fellow normal eye following enucleation of unilateral retinoblastoma is to treat a small peripheral white dot in the retina because of the possibility that it could be retinoblastoma. Small white dots are relatively common as part of the "bay complex." If they are treated before there is clear definite evidence of growth, the child will forever be labeled as having bilateral retinoblastoma. The consequences of that label are so devastating and far-reaching that an experienced ocular oncologist would make absolutely certain that the child did have an expanding mass before instituting treatment. The confidence to know that a 3-week delay in treating a lesion of this size would not have an adverse effect on the ability to control the tumor is essential to avoid the impulse to treat immediately.

The Children's Oncology Group (COG) has formed a Retinoblastoma Steering Committee to generate clinical trials in retinoblastoma. Questions under development at this time concern whether etoposide can be eliminated in the systemic regimen for the treatment of intraocular retinoblastoma that has not developed vitreous or subretinal seeding. At least four known cases of leukemia were induced by this drug when large doses were used to treat unilateral retinoblastoma. The value of local, sub-Tenon carboplatin as an adjunct to systemic chemotherapy in eyes with vitreous and/or subretinal seeding will also be evaluated. Finally, the role that intensity-modulated radiotherapy (IMRT), a technique that allows the radiotherapist to spread the entry dose over multiple sites, giving tighter isodose curves, will also be evaluated for efficacy as consolidation treatment in a protocol for bilateral advanced disease.

Once the COG protocols are in place pediatric ophthalmologists with an interest in retinoblastoma will be able to make application to COG as treating ophthalmologists on COG-approved protocols at their institutions. An ongoing part of such protocols will be Internet review of RetCam images for appropriateness of protocol entry and local treatment.

Consideration of a cyclosporine trial by the American College of Surgeons Oncology Group has been discontinued. A decision has been made by that group that any chemotherapy-based therapy would more appropriately be managed through the COG Intergroup mechanism. The data that high doses of cyclosporine significantly add to the efficacy of systemic chemotherapy by the proposed mechanism of blocking multiple drug resistance (p-glycoprotein) are awaiting confirmation.

UVEAL MELANOMA

Uveal melanoma is rare, but can occur, in children. The youngest reported case is an Australian infant who underwent enucleation at 5 days of age for a choroidal melanoma.[18] Only 1% of choroidal melanoma patients are less than 20 years of age and the majority of these patients are in their late teens.[3,4,34,66] An 11-year experience at the Wills Eye Institute was reported in 1975.[34] Among 378 patients with uveal melanoma, only 5 were less than 20 years of age. More recently, the Wills experience has been rereported. Of 3706 consecutive patients with intraocular melanoma, only 40 were patients less than 20 years of age.[57] Barr et al. reviewed uveal melanomas at the AFIP registry.[4] Of 6358 patients with the disease, 101 were less than 20 years of age. Choroidal melanoma in a child has been reported in association with dysplastic nevus syndrome.[26] In a few older teenagers and one 5-year-old child, choroidal mela-noma has been associated with ocular melanocytosis.[49,65] Although diffuse uveal melanomas comprise 4.5% to 5.0% of melanomas reported in adults, only one diffuse tumor has been reported in patients under 20 years of age, and this was in a 5-year-old child.[50]

The prevalence of uveal melanoma among male and female children appears to be equal in most series. Caucasian patients predominate, but there are at least four cases reported with choroidal and/or ciliary body melanomas in young black patients.[23] In the AFIP series of uveal melanoma, 78 of the 101 cases found in patients less than 20 years of age met the criteria of adequate historical information and at least 5 years follow-up.[4] Of these, 42 cases were of choroidal or ciliary body origin. Of the remaining tumors, 27 involved the iris and 9 additional iris lesions were reclassified as nevi. The relative incidence of iris melanomas in this series of young patients is higher than that generally reported for adults. In the recent Wills series of young patients, 12% of intraocular melanomas occurred exclusively in the iris.[57]

Presenting signs and symptoms of choroidal melanoma in children and adolescents are variable. Five of 42 patients in Barr's series came to ophthalmologic attention because of antecedent trauma.[4] Retinal reattachment or glaucoma surgery was performed in 6 of 42 patients before the correct diagnosis was made. A review of case reports of 6 children under age 6 years revealed that 3 presented with red eyes,[12,26,46] 1 with strabismus,[55] 1 with blurred vision,[23] and 1 with ocular enlargement.[18] Frequently, young patients have retinal detachment at the time of diagnosis.

The differential diagnosis of pigmented intraocular tumors in children includes choroidal nevus, melanocytoma, pigmented neurofibroma, juvenile xanthogranuloma (JXG), and RPE hamartoma. A diffuse choroidal melanocytoma mimicking a diffuse choroidal melanoma has been reported,[20] but both lesions are extremely rare in young patients. Patients with melanocytomas are usually over age 30. Moreover, these tumors usually arise adjacent to the optic disc. Intraocular neurofibromas may involve the iris and ciliary body and may be pigmented. Occasionally, a diktyoma is pigmented, but this is rarely confused with melanoma.

The diagnosis of uveal melanoma is made in the same manner as in adults. However, in children, retinal detachment and an inadequate view of the tumor may be more common.[4] Ultrasound is essential. Choroidal melanoma is rarely calcified on CT scan although eyes with long-standing disorganization may develop calcification. An index of suspicion regarding intraocular masses should be maintained as these tumors do occur in young people.

Malignant melanomas in children were once thought to have a more benign course than their adult counterparts. However, the review of Barr et al. demonstrated that the mortality at 5 years is similar to the adult population.[4] Of the 42 patients with choroidal or ciliary body tumors, 13 died of metastatic disease. Features that correlated with a poor outcome were a red painful eye at presentation, extraocular extension, basal tumor diameter greater than 10 mm, increased mitotic activity, and tumor necrosis. Their follow-up ranged from a minimum of 5 to a maximum of 47 years. In the recent Wills series, 23 cases of choroidal tumors had a basal diameter greater than 10 mm, and 1 patient had extraocular extension. Of the 27 patients with malignant iris tumors, 4 succumbed to metastatic disease. Fatal outcome in this group correlated with glaucoma, tumor invasion of the ciliary body and angle and scleral invasion, diffuse growth, and increased mitotic activity.

Uveal melanoma in children and adolescents, albeit rare, may be similar in behavior to the disease in adults.[3,4,34] However, children rarely complain of visual loss and, as a result, choroidal tumors may present at a more advanced stage. Treatment plans frequently include enucleation if the disease is advanced and the eye is blind. Modern diagnostic methods may permit earlier diagnosis and intervention with fewer diagnostic errors. Patient care in referral centers may also significantly improve survival rates. The COMS study, a 15-year multicenter trial comparing enucleation with Iodine 125 brachytherapy for medium choroidal melanomas in adults, found no difference in survival (approximately 80%) between the two groups.[9a] Pre-radiation of large melanomas before enucleation did not enhance survival.[9b] After plaque brachytherapy, 68% have poor acuity in one ten-year followup study.[59a]

MEDULLOEPITHELIOMA (DIKTYOMA)

Medulloepitheliomas are believed to be primary tumors of the nonpigmented ciliary epithelium that arise in childhood and are characterized by their embryonic appearance.[6] These tumors are uniocular and usually arise from the ciliary body or iris. They are rarer than retinoblastoma. Females and males are affected equally, and there is no racial predilection. There are no hereditary or systemic associations.

The median age of presentation is 5 years of age, but patients have presented as early as the first few months of life.[6] The oldest reported case occurred in a 78-year-old man.[13] Medulloepitheliomas are classified as either teratoid or nonteratoid and are further distinguished as benign or malignant. This spectrum of histopathology has been well described by Broughton and Zimmerman.[6] Their classification has been adopted by the World Health Organization. Their criteria for malignancy include composition by poorly differentiated neuroblastic cells, polymorphism, increased mitotic activity, and sarcomatous appearance.

The most common presenting symptoms are pain and poor vision. An anterior chamber cyst or mass, leukocoria, and pupil abnormalities are the most common presenting signs.[6] Frequent ocular associations include glaucoma [present at diagnosis in half the reported patients (Fig. 9-14)], cataract, and rubeosis.[6,8] Persistent hyperplastic primary vitreous (PHPV) was present in 11 of the 56 patients reported by Broughton and Zimmerman.[6]

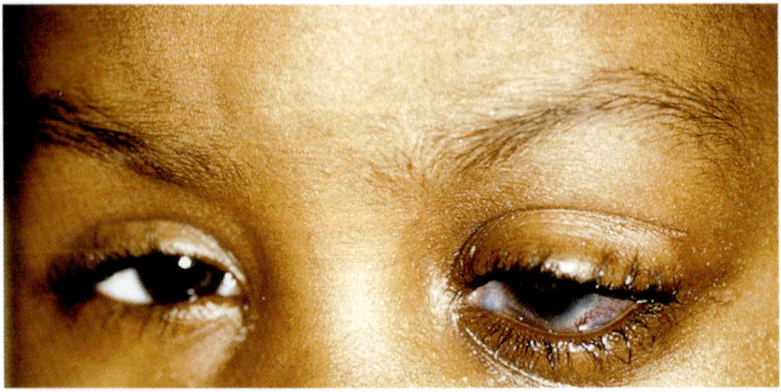

FIGURE 9-14. Unilateral buphthalmic eye and severe glaucoma.

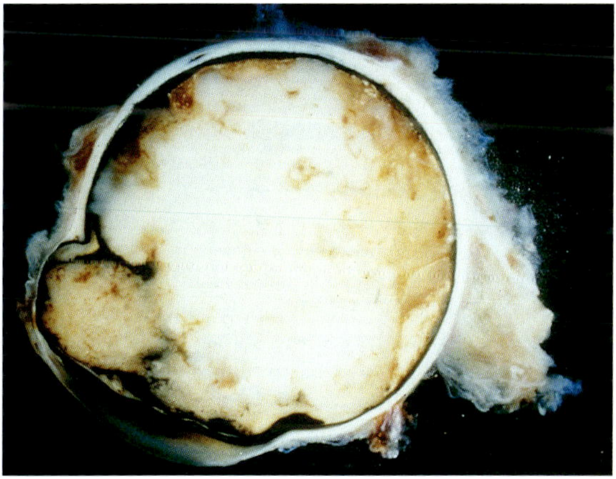

FIGURE 9-15. Enucleated eye showing medulloepithelioma filling the eye. (Courtesy of Dr. K.W. Wright, Los Angeles, CA)

Medulloepitheliomas usually appear as a grayish-white mass, often cystic, which arises from the iris or ciliary body. The tumor can be solid, fleshy pink, and occasionally pigmented (Fig. 9-15). In several case reports, the tumor consisted of almost flat, nondescript sheets over the iris. Thus, the differential may include JXG, iris melanoma, and leiomyoma. In the Broughton and Zimmerman series of 56 patients at the AFIP, 9 patients had undergone enucleation for blind and/or painful eyes.[6] In these 9 cases, the existence of intraocular tumor was not suspected preoperatively. In only 7 of these 56 cases was the diagnosis of medulloepithelioma made correctly preoperatively.

Rarely, these tumors can arise from the optic nerve and retina and simulate retinoblastoma.[22] In one case, the tumor involved the retrobulbar portion of the optic nerve and mimicked an optic nerve glioma.[17] A case report exists of an infant presenting with a medulloepithelioma that mimicked PHPV.[58] The presenting signs were leukocoria, a shallow anterior chamber, mild cataract, and retrolental fibrovascular tissue.

Delay of diagnosis of as much as 1 year from the onset of signs and symptoms is common.[6] CT and ultrasound may or may not be helpful. Frequently, the tumor is very anterior and may not have much mass effect. The diagnosis should be suspected in any blind or distorted eye in a child. Several case reports had an anecdotal history of trauma as a "red herring." The diagnosis should be considered particularly with ciliary body and iris lesions. In several cases, an anterior chamber (AC) tap has led to the correct diagnosis.[44] However, it is often contraindicated to enter the eye of a child with a needle, especially if the eye may harbor an active retinoblastoma.

Enucleation has been the preferred method of treatment in the majority of cases. In a few cases, iridocyclectomy has been curative.[6,8] In one report, however, a patient developed two recurrences following local excision that looked increasingly malignant histopathologically. Highly malignant histopathological features developed, and the eye was subsequently enucleated.[29]

The survival rate from this tumor is excellent. It is slow growing and only locally invasive. In the series of Canning et al., all 15 patients who were included survived.[8] From the AFIP series, 4 of 56 patients died of metastatic disease. The most important prognostic factor identified in their series was the presence of extraocular extension. All 4 tumor deaths were preceded by orbital spread.

LEUKEMIA

Leukemia is classified as acute or chronic, and in children acute leukemia predominates. The cell type most common among the acute leukemias in childhood is lymphoblastic (ALL). All ocular structures may be affected by the leukemia in these children.[28] Ocular tissue may be involved by direct infiltration of leukemic cells, hemorrhage, or infection.

In a series of 117 consecutive patients with acute leukemia reported by Guyer et al., 44 of the patients were pediatric.[19] Among the children in this series, 16 had some form of leukemic retinopathy at the time of diagnosis. Several authors have noted a much higher incidence of ocular involvement if the entire course of the disease is considered.[48]

Clinically, the retina is most commonly involved in leukemia, whereas histopathologically the choroid is most frequently infiltrated.[28] Leukemic retinopathy is more common in acute leukemia and is more common at diagnosis in adults than in children.[19] The retinopathy may be characterized by tortuous dilated veins, vascular sheathing, cotton wool spots, and exudates. Retinal hemorrhage is the most common feature of the retinopathy and usually occurs in the posterior pole. The hemorrhages may be white centered. In children, cotton wool spots are rare.[19,28,51] Guyer et al.[19] found an association between the presence of intraretinal hemorrhages and thrombocytopenia, as well as relatively lower hematocrit levels.

Leukemia may also manifest in the eye as conjunctival thickening, perilimbal infiltrate, ring corneal ulcers, hypopyon, iris infiltrate, nodular retinal infiltrate, vitreous invasion, optic nerve or peripheral neovascularization, exudative retinal detachment, RPE detachment, microaneurysms, and pre- or postlaminar optic nerve involvement.[1,10,24,52,54,61,67]

Ocular involvement is rarely the presenting sign of the underlying disease, but with longer-term survival, ocular disease is being reported in association with or following CNS relapse.[7] There are increasing numbers of case reports of ocular disease (hypopyon, iris infiltration, choroidal relapse, optic nerve leukemia) as isolated sites of extramedullary relapse in patients who are in remission and who have not had any antecedent or concurrent evidence of CNS or hematological relapse.[1,7,43,56]

Opportunistic infections are common in the immunocompromised host. Rarely, a leukemic retinal or choroidal infiltrate or leukemic hypopyon may be difficult to distinguish from infectious processes. In certain cases, an anterior chamber tap, posterior chamber aspirate, or biopsy of the choroid and retina may be necessary to distinguish direct leukemic infiltrate from an infectious process.[56,64]

There are many clinical ocular signs of the disease, but a significant number do not require treatment. The signs are often noted by the oncologist and not referred to the ophthalmologist. A red eye associated with pain can be an indication of opportunistic infection or direct conjunctival or anterior chamber infiltrate by leukemia. An infiltrative conjunctival process, a leukemic hypopyon, or pre- or postlaminar optic nerve disease can certainly result in visual loss. In the case of conjunctival, anterior chamber, or iris involvement, after cytological diagnosis external beam radiation has been very effective in eliminating the infiltrative process (400–2000 cGy over 2 weeks).[28] A mild anterior chamber reaction in a leukemic patient may represent active ocular leukemia. There are case reports of this type of active disease responding temporarily to topical steroids when treated as a "uveitis."[1]

Prelaminar optic nerve infiltrations are most common in children with ALL and must be distinguished from papilledema secondary to CNS relapse.[51] Postlaminar nerve invasion more frequently results in significant visual loss and also may have concurrent disc edema.

References

1. Abramson DH, Wachtel A, Watson CW, Jereb B, Wollner N. Leukemic hypopyon. J Pediatr Ophthalmol Strabismus 1981;18:42.
2. Adler R, Lappe M, Murphree AL. Pupil dilatation at the first well-baby examination for documenting choroidal light reflex. J Pediatr 1991;118:249–252.
3. Apt L. Uveal melanomas in children and adolescents. Int Ophthalmol Clin 1962;2:403–410.
4. Barr CC, McLean IW, Zimmerman LE. Uveal melanoma in children and adolescents. Arch Ophthalmol 1981;99:2133.
5. Bhatnagar R, Vine AK. Diffuse infiltrating retinoblastoma. Ophthalmology 1991;98:1657–1661.
6. Broughton WL, Zimmerman LE. A clinicopathologic study of 56 cases of intraocular medulloepitheliomas. Am J Ophthalmol 1978; 85:407–418.
7. Bunin NJ, Pui CH, Hustu O, Rivera GK. Unusual extramedullary relapses in children with acute lymphoblastic leukemia. J Pediatr 1986;109:665–669.
8. Canning CR, McCartney AC, Hungerford J. Medulloepithelioma (diktyoma). Br J Ophthalmol 1988;72:764–767.
9. Cavenee WK, Dryja TP, Phillips RA, et al. Expression of recessive alleles by chromosomal mechanisms in retinoblastoma. Nature (Lond) 1983;305:779–784.

9a. Collaborative Ocular Melanoma Study Group. The COMS randomized trial of Iodine 125 Brachytherapy for choroidal melanoma, III: Initial Mortality findings: COMS report number 18. Arch Ophthalmol 2001;119:969–982.

9b. Collaborative Ocular Melanoma Study Group. The COMS randomized trial of pre-enucleation radiation of large choroidal melanoma, II: inital mortaliy findings: COMS report number 10 Am J Ophthalmol 1998;125:779–796.

10. De Juan E, Green WR, Rive TA, Erozan YS. Optic disc neovascularization associated with ocular involvement in acute lymphocytic leukemia. Retina 1982;2:61–64.
11. Devesa SS. The incidence of retinoblastoma. Am J Ophthalmol 1975; 80:263–265.
12. Fledelius H, Land AM. Malignant melanoma of the choroid in an 11-month-old infant. Acta Ophthalmol 1975;53:160–166.
13. Floyd BB, Minckler DS, Valentin L. Intraocular medulloepithelioma in a 79-year-old man. Ophthalmology 1982;89:1088–1094.
14. Friend SH, Bernards R, Rogeli S, et al. A human DNA segment with properties of the gene that predisposes to retinoblastoma and osteosarcoma. Nature (Lond) 1986;323:643–646.

15. Fung YKT, Murphree AL, Zhang FH, et al. The Rb gene suppresses the growth of normal cells. Oncogene 1993;8(10):2659–2672.
16. Gallie BL. Retinoblastoma gene mutations in human cancer [Letter, Comment]. N Engl J Med 1994;330(11):786–787.
17. Green WR, Iliff WJ, Trotter RR. Malignant Teratoid Medulloepithelioma of the Optic Nerve. Arch Ophthalmol 1974;91:451–454.
18. Greer CH. Congenital melanoma of the anterior uvea. Arch Ophthalmol 1966;76:77–78.
19. Guyer DR, Schachat AP, Vitale S, et al. Leukemic retinopathy. Relationship between fundus lesions and hematologic parameters at diagnosis. Ophthalmology 1989;96:860–864.
20. Haas BD, Jakobiec FA, Iwamoto T, Cox M, Bernacki EG, Pokorny KL. Diffuse choroidal melanocytoma in a child. A lesion extending the spectrum of melanocytic hamartomas. Ophthalmology 1986;93: 1632–1638.
21. Haik BG, Siedlecki A, Ellsworth RM, Sturgis–Buckhout L. Documented delays in the diagnosis of retinoblastoma. Ann Ophththalmol 1985;17:731–732.
22. Hamburg A. Medulloepithelioma arising from the posterior pole. Ophthalmologica 1980;181:152–159.
23. Hill JC, Stannard C, Bowen RM. Ciliary body malignant melanoma in a black child. J Pediatr Ophthalmol Strabismus 1991;28:38–40.
24. Holbrook CT, Felsas FJ, Crist WM, Castleberry RP. Acute leukemia and hypopyon. J Pediatr 1978;93:626–628.
25. Hungerford J. Personal communication, Los Angeles, January 1992.
26. Jensen OA, Movin M, Mueller J. Malignant melanoma of the choroid in an infant with the dysplastic naevus syndrome. Acta Ophthalmol Copenh 1987;65:91–100.
27. Kallioneimi A, Kallioneimi OP, Waldman F, et al. Detection of retinoblastoma gene deletions in metaphase chromosomes and interphase nuclei by fluorescence in situ hybridization. Cytogenet Cell Genet 1992;60(3-4):190–193.
28. Kincaid MC, Green WR. Ocular and orbital involvement in leukemia. Surv Ophthalmol 1983;27:211–232.
29. Kivela T, Tarkkanen A. Recurrent medulloepithelioma of the ciliary body. Immunohistochemical characteristics. Ophthalmology 1988; 95:1565–1575.
30. Knudson AG Jr. Genetics of human cancer. J Cell Physiol (Suppl) 1986;4:7–11.
31. Knudson AG Jr. Hereditary cancer, oncogenes, and antioncogenes. Cancer Res 1985;45:1437–1443.
32. Knudson AG Jr. Mutation and cancer: statistical study of retinoblastoma. Proc Natl Acad Sci USA 1971;68:820–823.
33. Kock E, Naeser P. Retinoblastoma in Sweden 1958–1971: a clinical and histopathological study. Acta Ophthalmol 1979;57:344–350.
34. Leonard BD, Shields JA, McDonald PR. Malignant melanomas of the uveal tract in children and young adults. Can J Ophthalmol 1975;10: 441–449.

35. Los G, Smals OAG, van Vugt MJH, et al. A rationale for carboplatin treatment and abdominal hyperthermia in cancers restricted to the peritoneal cavity. Cancer Res 1992;52:1252–1258.
36. Messmer EP, Fritze H, Mohr C, et al. Long-term treatment effects in patients with bilateral retinoblastoma: ocular and mid-facial findings. Graefe's Arch Clin Exp Ophthalmol 1991;229:309.
37. Murphree AL. Personal observation, 1992.
38. Murphree AL. Unpublished data, 1992.
39. Murphree AL, Benedict WF. Retinoblastoma: clues to human oncogenesis. Science 1984;223:1028–1033.
40. Murphree AL, Gomer CJ, Sato J. Transpupillary diode laserthermia is synergistic with systemic carboplatin in the treatment of focal retinoblastoma. J Pediatr Ophthalmol Strabismus. Submitted.
41. Murphree AL, Rother C. Retinoblastoma. In: Ryan SJ (ed) Retina, vol VI. Part II. St. Louis: Mosby, 1989:529–530.
42. Nadol JB Jr. Pseudocellulitis of the orbit: a case report of retinoblastoma masquerading as orbital cellulitis. Ann Otol 1977;86:86–88.
43. Ninane J. The eye as a sanctuary in acute lymphoblastic leukemia. Lancet 1980;1:452–453.
43a. Orjuela M, Castaneda VP, Ridaura C, et al. Presence of human papilloma virus in tumor tissue from children with retinoblastoma: an alternative mechanism for tumor development. Clin Cancer Res 2000;6(10):4010–4016.
44. Orellana J, Moura RA, Font RL, Boniuk M, Murphy D. Medulloepithelioma diagnosed by ultrasound and vitreous aspirate: electron microscopic observations. Ophthalmology 1983;90:1531–1539.
45. Pendergrass TW, Davis S. Incidence of retinoblastoma in the United States. Arch Ophthalmol 1980;98:1204–1210.
46. Reeh MJ, Petersen P, Kobrin JG, Chenoweth RG. Malignant melanoma of choroid developing in the eye of a three-year-old boy. Ann Ophthalmol 1979;11(1):57–70.
47. Reese AB. Tumors of the Eye. New York: Harper and Row, 1976.
48. Robb RM, Ervin LD, Sallan SE. A pathological study of eye involvement in acute leukemia of childhood. Trans Am Ophthalmol Soc 1978;76:90–101.
49. Roldan M, Llanes F, Negrete O, Valverde F. Malignant melanoma of the choroid associated with melanosis oculi in a child. Am J Ophthalmol 1987;104:662–663.
50. Rosenbaum PS, Boniuk M, Font RL. Diffuse uveal melanoma in a 5-year-old child. Am J Ophthalmol 1988;106:601–606.
51. Rosenthal AR. Ocular manifestations of leukemia. A review. Ophthalmology 1983;90:899–905.
52. Rowan PJ, Sloan JB. Iris and anterior chamber involvement in leukemia. Ann Ophthalmol 1976;8(9):1081–1085.
53. Saraux H, Dhermy P, Bechetoille A, Nou B. Les hyphemas revelateurs de retinoblastome. Bull Soc Ophthalmol (Fr) 1974;74(3):301–304.

54. Schachat AP, Jabs DA, Graham ML, Ambinder RF, Green WR, Saral R. Leukemic iris infiltration. J Pediatr Ophthalmol Strabismus 1988; 25:135–138.
55. Scheffer CH, Binkhorst PG, Hamburg A. Malignant melanoma of the choroid in a 2-year-old infant. Ophthalmologica 1974;169:401–410.
56. Schmiegelow K, Scherfig E, Prause JU, Jensen OA. Isolated leukemic choroidal relapse in a child with acute lymphoblastic leukemia, one year off therapy, diagnosed through transvitreal retinochoroidal biopsy. Acta Ophthalmol Copenh 1988;66:33–37.
57. Shields CL, Shields JA, Milite J, De Potter P, Sabbagh R, Menduke H. Uveal melanoma in teenagers and children. A report of 40 cases. Ophthalmology 1991;98:1662–1666.
58. Shields JA, Shields CL, Schwartz RL. Malignant teratoid medulloepithelioma of the ciliary body simulating persistent hyperplastic primary vitreous. Am J Ophthalmol 1989;107:296–298.
59. Shields JA. Diagnosis and management of intraocular tumors. St. Louis: Mosby, 1983.
59a. Shields C, et al. Plaque radiotherapy for uveal melanoma: Long term visual outcome in 1106 consecutive patients. Arch Ophth 2000; 118(9):1219–1228.
60. Stafford WR, Yanoff M, Parnell BL. Retinoblastomas initially misdiagnosed as primary ocular inflammations. Arch Ophthalmol 1969; 82:771–773.
61. Stewart MW, Gitter KA, Cohen G. Acute leukemia presenting as a unilateral exudative retinal detachment. Retina 1989;9:110–114.
62. Suckling RD, Fitzgerald PH, Stewart J, Wells E. The incidence and epidemiology of retinoblastoma in New Zealand: a 30-year survey. Br J Cancer 1982;46:729–736.
63. T'Ang A, Varley JM, Chakraborty S, Murphree AL, Fung YKT. Structural rearrangement of the retinoblastoma gene in human breast carcinoma. Science 1988;242:263–266.
64. Taylor D, Day S, Tiedemann K, Chessels J, Marshall WC, Constable IJ. Chorioretinal biopsy in a patient with leukaemia. Br J Ophthalmol 1981;65:489–493.
65. Velazquez N, Jones IS. Ocular and oculodermal melanocytosis associated with uveal melanoma. Ophthalmology 1983;90:1472–1476.
66. Verdaguer J. Prepubertal and pubertal melanomas in ophthalmology. Am J Ophthalmol 1965;60:1002–1011.
67. Zakka KA, Yee RD, Shorr N, Smith GS, Pettit TH, Foos RY. Leukemic iris infiltration. Am J Ophthalmol 1980;89:204–209.

10

Retinopathy of Prematurity

Richard R. Ober, Earl A. Palmer, Arlene V. Drack, and Kenneth W. Wright

Retinopathy of prematurity (ROP) is a disease that occurs in premature infants and affects the blood vessels of the developing retina. It results in the development of vascular shunts, neovascularization, and, in its more severe forms, traction retinal detachment. The development of retinal vascular shunts and neovascularization in ROP is believed to be related to local ischemia, which is a predominant feature of other proliferative retinopathies such as sickle cell and diabetic retinopathy. The unique feature of ROP relates to its occurrence only in premature infants with immature and incompletely vascularized retina. ROP is mild and undergoes spontaneous regression with no visual sequelae in the majority of affected infants. However, progression to advanced ROP does occur in a significant number of infants and can lead to severe visual impairment and even complete unilateral or bilateral blindness in some cases. Recent technological advances in neonatology have increased the survival rate of very low birth weight infants, which has led to a correspondingly increased incidence of ROP. This, in turn, has provided a major challenge to all physicians treating the premature infant and has created renewed interest in the pathogenesis, prevention, and treatment of ROP.

HISTORICAL CONSIDERATIONS

The original description and first correlation of this disease with prematurity was made by Terry in 1942 and 1943.[166,167] Terry's initial impressions were based on his observations of a retrolental proliferation of the embryonic hyaloid system, therefore, the condition was designated as "retrolental fibroplasia." As the pathoanatomy became more fully appreciated and improved classification systems were developed, the term *retinopathy of prematurity* was adopted. During the 10 years following Terry's observations, ROP was seen in epidemic proportions and became the largest cause of blindness in children in the United States and a major cause of blindness throughout the developed world; approximately 7000 children in the United States alone were blinded by ROP.[150] In the late 1950s and 1960s, oxygen therapy was curtailed because of its incrimination as the principal cause of ROP, and this led to a dramatic decline in the incidence of ROP. This decline was, however, associated with an adverse effect on premature infant morbidity and mortality rates.[7,103] Cross[25] estimated that for each case of blindness prevented approximately 16 babies died as a result of inadequate oxygenation. In the 1970s, developments in arterial blood gas monitoring made possible more careful documentation of the premature infant's oxygen needs. However, despite improvement in oxygen tension monitoring, a "second epidemic" of ROP resulted from survival of younger and smaller preterm infants. Their lower birth weight and gestational age became recognized as ROP risk factors. The 1980s and early 1990s can be considered to be a period of progress in terms of reducing the complications from ROP, and there were numerous clinical trials of treatment with reduced nursery light levels, vitamin E, cryotherapy, and laser photocoagulation.

INCIDENCE AND NATURAL HISTORY

ROP reached epidemic proportions between 1948 and 1954.[127] However, after excess oxygen was implicated as the principal cause of ROP in the 1950s, a marked decrease in the incidence of ROP occurred after curtailment of oxygen. Beginning in the mid-1960s, because of technological advances in neonatology associated with the increased survival of low birth weight infants, a steady increase in the incidence of ROP was noted.[127] A report[131] of survival rates specific for birth weight and gestational age for 6676 inborn neonates registered during the CRYO-ROP study in 1986 and 1987 who weighed less than 1251 g at birth demonstrated that overall 28-day survival increased with gestational age and birth weight, from 36.5% at 24 weeks gestation to 89.9% at 29 weeks gestation. Survival increased from

30.0% for neonates of 500 through 599g birth weight to 91.3% for neonates of 1200 through 1250g.

Reports of the incidence of ROP from the 1950s and 1960s are difficult to compare with those of the 1970s and 1980s due to variations in patient selection, the lack of a standard classification system, and the lack of appreciation of mild forms of ROP, which became possible with the availability of indirect ophthalmoscopy in the 1970s.[29] In the 1980s, several large studies[15,47] provided information on the incidence of ROP and reaffirmed that the incidence was inversely related to gestational age and birth weight. Flynn[47] performed multivariate risk analysis techniques and concluded that birth weight was the strongest and most consistent predictor of acute ROP in a population of 639 infants with birth weight ranging from 600 to 1500g. Campbell et al.[15] determined the incidence of acute ROP in 2958 admissions to a tertiary hospital neonatal intensive care unit (NICU). Among 2484 survivors, acute ROP developed in 72 (2.9%); 60 (83%) of these newborns had birth weights less than 1500g. The incidence of acute ROP among survivors with birth weights of less than 1000g (28%) was approximately three times that of survivors with birth weights between 1001 and 1500g (10.1%).

Accurate estimations of the incidence of blindness secondary to ROP are lacking because of the absence of an organized reporting system in the United States. Campbell et al.[15] reported an overall incidence of blindness in 4.5% of 2484 surviving infants in a tertiary NICU with birth weights less than 1000g and 1.2% of those surviving with birth weights of 1000 to 1500g. Phelps[128] estimated that approximately 546 infants were blinded from ROP in the United States during 1979 and that approximately 2100 infants would be affected annually with cicatricial sequelae including myopia, strabismus, blindness, and late retinal detachment.

Prospective studies[29,42] have provided new information regarding the current incidence of various stages of ROP and have relevance in determining ROP screening protocols. Fielder et al.[42] studied 572 infants weighing 1700g, or less and noted development of acute ROP in 50.9%. All ROP stages 1 and 2 underwent complete resolution and of the 27 (4.7%) infants with stage 3–4 disease, cicatricial sequelae developed in 6. Incidence and severity increased with decreasing birth weight and gestational age.

Among premature infants, the high-risk group that was selected for the Multicenter Trial of Cryotherapy for Retinopathy of Prematurity (CRYO-ROP) was the cohort with birth weights less than 1251 g, referred to herein as *very low birth weight* (VLBW).[29] Sequential ophthalmic examination was performed on 4099 infants beginning at age 4 to 6 weeks to monitor the incidence and course of ROP. Overall, 65.8% of the infants developed some degree of ROP, 81.6% for infants less than 1000 g birth weight. The lower the birth weight, the higher the risk of ROP, such that for the subgroup weighing below 750 g at birth, 90% developed some degree of ROP (Table 10-1).

The median time of onset of stage 1 ROP, for infants whose ROP did not progress any further than stage 1, is 34.3 weeks postconception (gestational age at birth plus postnatal age); that of onset of stage 2 (maximum) is 35.4 weeks, and that of stage 3 is 36.6 weeks.[29] (See later sections for further description of the International Classification of ROP and the CRYO-ROP study.)

Moderately severe ROP that had not reached the threshold for randomization into the CRYO-ROP study was categorized as *prethreshold* if any of the following criteria were met: any zone I ROP, zone II ROP at stage 2+, stage 3 without plus, or stage 3+ with less than the requisite clock-hours of circumferential involvement to qualify as threshold[26] (severity categories are summarized in Table 10-2). Prethreshold ROP occurred in 17.8% of VLBW infants between 32 and 42 weeks postconception in 90% of the cases (median onset, 36.1 weeks).[29]

In the CRYO-ROP study, *threshold* ROP was defined as stage 3+, located in zone I or II, and extending five to eight 30° clock-hour sectors of the circumference of the eye (five sectors if contiguous and eight if cumulative) (Table 10-2). If untreated, 47.4% of the eyes developed adverse structural outcomes (retinal detachment or fold within zone I, or retrolental membrane obscuring the view of the fundus) 12 months after ran-

TABLE 10-1. Percent of Patients with Various Categories of Retinopathy of Prematurity (ROP).

Wt. in grams	*Any ROP*	*Stage 3*	*Prethreshold*	*Threshold*
<750	90.0	37.4	39.4	15.5
750–999	78.2	21.9	21.4	6.8
1000–1250	46.9	8.5	7.3	2.0
Total group	65.8	18.3	17.8	6.0

Source: From Cryotherapy for Retinopathy of Prematurity Group. Arch Ophthalmol 1991;98: 1628–1640, with permission.

TABLE 10-2. Definitions of Retinal Vascular Development in Premature Infants, Stages of ROP, and Criteria for Enrollment in CRYO-ROP Study.

Terms	*Definitions*
Normal premature retina	An area of nonvascularized retina extends posteriorly from the ora serrata, gradually showing vascularization inroads at the anterior edge of the vascularized retina. Choroidal vessels may or may nor be readily visible through the avascular retina, but are normally visible through the vascularized retina.
Stage 1	A thin, relatively flat, white demarcation line separates the avascular retina anteriorly, from the vascularized retina posteriorly. Vessels that lead up to the demarcation line are abnormally branched and/or arcaded.
Stage 2	The demarcation line has visible volume and extends off the retinal surface as a ridge, which may be white or pink. Retinal vessels may appear stretched locally, and vault off the surface of the retina to reach the peak of the ridge. Tufts of neovascular tissue may be present posterior to, but not attached to, the ridge.
Stage 3	Extraretinal fibrovascular (neovascular) proliferative tissue emanates from the surface of the ridge, extending posteriorly along the retinal surface, or anteriorly toward the vitreous cavity; this gives the ridge a ragged appearance.
Plus Disease	ROP in the presence of progressive dilatation and tortuosity of the retinal vessels, not only adjacent to the ROP line or ridge, but also in the posterior fundus. When present, a plus (+) sign is added to the staging number.
Prethreshold ROP	Zone I ROP of any stage less than threshold, zone II ROP at stage 2+, stage 3 without plus, stage 3+ with fewer than the threshold number of clock-hour sectors of stage 3+.
Threshold ROP	Five or more contiguous or eight cumulative clock hours (30° sectors) of stage 3+ ROP in either zone I or II; an eligibility criterion for enrollment in the multicenter randomized clinical trial of cryotherapy.

domization.[28] Threshold ROP occurred in 6% of VLBW infants between 34 and 42 weeks postconception 90% of the time (median onset, 36.9 weeks).[29] Thus, ROP appears, runs its course, and reaches its most damaging stages within a specific developmental time frame; in VLBW infants, this corresponds to approximately 1 to 3 months postpartum.

Of the eyes that reached threshold ROP and were randomized to no treatment, 12% developed subtotal retinal detachment (stage 4), 32.4% total retinal detachment (stage 5), and 6.9% a posterior retinal fold (grade III, Reese Classification[141]) 3 months after randomization.[27] In eyes treated according to the CRYO-ROP study protocol, these figures were reduced to 9.9% for stage 4, 18% for stage 5, and 3.2% for a posterior retinal fold affecting the macula (as judged by masked grading of retinal photographs).[27]

This prospective study[29] provided new insight into the development of ROP and again confirmed that ROP incidence and severity were higher in lower birth weight and gestational age categories. The timing of retinal vascular events correlated more closely with postconceptional age than with postnatal age, implicating the level of maturity more than postnatal environmental influences in governing the timing of these vascular events.

PATHOGENESIS

Normal Vascular Development

In infants, retinal vascular development begins at 16 weeks gestation with mesenchyme, the blood vessel precursor, growing from the disc to reach the ora nasally at 8 months and the ora temporally shortly after birth.[4,48,57] On the posterior edge of the advancing mesenchyme, a primitive immature network of capillaries develops according to Ashton's theory.[4] This delicate, chicken-wire meshwork undergoes absorption and remodeling to form mature retinal arteries and veins that are surrounded by the capillary meshwork.[4,48,53]

The Role of Oxygen in ROP

Clinical Findings

Campbell,[14] in 1951, observed a relationship of ROP to oxygen exposure. Patz and coworkers[126] confirmed the apparent role of supplementary oxygen in a controlled nursery study. In 1956, the results of the 18-hospital collaborative study chaired by Dr. V.E. Kinsey confirmed the role of oxygen as an important factor in the production of ROP.[84]

EXPERIMENTAL FINDINGS

Hyperoxic animal models[5,125] have clearly demonstrated that the immature and incompletely vascularized retina is susceptible to oxygen toxicity, providing experimental support for the initial clinical studies implicating oxygen as a major cause of ROP. Lesions closely resembling the early stages of human ROP have been produced in the kitten, mouse, rat, and puppy models.[5,125] Rearing newborn rats in variable, fluctuating supplemental oxygen also causes retinopathy.[100] The immature retinal vasculature of a term newborn kitten is comparable to a 6.5-month gestational human fetus, offering the unique advantage of studying a healthy term animal subject.[5]

The primary effect of oxygen on the incompletely vascularized retina of the experimental animal is retinal vasoconstriction, and vaso-obliteration which may be reversible with a short duration of oxygen exposure.[5,124,125] However, permanent occlusion of peripheral immature retinal vessels can occur as a result of exposure to significantly elevated arterial oxygen partial pressure for an extended period of several days.[57a] After sustained hyperoxia and subsequent removal of the kitten animal model to ambient air, nodules of endothelial proliferation arise from the residual vascular complexes adjacent to retinal capillaries closed during hyperoxia and canalize to form new vessels. These new vessels, similar to other proliferative retinopathies, penetrate through the internal limited membrane and proliferate on the inner retinal surfaces.

PATHOPHYSIOLOGY OF ROP

Fundamental to understanding the pathophysiology of ROP is knowledge that, in utero, the fetus is in a hypoxic state with a stable PaO_2 of 22 to 24 mm Hg. This is in contrast to a full-term baby and a normal adult where the PaO_2 is dramatically higher—ranging from 70 to 90 mm Hg. The developing retinal vessels grow from the optic nerve to the peripheral avascular retina. In animal models, this growth of immature retinal vessels into the peripheral avascular retina is stimulated by *vascular endothelial growth factor* (*VEGF*) (Fig. 10-1). Physiologic levels of VEGF are required to maintain vessel integrity of existing retinal vessels and to stimulate vessel growth.[57a] The amount of oxygen in the retinal tissue determines the amount of VEGF produced. Low tissue oxygen, or ischemia, stimulates VEGF production;

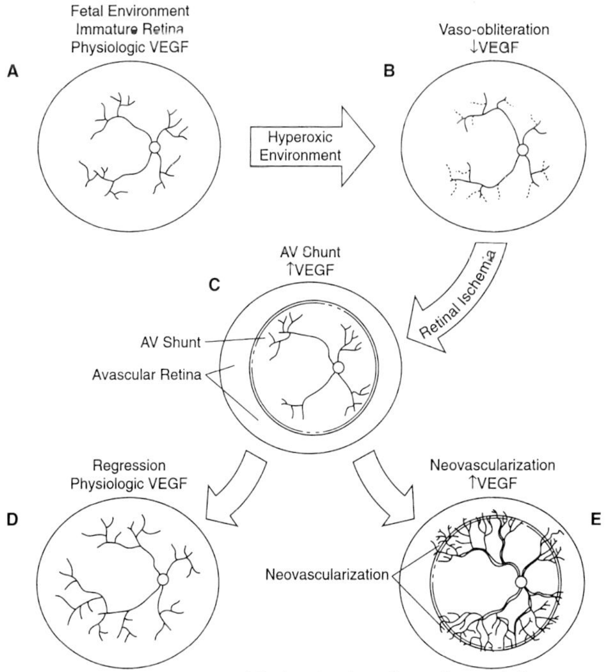

FIGURE 10-1A–E. VEGF model of pathophysiology of ROP. **(A)** Drawing of immature retinal vessels in a premature infant approximately 25–28 weeks gestational age. Note that the vessels have the normal tree-branching architecture. **(B)** Premature infant exposed to high oxygen, causing VEGF to be downregulated. The drawing shows constriction and vaso-obliteration of small vessels. **(C)** Over time, the peripheral avascular retina becomes ischemic from the lack of blood supply. Peripheral retinal ischemia causes an increase in local VEGF, stimulating arteriolar venous shunt formation at the junction between avascularized and vascularized retina. This represents Stage 1 to Stage 2 ROP. Note the vascular pattern of peripheral vessel straightening, or Broom-bristle pattern, indicative of a shunt associated with ROP. **(D)** Retinal vessels show pattern of regression as physiologic levels of VEGF stimulate normal vessel growth into the area of avascular retina. Note the normal vascular pattern of tree branching. **(E)** Drawing shows the effects of sustained peripheral retinal ischemia causing abnormally high levels of local VEGF. Consistently high levels of VEGF results in neovascularization (Stage 3 ROP) and dilated, tortuous posterior pole vessels (plus disease).

whereas high tissue oxygen levels down-regulate VEGF production and halt vessel growth. If the immature retina is exposed to persistent hyperoxia, the immature vessels will stop growing. The more immature the infant, the larger the area of avascular retina. Prolonged exposure to high levels of oxygen will result in vasoconstriction and, eventually, vaso-obliteration as the vessels involute due to lack of VEGF.[57a] This lack of normal vessel growth leaves the peripheral retina without adequate blood supply.

Over time, usually several weeks, the avascular retina becomes ischemic and stimulates VEGF production. If the area of avascular retina is relatively small, physiologic VEGF levels are produced and stimulate normal retinal vessel growth. If, on the other hand, the area of avascular retina is large and large amounts of VEGF are produced, this induces the immature retinal vessels to sprout *arterial venous (AV) shunts* at the border between the vascularized and avascular retina (ROP Stages 1 and 2). Regression occurs if VEGF stimulates normal vascularization past the AV shunt into the avascular retina. Extremely large areas of avascular retina, on the other hand, upregulates VEGF stimulating neovascularization of the AV shunt (ROP Stage 3). Sustained high levels of VEGF can even cause vasodilatation and tortuosity of existing posterior pole vessels (*PLUS disease*), iris vessel dilatation, and rubeosis iridis. Treatment of Stage 3 ROP with cryotherapy or laser therapy is directed at obliterating the peripheral avascular retina, thus lowering levels of VEGF.[57a] Reducing VEGF levels will result in regression of neovascularization and reduce the chances of an unfavorable outcome. Extensive neovascularization of the retina can cause retinal fibrovascular proliferation, scarring, and retinal detachment (ROP Stages 4 and 5).

Despite environmental risk factors, or a genetic predisposition that contributes to the development of ROP, hyperoxia in very low birth weight premature infants early in the NICU course remains a possible risk factor for ROP.[6,30a,39a,40,49,57a,59,79a,97,110,140a,143a,144,147c] Tin et al.[79a] reported ROP outcomes on premature infants less than 28 weeks gestation and showed that by strictly curtailing the oxygen dose, the incidence of threshold ROP was reduced four-fold. Hong, Wright, et al.[30a] reported a significant decrease in severe ROP after institution of a protocol for strict curtailment of oxygen in premature infants under 1500 grams. Oxygen was kept between 83% to 90% O_2 saturation, and oxygen curtailment was started in the delivery room. Over the last 3 years in this level III NICU, over 300 premature infants were examined for ROP and none of the premature infants on the new protocol for curtailed oxygen developed threshold ROP. Perhaps with the use of low stable oxygen delivery, severe ROP can be reduced.[30a] Careful attention to mortality and morbidity in clinical trials will be needed to determine if this is feasible. Fluctuating arterial oxygen tension has also been associated with a greater risk of developing progressive ROP.[144a]

Risk Factors

Many reports have confirmed that gestational age and birth weight are key risk factors for the development of ROP.[15,19,29,33,51,65,84,100,131] Although oxygen supplementation has been recognized as a risk factor for the development of ROP since the 1950s, this association has been difficult to define in terms of the duration and concentration of oxygen. Shohat et al.[148] could not demonstrate a significant association between babies with ROP and the duration of supplemental oxygen or the mean maximum oxygen concentration required. A multicentered cooperative study[84] found an association between ROP and oxygen supplementation but could not relate the incidence of ROP to arterial PO_2 levels. However, Flynn et al.[50,52] correlated the incidence and severity of ROP with the duration of exposure to different ranges of oxygen tension as measured by transcutaneous oxygen monitoring ($tcPO_2$) in 101 premature infants with birth weights between 500 and 1300 g. There was a significant association between the amount of time that the $tcPO_2$ was greater than or equal to 80 mm Hg and the incidence and severity of ROP.[52]

Because ROP has occurred in the absence of supplemental oxygen,[100,148] in association with cyanotic heart disease,[78] and in anencephalic infants,[1] these observations suggest determinant factors other than supplemental oxygen as the etiology for ROP. Shohat et al.[148] examined 32 possible risk factors in 34 infants with ROP and noted the following factors significantly associated with ROP: apnea with mask and bag ventilation; prolonged parenteral nutrition; number of blood transfusions; and episodes of hypoxemia, hypercarbia, and hypocarbia. Gunn et al.[63] found several factors significantly associated with ROP in 27 infants, including apnea requiring bag and mask resuscitation with oxygen, septicemia, degree of illness, blood transfusion, and mechanical ventilation. Hammer et al.[65] reviewed 47 potential risk factors in a prospective study of 328 high-risk neonates. Only 4 were significant: ventilator hours, xanthine administration, birth weight, and maternal bleeding. Darlow et al.[36] prospectively determined risk factors in 69 infants with acute retinopathy. On multiple logistic regression analysis, three variables made statistically significant independent contributions to the risk of any acute retinopathy: gestational age, principal hospital caring for the infant, and treatment with indomethacin. They speculated that the larger level III units obtained better results because their size and experience enabled them to provide a better overall quality of care. Charles et al.[19] reported a 72% incidence of ROP in infants under 1200g from a low-income, inner-city population. Significant risk factors observed were low birth weight, short gestation period, extended supplemental oxygen administration, intraventricular hemorrhage, respiratory distress syndrome, and sepsis. In addition, they speculated that limited prenatal care and other maternal factors such as inadequate nutrition may have contributed to the high incidence of ROP in their study. Sieberth and Linderkamp confirmed that low birth weight, low gestational age, artificial ventilation longer than 7 days, high-volume blood transfusion, and surfactant increased risk of ROP in 402 infants less than or equal to 1500gm.[147a] Maternal preeclampsia, antepartum betamethasone, and vitamin E therapy decreased risk.

In the CRYO-ROP study,[33] an increased risk of reaching threshold ROP was found associated with lower birth weight, younger gestational age, white race, multiple births, and being born outside a study center nursery. The risk of an unfavorable macular outcome was increased with zone I ROP, "plus" disease, the severity of the stage, and the amount of circumferential involvement. A higher risk also was associated with a rapid rate of progression of ROP to prethreshold disease, but not with the postconceptional age at which ROP was first noted.

Light has also been discussed as a possible risk factor for ROP.[6,59,144] One prospective study[59] concluded that the high level of ambient illumination commonly found in the hospital nursery may be one factor contributing to ROP. However, the multi-center, randomized light–ROP study found no difference in incidence or severity of ROP between infants fitted with light-blocking goggles shortly after birth and those exposed to ambient nursery light.[39a,143a] In addition, an infant with complete cataracts was noted to have threshold ROP immediately after cataract surgery.[140c] Because very little light had ever reached this infant's retinas, at most light may play a mild cofactor role. Some authors have found a correlation between mutations in the Norrie disease gene, the full expression of which leads to congenital retinal detachment, and severe ROP.[147c]

INTERNATIONAL CLASSIFICATION OF ROP

Because of significant observations during the past three decades, it became evident that the Reese[141] and other classification systems did not adequately describe the early active stages of ROP. The traditional term, *retrolental fibroplasia*, described only the severe late cicatricial changes and was inappropriate for the acute phase of this disease. In 1984, 23 ophthalmologists from 11 countries formed a committee and cooperated in developing the International Classification of Retinopathy of Prematurity (ICROP).[173] This new classification involves three parameters: (1) the location (zone) of the disease in the retina, (2) the extent (clock hours) of the developing vasculature involved, and (3) the severity (stage) of abnormal vascular response observed. The development of a uniform anatomic classification system allowed the results of treatment techniques to be compared by clinicians and researchers worldwide.

The location of ROP is described by three zones (Fig. 10-2). Zone I (posterior pole or inner zone) is a posterior circle centered on the disc, and extends twice the distance from the disc to the center of the macula in all directions. The zone is defined by the most posterior location of disease. If, therefore, *any* ROP is found in zone I, the eye is a "zone I eye." A circle, centered on the disc, with a radius equal to the distance to the nasal ora serrata, defines the boundary between zone II and zone III. We like the CRYO-ROP study approach whereby zones II and III are divided by a convention, rather than by a structure. The convention is that zone II extends all the way from the zone I perimeter to the ora serrata on the nasal side. There is no zone III at the nasal meridian, and only a sliver of it in the oblique nasal quadrants. Zone III is basically a temporal crescent, yet is defined by what is observed nasally. If ROP is present nasally, then the eye cannot be a "zone III eye." On the other hand, if vessels reach the ora nasally and there is no ROP there, but ROP

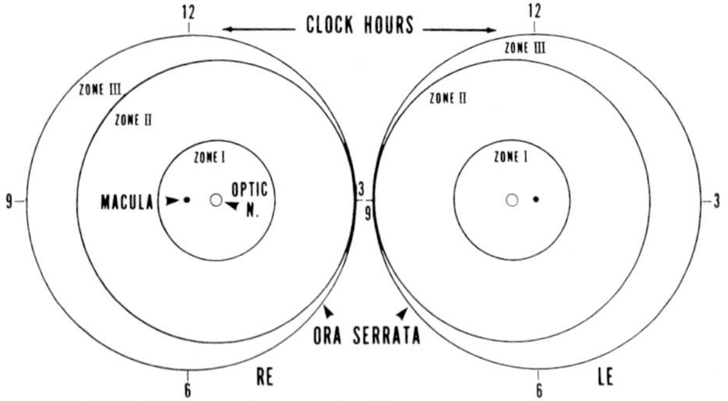

FIGURE 10-2. Scheme of retina of right eye (*RE*) and left eye (*LE*) shows zone borders and clock hours employed to describe location and extent of retinopathy of prematurity. (From The Committee for the Classification of Retinopathy of Prematurity. An international classification of retinopathy of prematurity. Arch Ophthalmol 1984;102:1130–1134, with permission.)

is present temporally, this is apparently categorized as "zone III ROP," no matter where it is located. This convention is only implied in the International Classification, but it is not entirely clear whether it would be still called zone III even if the temporal ROP were located very far posteriorly. In practice, this rarely, if ever, occurs and in the CRYO-ROP study, whenever the vessels were maturely developed on the nasal side and no ROP was located there, all such eyes were categorized as zone III eyes.[26]

The extent of the disease is specified as hours of the clock (see Fig. 10-2). As the observer looks at each eye, the 3-o'clock position is to the right and nasal in the right eye and temporal in the left eye, and the 9-o'clock position is to the left and temporal in the right eye and nasal in the left eye.

The severity of ROP is defined by five stages. Stage 1 is defined as a thin whitish demarcation line abruptly separating vascularized retina posteriorly from the more peripheral avascular retina, which usually has a blanched or opalescent appearance (Tables 10-3 and 10-4). The demarcation line is within the plane of the retina and is usually associated with abnormal branching or arcading of retinal vessels leading up to it (Fig. 10-3). If the demarcation line takes on height and width, occupies a volume, and extends out of the plane of the retina it is termed

TABLE 10-3. Stages of Retinopathy of Prematurity.

Stage number	*Characteristic*		
1	Demarcation line		
2	Ridge		
3	Ridge with extraretinal fibrovascular proliferation		
4	Subtotal retinal detachment		
	A. Extrafoveal		
	B. Retinal detachment including fovea		
5	Total retinal detachment		
	Funnel:	Anterior	Posterior
		Open	Open
		Narrow	Narrow
		Open	Narrow
		Narrow	Open

Source: From Committee for the Classification of Retinopathy of Prematurity. Arch Ophthalmol 1987;105:906–913, with permission.

TABLE 10-4. Regressed Retinopathy of Prematurity.

Peripheral changes

- Vascular
  1. Failure to vascularize peripheral retina
  2. Abnormal, nondichotomous branching of retinal vessels
  3. Vascular arcades with circumferential interconnection
  4. Telangiectatic vessels
- Retinal
  1. Pigmentary changes
  2. Vitreoretinal interface changes
  3. Thin retina
  4. Peripheral folds
  5. Vitreous membranes with or without attachment to retina
  6. Lattice-like degeneration
  7. Retinal breaks
  8. Traction/rhegmatogenous retinal detachment

Posterior changes

- Vascular
  1. Vascular tortuosity
  2. Straightening of blood vessels in temporal arcade
  3. Decrease in angle of insertion of major temporal arcade
- Retinal
  1. Pigmentary changes
  2. Distortion and ectopia of macula
  3. Stretching and folding of retina in macular region leading to periphery
  4. Vitreoretinal interface changes
  5. Vitreous membrane
  6. Dragging of retina over disc
  7. Traction/rhegmatogenous retinal detachment

Source: From Committee for the Classification of Retinopathy of Prematurity. Arch Ophthalmol 1987;105:906–913, with permission.

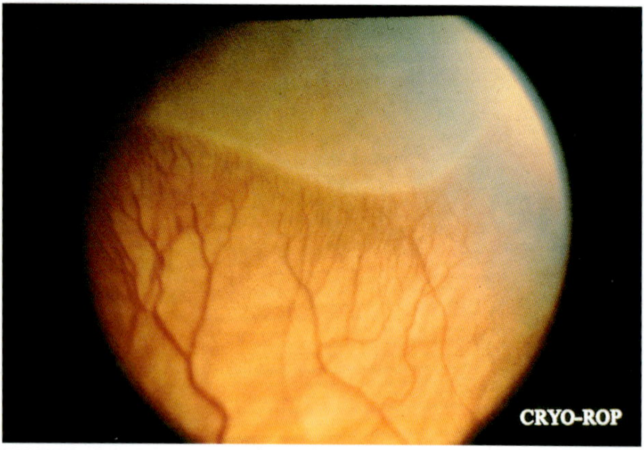

FIGURE 10-3. Demarcation line of stage 1. (Courtesy of Cryotherapy for Retinopathy of Prematurity Cooperative Group.)

a "ridge," which is defined at stage 2 ROP (Fig. 10-4). Small isolated tufts of new vessels may be seen posterior to this ridge structure. When extraretinal fibrovascular proliferative tissue is added to the ridge of stage 2 it appears velvety, frayed, or

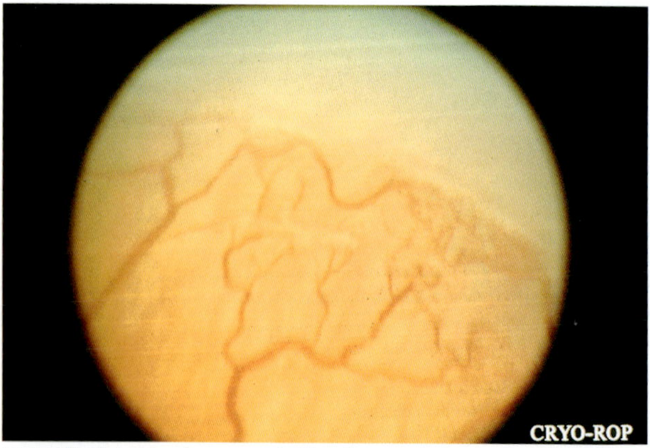

FIGURE 10-4. Development of ridge characteristic of stage 2. Small isolated tufts of new vessels lying on the surface of the retina are seen posterior to the ridge structure. (Courtesy of Cryotherapy for Retinopathy of Prematurity Cooperative Group.)

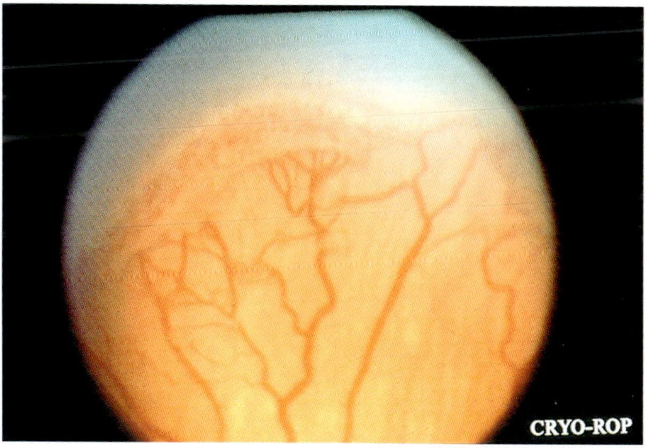

FIGURE 10-5. Extraretinal fibrovascular proliferative tissue of stage 3. (Courtesy of Cryotherapy for Retinopathy of Prematurity Cooperative Group.)

"ragged" and is termed stage 3 ROP (Fig. 10-5). The eye is evaluated in terms of twelve 30° "clock-hour" sectors, and the predominant stage in each sector is noted and the eye is categorized according to the highest stage of ROP observed. Thus, for example, if there are 10 sectors of stage 2 and 2 sectors of stage 3, the eye is categorized as a "stage 3 eye." The unifying principle underlying ICROP is that the more posterior the disease and the greater the amount of retinal vascular involvement, the more serious the disease.

Progressive vascular incompetence, occurring along with the changes described at the edge of the abnormally developing retinal vasculature, is noted by increasing dilation and tortuosity of the peripheral retinal vessels, iris vascular engorgement, pupillary rigidity, and vitreous haze. If this progressive vascular incompetence is so marked that the posterior veins are enlarged and arteries tortuous, this characterizes "plus" disease, and a plus sign (+) is added to the ROP stage number (Fig. 10-6). Progression of ROP may be rapid if plus disease involves zone I or posterior zone II.

The first publication in 1984 by the International Committee defined stage 4 ROP as an unequivocal detachment of the retina caused by exudation, traction, or both.[173] In 1987, another

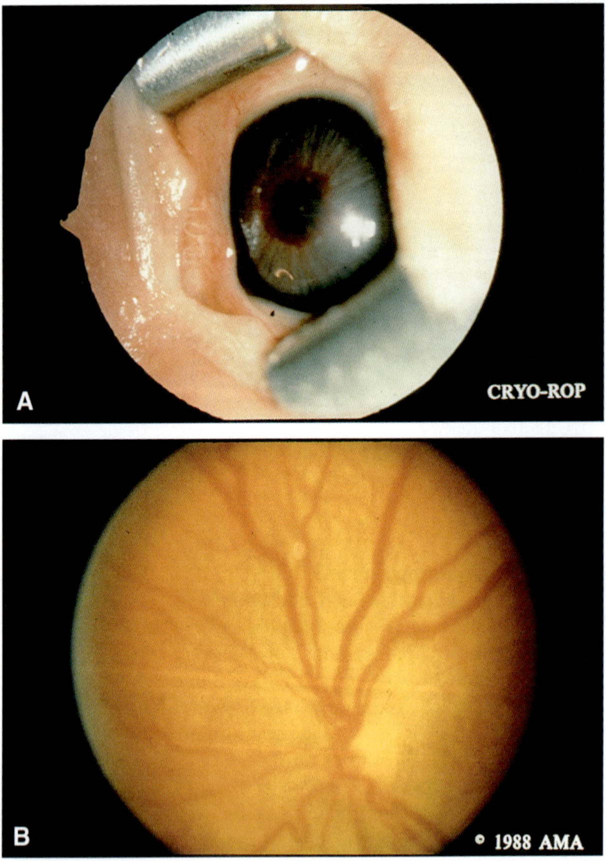

FIGURE 10-6A,B. (A) External photograph of marked iris vascular engorgement that may be part of "plus" disease representing progressive vascular incompetence. (Courtesy of Cryotherapy for Retinopathy of Prematurity Cooperative Group.) **(B)** Standard photography of "plus" disease used for the CRYO-ROP study. Degree of vascular dilatation and tortuosity shown here represented minimum acceptable abnormality to categorize a fundus as plus disease for the study. (From Cryotherapy for Retinopathy of Prematurity Cooperative Group. Multicenter trial of cryotherapy for retinopathy of prematurity: preliminary results. Arch Ophthalmol 1988;106:471–479, with permission.)

international committee expanded the description of the features of the retinal detachment (stage 4).[174] This elaboration was based on further surgical observations and study of pathological specimens.[101] Stage 4A was defined as a concave, tractional type of subtotal retinal detachment occurring in the periphery without involvement of the macula (extrafoveal). The detachment may be circumferential, extending for 360°, or segmental, and extending for less than 360°. The prognosis for vision for this type of detachment is good providing there is no extension into the macula. If the partial detachment extended posteriorly to involve the macula, this was termed stage 4B, and the prognosis for vision for this type of subtotal detachment is poor. Stage 5 is a total funnel-shaped retinal detachment. For descriptive purposes the retinal detachment can be subdivided into an anterior and posterior part based on the configuration of the funnel (see Table 10-3). The most common configuration is a concave detachment with the funnel open both anteriorly and posteriorly. The other configurations in decreasing order of frequency are narrow–narrow, open–narrow, and narrow–open. If opaque retrolental membranes prevent visualization of the fundus, ultrasonography may be helpful in defining the configuration of the funnel.[38,137]

Although regression with or without vascular or cicatricial sequelae is the most common outcome of ROP, the International Committee decided that classification of such a wide variety of changes was impossible. However, they realized the importance of identifying these changes and recommended recording the broad spectrum of peripheral and posterior retinal and vascular changes (Table 10-4). The vascular changes include retinal avascularity, abnormal retinal branching, and telangiectatic retinal vessels (Fig. 10-7). The retinal changes include pigmentary changes, vitreoretinal interface changes, and tractional forces that may cause dragging and displacement of retinal vessels and ectopia of the macula (Fig. 10-8). Traction and rhegmatogenous retinal detachment may also develop as late complications of regressed ROP. In general, the more severe the acute disease in terms of location, extent, and stage, the more serious the resulting regressed peripheral and posterior retinal and vascular sequelae.

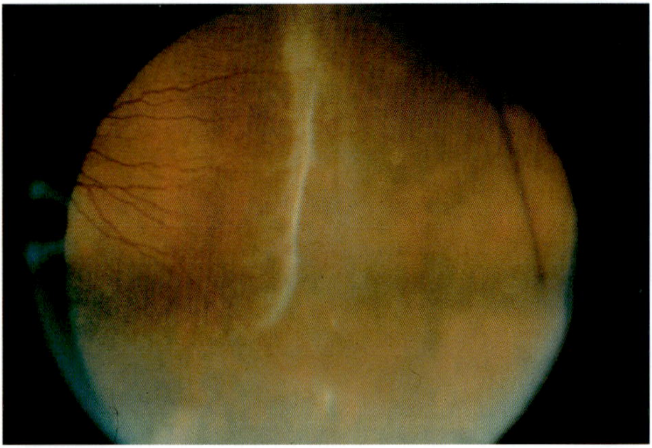

FIGURE 10-7. Regressed ROP: peripheral retinal avascularity, abnormal retinal branching, and retinovitreous interface changes. (From The International Committee for the Classification of the Late Stages of Retinopathy of Prematurity. An international classification of retinopathy of prematurity. II. The classification of retinal detachment. Arch Ophthalmol 1987;105:906–913, with permission.)

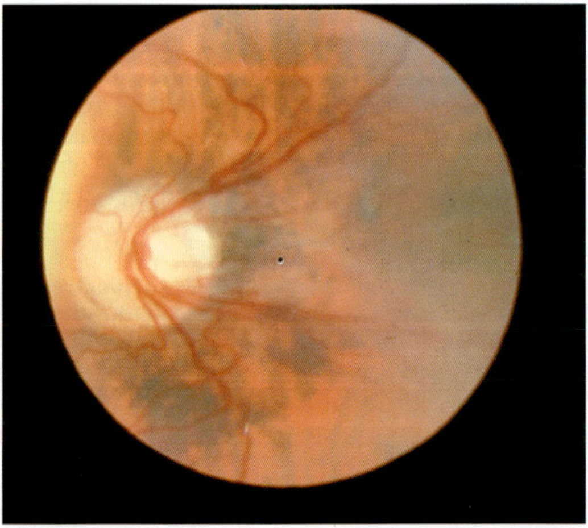

FIGURE 10-8. Regressed ROP: macular pigmentary changes and ectopia. (From Watzke RC, et al. Photographic grading in the retinopathy of prematurity trial. Arch Ophthalmol 1990;108:950–955, with permission.)

CLINICOPATHOLOGICAL CORRELATION OF ROP STAGES

Stage 1: Demarcation Line

This stage represents a thickened exaggeration of the line of normal advancing vasculature and comprises two distinct zones.[54,56] The anterior vanguard zone is formed by a sheet of spindle-shaped cells that are the precursors of the differentiated vascular endothelium. It corresponds to the primitive mesenchyme (spindle cells) seen in normal fetal development, but the cells are hyperplastic, causing the demarcation line to be clinically visible (Fig. 10-9). Behind the proliferating spindle cells is a rear guard zone comprised of endothelial cells that have differentiated from the vanguard mesenchymal cells and are forming a primitive capillary meshwork. This zone is not clinically discernible until stage 2.

Stage 2: Ridge

The ridge represents a further thickening of the line in stage 1 because of continued proliferation of spindle cells in the vanguard zone.[54–56] In addition, a thin white line behind the vanguard is separated by a lucent line of approximately the same width. The white line (ridge) is the predominant feature of this stage and histologically corresponds to proliferation of the endothelial cells of the rear guard zone (Fig. 10-10). The ridge has increasing height, width, and volume and extends up out of the plane of the retina. The ridge may turn from white to pink, which corresponds to an arteriovenous shunt of primitive vascular channels that has been shown clinically to leak fluorescein dye by Flynn et al.[53] The retinal lesions in stage 1 and 2 regress in most cases, leaving few, if any, residual signs.

Stage 3: Ridge with Extraretinal Fibrovascular Proliferation

Stage 3 involves neovascular proliferation of vessels that are continuous with the posterior aspect of the ridge and that extend into the vitreous perpendicular to the plane of the retina.[54–56] Foos[56] referred to these new vessels as "extraretinal vascular-

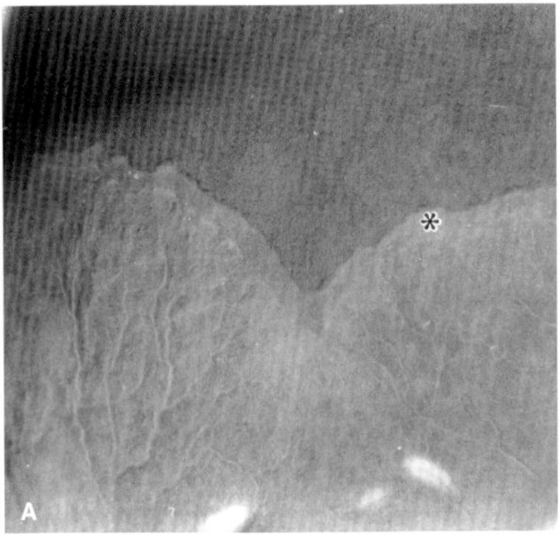

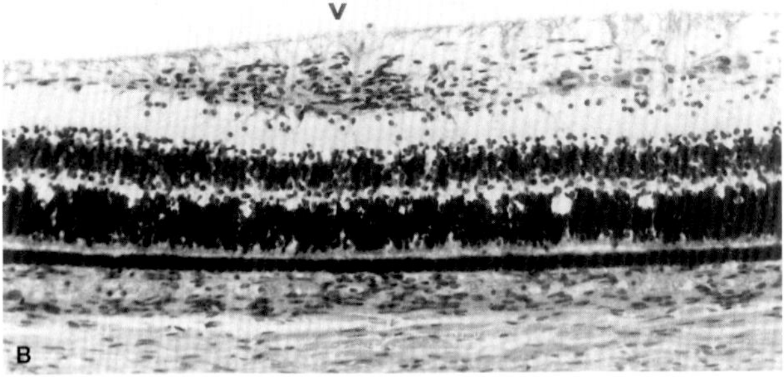

FIGURE 10-9A,B. **(A)** ROP, stage 1: macroscopic demarcation line (*asterisk*) represents a thickened exaggeration of normal vanguard. Vasodilation is evident posterior to the demarcation line. (From Foos RY. Retinopathy of prematurity: pathologic correlation of clinical stages. Retina 1987;7:260–276, with permission.) **(B)** ROP, stage 1: microscopic demarcation line demonstrates thickening of retina that is related to proliferation of spindle cells in vanguard (*V*). H&E, ×300. (From Foos RY. Retinopathy of prematurity: pathologic correlation of clinical stages. Retina 1987;7:260–276, with permission.)

ization" and described three fairly distinct forms: placoid, polypoid, and pedunculated. The placoid form is the most common and has a circumferential orientation because of its occurrence in the region of the ridge (Fig. 10-11). It is also the most impor-

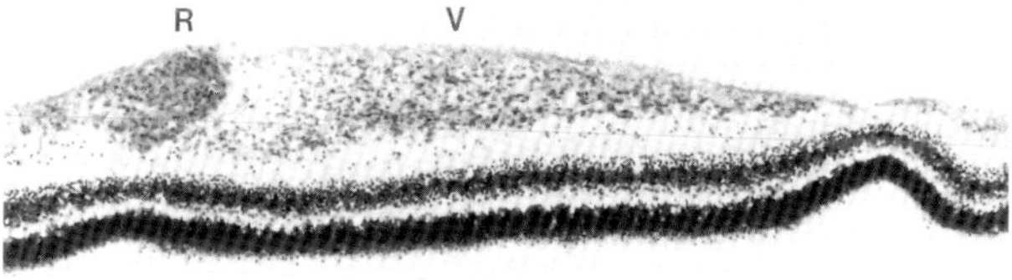

FIGURE 10-10. ROP, stage 2: meridional microsection through retinal ridge, with thick layer of spindle cells that tapers anteriorly (*to the right*), representing the proliferative vanguard zone (*V*), and a round profile of proliferating endothelial cells in the rear guard zone (*R*). H&E, ×250. (From Foos RY. Retinopathy of prematurity: pathologic correlation of clinical stages. Retina 1987;7:260–276, with permission.)

tant type by virtue of its relationship to the early stages of retinal detachment. The polypoid form is uncommon and occurs behind the ridge as isolated sessile mounds. The least common form is the pedunculated type, resembling a sea fan and arising

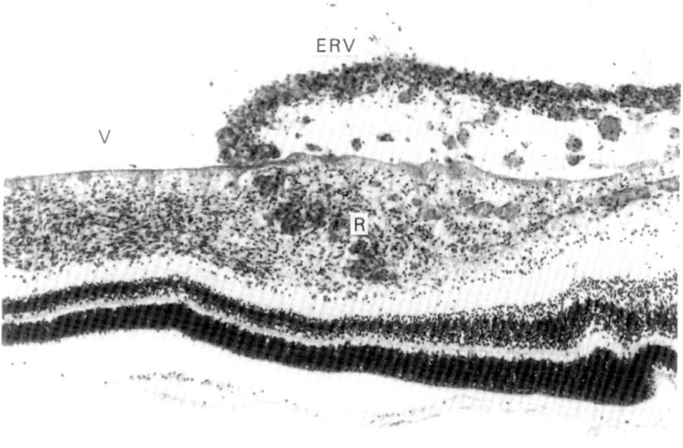

FIGURE 10-11. ROP, stage 3: microsection through placoid extraretinal vascularization shows a portion of vanguard zone (*V*), aggregation of endothelial cells in rear guard zone (*R*), and cords of endothelial cells and delicate vessels extending into a plaque of vasoproliferative tissue (*ERV*) in overlying vitreous. H&E, ×250. (From Foos RY. Retinopathy of prematurity: pathologic correlation of clinical stages. Retina 1987;7:260–276, with permission.)

from the retina behind the ridge. Foos[55,56] has demonstrated microscopically proliferation of solid cords of endothelial cells from the region of the rear guard (ridge) through the retinal surface into the vitreous cavity. Based upon Factor VIII preparations, Foos[56] confirmed that these vessels are derived from proliferating endothelial cells, not from vasoformative mesenchymal cells, as in normal retinal angiogenesis. Serous exudate may accumulate under the retina during stage 3, and alterations of the vitreous also become evident. The changes in the vitreous body take two major forms: synchysis and condensation. Foos[56] suggested that synchytic destruction of the vitreous body was related to the release of lytic substances by incompetent vessels within the retina or vitreous body and that condensation of the vitreous body over the ridge was related to depolymerization of hyaluronic acid and collapse of the collagenous framework into optically visible structures.

Stage 4: Subtotal Retinal Detachment

The retina begins to buckle and fold at the ridge and is drawn anteriorly toward the lens margin by vitreous condensation (Fig. 10-12). Although tractional forces are predominant, the detachment may have a serous component. Commonly, radial tractional forces limited to the temporal quadrants draw the nasal retina temporally, resulting in a meridional fold extending from the region of the disc to the temporal periphery. The contraction process may be so strong that finally all vessels will pass in a straight line from the optic nerve head toward the temporal periphery and nasal retina may overlie the nerve head.

Stage 5: Total Retinal Detachment

As the retina becomes folded and progressively drawn anteriorly and centrally, it becomes pleated or rolled, like a scroll, resulting in foreshortening and progressive detachment of the posterior retina (Fig. 10-13). Subsequently the "V" or funnel shape of the detachment becomes altered in shape by both anterior and posterior closure. Machemer[101] explains the pattern of the retinal detachment based on proliferation and contraction of tissue originating from the shunt area. When the shunt area forms a ring the pattern of the retinal detachment may vary according to whether the shunt area is anterior, equatorial, or posterior in location. For example, with equatorial or posterior

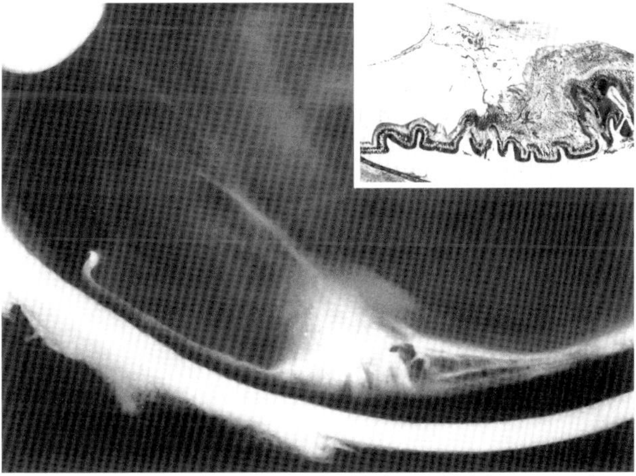

FIGURE 10-12. ROP, late stage 3: buckled and folded retina is being drawn anteriorly toward the lens margin by vitreous condensations emanating from the highly elevated ridge. ×6. *Insert:* microscope features. H&E, ×25. (From Foos FY. Chronic retinopathy of prematurity. Ophthalmology 1985;92:563–574, with permission.)

shunts the avascular peripheral retina stretches and stays attached forming a "trough" at its juncture with the detached nonstretchable vascularized retina. The vitreous undergoes further central synchysis and condensation of vitreous sheets on the retinal surface, but posterior vitreous detachment is rare. Extraretinal proliferation of nonvascular tissue is usually present at this stage, which includes retinal glial processes extending into the vitreous, epithelial membranes, and pigmented and nonpigmented retroretinal membranes.[55,56]

The vitreoretinal traction forces that cause the unique, progressive retinal detachment seen in ROP are poorly understood, especially because some features that characterize proliferative vitreoretinopathy associated with rhegmatogenous retinal detachment in adults are not conspicuous, for example, cell-mediated proliferation along the surface of the detached posterior vitreous.[56] However, the process is multifactorial and includes both intraretinal and extraretinal factors. Intraretinal factors may include contractile proteins in the vanguard cells, contraction of the rear guard endothelial cells, and astrogliosis of the superficial retina[56] Extraretinal factors include contraction

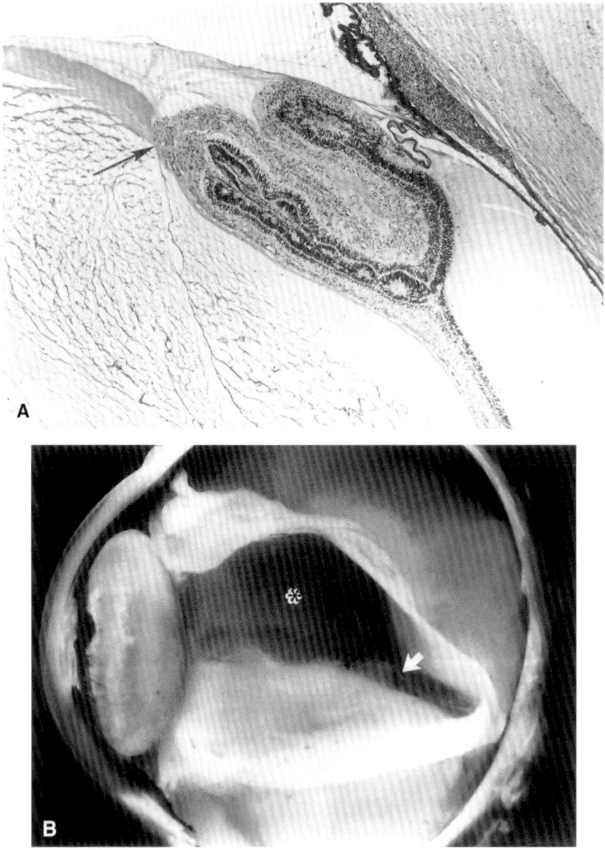

FIGURE 10-13A,B. **(A)** ROP, stage 5: microscopic features of peripheral retina, which is folded and rolled like a scroll. Extraretinal vascularization is notable only at the summit of some of the folds (*arrow*). Posteriorly, the foreshortened retina is detached, and serous exudate is present in retroretinal space and overlying vitreous body. Epiretinal and retroretinal membranes are lacking. H&E, ×60. (From Foos RY. Chronic retinopathy of prematurity. Ophthalmology 1985;92:563–574, with permission.) **(B)** ROP, stage 5: folding and rolling of peripheral retina, foreshortened totally detached retina, retroretinal serous exudate, serous exudate in vitreous, central synchysis of vitreous (*asterisk*), and sheets of condensed vitreous on the retinal surface throughout the fundus (*arrow*). (From Foos RY. Chronic retinopathy of prematurity. Ophthalmology 1985;92:563–574, with permission.)

of the extraretinal vasoproliferative tissue and synchytic destruction of the vitreous body, which provides a scaffold for growth of the extraretinal vessels.[56]

OCULAR FINDINGS IN REGRESSED ROP

Myopia, Astigmatism, and Anisometropia

Myopia is a common finding in the newborn premature infant even without ROP with a tendency toward less myopia by the latter half of the first year after birth.[46,60,72a] Myopia that is of higher degree and persists into later life is usually associated with prematurely born children afflicted with ROP.[30] The incidence of myopia was determined in a large group of premature infants with birth weights of less than 1251 g followed as part of the multicenter study of Cryotherapy for Retinopathy of Prematurity.[30] These eyes, which did not undergo cryotherapy, were refracted at 3, 12, and 24 months. Myopia was observed in approximately 20% of the children at each test age, and the percentage of high myopia (≥5 diopters) doubled from 2% to 4.6% between 3 and 12 months and remained stable thereafter. Lower birth weight and increasing severity of ROP were predictors of myopia and high myopia. In addition, anisometropia, astigmatism, and the presence of macular heterotopia and retinal folds also were associated with a higher incidence of myopia and high myopia. The exact mechanism of the myopia associated with ROP is unknown and may be due to an elongation of the globe, alteration of the lens or the corneal curvature, or a combination of all of these factors.[30,34,46,81,140a] More severe ROP results in a higher risk of myopia.[82a,140a] The degree of myopia at age 3 months predicts the presence of high myopia at 5.5 years; between 3 months and 1 year of age, a decrease in the proportion of eyes with hyperopia and an increase in the proportion with myopia occurs.[140a] Eyes with ROP treated with laser develop less myopia, on average, than do those treated with cryotherapy.[85a] Further animal model work, more studies of biometric measurements in the developing eye, and further observations on the effects of light on the developing eye may help clarify the factors underlying the development of abnormal refractive errors in infants with ROP.[30]

Other studies[34,89,91,98,147] performed in infants with regressed ROP have noted a higher incidence of strabismus, amblyopia, anisometropia, and high refractive errors compared with control groups of infants who did not have ROP. Gallo et al.[58] noted an increased incidence of refractive errors, strabismus, and retinal complications in children with regressed ROP. Microcornea and microphthalmos have also been associated with ROP.[31,81]

Foveal Avascular Zone

Ibayashi et al.[74] studied vascular patterns using fluorescein angiography in patients aged 5 to 15 years with cicatricial retinopathy of prematurity and found a high incidence of incomplete development of avascular zones in the macula when compared to a control group. They concluded that underdevelopment of the foveal avascular zone was an important feature of cicatricial ROP and had a significant correlation with active disease but had no relationship to visual prognosis in most cases. Isenberg[75] demonstrated a delayed macular development in infants with ROP, and he speculated that this possibly could engender amblyopia, which could lead to strabismus.

LATE COMPLICATIONS OF REGRESSED ROP

Glaucoma

Kwitko[94] estimated that secondary glaucoma developed in 30% of eyes with severe retinopathy of prematurity. Young infants or children with severe advanced ROP are most often affected; however, acute angle closure has been reported in adults.[108,151] The mechanism most likely causing secondary angle-closure glaucoma is an anterior displacement of the lens–iris diaphragm secondary to contraction of a retrolental fibroglial mass.[108] However, other mechanisms have been proposed. In adult eyes with ROP and no retrolental mass, possible mechanisms include both pupillary block and ciliary block.[90,108] Increased lens thickness has been documented in ROP patients and may also play a role in a pupillary block mechanism.[108] Progressive very high myopia maybe a sign that the large lens is crowding the angle, and glaucoma is a risk. Other mechanisms to explain secondary angle-closure glaucoma seen in ROP include inflammation[93] and anterior segment neovascularization.[108] Hartnett et al.[68] prospectively examined the anterior segment of 27 eyes of 17 premature infants with stage 4 and 5 ROP to identify and classify structural characteristics that could predispose the premature infant with ROP to glaucoma. In addition to identifying pathological changes, for example, anterior and posterior synechiae, they noted changes that may have a developmental origin such as corneal dystrophy, Barkan's-like membrane, and large tunica vasculosa-like vessels. Thus, abnormal development of the angle and inadequate outflow could possibly contribute to the pathogenetic mechanism of glaucoma seen in eyes with advanced ROP.[68]

The choice of therapy for secondary glaucoma in ROP may include medical or surgical measures and is based on the initial intraocular pressure and vision, degree of lens opacity and intumescence, presence of anterior segment neovascularization, and the gonioscopic appearance of the anterior chamber angle.[108] Acute angle-closure glaucoma occurring in adults may respond to medical treatment, including miotic therapy. Following stabilization of intraocular pressure, laser iridotomy or surgical peripheral iridectomy can be performed.[108,151] Kushner[90] reported the successful relief of apparent ciliary block glaucoma in two children and one adult with cicatricial ROP using cycloplegic therapy after failure of miotic therapy. Two of these patients later required either lensectomy or vitreous aspiration. Pars plana lensectomy and anterior vitrectomy or lensectomy via the limbal approach has been advocated by Pollard[135,136] to treat secondary angle-closure glaucoma with severe advanced cicatricial ROP. Most of these patients presented after the age of 2 years. Although patients had final vision of only light perception to hand motion, his rational was to retain a painfree eye and avoid enucleation. Kushner and Sondheimer[93] treated seven children with cicatricial grade 5 ROP and secondary glaucoma with shallow anterior chambers with corticosteroids. They were able to control intraocular pressures and avoid enucleation. Inflammation in these eyes secondary to either phacolytic glaucoma, blood or blood breakdown products, or neovascular glaucoma responded to topical corticosteroids. Filtering surgery for late-onset acute or chronic angle-closure glaucoma may be necessary if intraocular pressure cannot be controlled with either medical treatment or peripheral iridectomy.[108] Alloplastic tube shunt implantation may be the treatment of choice for neovascularization-induced secondary angle closure in eyes with useful vision potential.[108] Ciliodestructive procedures are recommended for blind and painful eyes.[108]

Late-Onset Retinal Detachment

Retinal detachment is a complication of regressed ROP in the childhood or teen years, or even later in life. Eyes at risk for late-onset retinal detachment have changes described by the committee for the classification of ROP[174] that include abnormal peripheral vascular changes, avascular peripheral retina, straightening of the temporal blood vessels, vascular tortuosity, retinal pigment epithelial changes, vitreoretinal interface changes, retinal folds, vitreous membranes, retinal breaks, and lattice-like degeneration. Because ROP represents a lifelong threat to vision, afflicted patients should be examined at least once each year for life. Additionally, these eyes often have high myopia.[158–160] Tasman[160] reported a greater than 80% incidence of myopia, usually greater than 6 diopters, in regressed ROP. It is uncertain whether retinal breaks and retinal detachment in regressed ROP are secondary to ongoing changes of ROP, to abnormal vitreoretinal interface changes due to ROP, or to some other unrecognized factor.[152] The high myopia and the lattice-like changes seen in regressed ROP may also place these eyes at high risk for development of retinal detachment.[152]

Previously reported series using standard scleral buckling procedures in the management of retinal detachment associated with regressed ROP showed a final success rate ranging from 63% to 100%.[41,66,158,163] Because retinal detachments associated with regressed ROP can be associated with significant vitreoretinal traction and/or posterior retinal breaks, vitrectomy techniques in conjunction with scleral buckling may be required for optimal management to achieve long-term reattachment. Sneed et al.[152] successfully reattached 14 (88%) of 16 eyes with retinal detachment associated with regressed ROP. A pars plana vitrectomy was required in 8 eyes; 4 eyes either initially presented with proliferative vitreoretinopathy, posterior retinal breaks, subretinal fibrosis, or vitreoretinal traction bands, and the remaining 4 eyes had posterior vitreoretinal traction after failed scleral buckling procedures. Visual acuity stabilized or improved in 13 of the 14 eyes with successful retinal reattachment. In a series of 29 pediatric eyes with retinal detachment, Fivgas and Capone[44a] noted that 34% were related to Stickler syndrome or ROP, another 34% to prior ocular surgery. Average age of presentation was 9.6 years, but late diagnosis was a problem. In this heterogeneous group, which included late-onset detachment from ROP, 72% were reattached after 2.2 surgeries per eye.[44a]

DIFFERENTIAL DIAGNOSIS

In early stages of ROP, the principal condition to differentiate is familial exudative vitreoretinopathy[24,117] (FEVR), which has features in both the acute and late forms of the disease that may be indistinguishable from ROP. Familial exudative vitreoretinopathy may be autosomal dominant, X-linked recessive, or autosomal recessive.[147b] It occurs in infants who are otherwise normal and may be full term. Clinical findings in the acute form include peripheral retinal avascularity, retinal exudates, and extraretinal neovascularization. Progression may occur slowly, and late changes include temporal dragging of the macula, organized vitreous membranes, vitreo-retinal traction, retinal breaks, and retinal detachment. Severe changes are often asymmetrical, and may not be detected until several years after birth.[117] Criswick and Schepens[24] have observed that familial exudative vitreoretinopathy cannot only mimic features of ROP, but also Coat's disease, peripheral uveitis or pars plantis, and other posterior segment abnormalities. Interestingly, mutations in the gene that causes congenital RD in Norrie disease have also been implicated as causative in FEVR and may be related to the severity of some ROP cases.[147c]

The differential diagnosis of advanced ROP includes other conditions associated with leukocoria including persistent hyperplastic primary vitreous, retinoblastoma, and Norrie disease. Persistent hyperplastic primary vitreous is a congenital anomaly, usually unilateral, and occurring in the term infant.[139] Anterior segment abnormalities are common and include microcornea, shallow anterior chamber, and elongated ciliary processes. The posterior segment findings may include vitreous membranes and a stalk containing hyaloid artery remnants. The retina can be incorporated into the vitreous membranes and pulled forward, forming a retinal fold that may extend to the periphery.

Although retinoblastoma is rarely confused with ROP, it should be considered in the differential diagnosis. Infants with retinoblastoma, in general, have a history of term birth, and no supplementary oxygen use. There may be a positive family history of retinoblastoma. Although ROP is usually bilateral and fairly symmetrical[35,42] retinoblastoma is often unilateral and if bilateral, is asymmetrical. Ultrasonography and computed tomography (CT) scans are usually helpful in differentiating the large mass lesion of retinoblastoma, which usually demonstrates calcium, from the complex retinal detachment associated with vitreoretinal membranes in advanced ROP.

Norrie disease is a rare syndrome of retinal dysplasia, deafness, and mental retardation and/or deterioration that can mimic advanced ROP.[99] Norrie disease has an X-linked recessive pattern of inheritance and is not associated with prematurity. Patients with Norrie disease demonstrate leukocoria considerably earlier than those with ROP.

Infants with congenital cataract may present with leukocoria, however, the diagnosis is easily made by slit lamp examination; when the retina is visualized despite the presence of the cataract, it is normal.

Cases of ROP have been reported[86,92,149] in full-term infants of normal birth weight and with no history of supplemental oxygen use. At least some of these may have represented sporadic cases of familial exudative vitreoretinopathy, or cases in which either family members were not examined or a family history could not be obtained because of asymptomatic, mild disease. Given the pathogenesis of ROP, it seems unlikely that this form of retinopathy could occur to any serious degree in full-term infants.

EXAMINATION PROCEDURES IN THE NURSERY

Selection of Patients for Screening

The demonstration that cryotherapy of the peripheral retina in advanced stage 3+ ROP can significantly reduce the chances of an unfavorable outcome mandates the following: all infants at high risk of developing "threshold" disease must be screened.[26–28,32] A comprehensive ROP screening program should be developed and a close working relationship established between ophthalmologists and the medical and nursing staffs of NICUs. An ideal screening program should be able to detect all cases of ROP when they commence and, at the same time, reduce unnecessary retinal examinations.

Unfortunately, although many recommendations have been made,[154] a universally accepted set of indications for screening examinations has not been established due to an inadequate database concerning the onset, progression, resolution, and outcome of ROP. Although it is agreed that the risk of ROP increases inversely with birth weight, the establishment of an upper "limit" of birth weight is controversial. Although the CRYO-ROP study did not collect data on infants greater than 1250g, other studies have reported that stage 3 does not develop in infants weighing more than 1500g[42] or 1600g.[12] However, some clinicians still use 2000g as an upper "limit" of birth weight.

Because ROP is also inversely related to gestational age, the timing of the examination is also critical. Although a universally accepted indication for the timing of the exam has not been adopted, there are good guidelines available.[22,26,29,119,120] Palmer[119,120] suggested that the optimal age for the initial examination for acute ROP is between 7 and 9 weeks of age. His data, additionally, suggested that screening examinations performed during the first month of life have a low yield of positive findings and are insufficient. In the wake of the proof that treatment is beneficial, the authors of the CRYO-ROP study recommended that initial eye examinations begin at 4 to 6 weeks of age.[26] A more recent report from the CRYO-ROP study[29] indicated that postconceptional age (gestational plus postnatal age) of the infant correlated better with the time of onset of either prethreshold or threshold ROP than does the postnatal age. A British study[42] determined that ROP is rarely seen before 31 weeks postconceptual age. Screening guidelines have, therefore, been drawn up by the British Association for Perinatal Medicine and the College of Ophthalmologists, which confines screening to infants weighing less than 1500g at birth with the fundus examination(s) carried out between 32 and 36 weeks postconceptional age.

In the United States, screening guidelines have been recommended in a joint statement from the American Academy of Pediatrics, the American Association for Pediatric Ophthalmology and Strabismus, and the American Academy of Ophthalmology.[3] These recommendations are as follows:

1. Infants with a birth weight of less than 1500g or with a gestational age of 28 weeks or less, as well as selected infants between 1500 and 2000g with an unstable clinical course who are believed to be at a high risk by their attending pediatrician or neonatologist, should have at least two fundus examinations performed after pupillary dilation using binocular indirect ophthalmoscopy to detect ROP. One examination is sufficient only

if it unequivocally shows the retina to be fully vascularized bilaterally.

2. Examination for ROP should be performed by an ophthalmologist with sufficient regular experience and knowledge in the examination of preterm infants for ROP to identify the location and sequential retinal changes in this disorder using binocular indirect ophthalmoscopy. The location and sequential retinal changes, if any, should be recorded using the International Classification of Retinopathy of Prematurity.

3. The first examination should normally be performed between 4 and 6 weeks of chronological age or, alternatively, within the 31st to 33rd week of postconceptional or postmenstrual age (gestational age at birth plus chronological age), whichever is later, as determined by the infant's attending pediatrician or neonatologist. If using the postconceptional age guideline, examinations are generally not needed in the first 4 weeks after birth. Treatment should generally be accomplished within 72h of determination of the presence of threshold ROP to minimize the risk of retinal detachment before treatment.

Beyond these national guidelines, "local" standards should be developed in cooperation with the neonatologist to identify possible special risk factors in infants with birth weights heavier than the guideline weight, for example, very ill infants, postasphyxia infants, or fetal hydrops. Trese and Batton[172] reported the isolated occurrence of bilateral stage 5 ROP in an infant with fetal hydrops weighing 1840g, indicating that birth weight alone may not be a sufficient criterion.

The results of the CRYO-ROP study[26,27] provided guideline information on which to base a follow-up schedule, once the initial screening examination is completed. Eyes with any zone II disease that is not prethreshold were examined at 2-week intervals. Prethreshold eyes (zone I, any stage; zone II, stage 2+; stage 3 or 3+ with less than required "clock hours" of involvement) were seen at least weekly. If an eye is seen with severe zone I involvement, but is still prethreshold, examinations should be considered at intervals less than 1 week; these eyes that are referred to as "rush"-type ROP can progress very rapidly.[114] Eyes with zone III involvement develop threshold ROP extremely rarely, if ever; therefore, these eyes, with or without ROP, can be examined 4 weeks later. However, the examiner must be cautious in determining zone III. If retinal vessels are not fully mature on the nasal side, the eye should still be considered a zone II eye. Eyes with no ROP, but immature retinal vasculature, should be seen in 1 to 2 weeks with zone I, 2 weeks with zone II involvement, but zone III eyes can be seen in 3 to 4 weeks. Premature eyes should be followed until retinal vascularization is mature and extends to the ora, which usually occurs between 37 and 40 weeks postconception.[4,48,57] In 90% of patients, involution begins by 44 weeks.[142a] Eyes with mild ROP or prethreshold ROP must be followed until threshold criteria are reached or until evidence of regression and stabilization occurs. Care should be exercised because, even if regression is noted, ROP can rarely reactivate resulting in double-demarcation lines.[56] In eyes that have mild ROP and have reached complete regression, the motility and refractive status should be checked at 6 to 12 months of age because of the increased incidence of astigmatism, strabismus, and myopia.[30,34,48,89,91,147] Even in the absence of need for continuing early eye care, annual examination should be continued indefinitely in individuals with vitreoretinal sequelae of ROP because of the risk of late-onset complications such as glaucoma[108] and retinal detachment.[158–160]

Mode of Examination

A timely and efficient examination can result if the NICU nursing staff anticipates the physician's arrival and arranges the infant's feeding schedule and any testing or procedures accordingly. Pupils may be effectively dilated in most infants with Cyclomydril eyedrops (cyclopentolate 0.2% and phenylephrine 1%) or a combination mixture that can be prepared by the hospital pharmacy and includes 7.5 ml cyclopentolate 1%, 7.5 ml tropicamide 1%, and 0.625 ml phenylephrine 10%. The final concentration of this solution, respectively, is 0.48%, 0.48%, and 0.4%. Cyclopentolate 0.5% may also be used. Carpel and Kalina[17] demonstrated the value of dilute phenylephrine to supplement mydriasis for these examinations. Eyedrops are instilled twice at 5-min intervals. We do not routinely occlude puncta, but do blot excess drops immediately from the lids. Although the systemic risks of dilating a premature infant in this way are minimal, awareness of possible side effects such as hypertension and intestinal ileus is important.[121] The examination in VLBW infants may be extremely difficult due to poor pupillary dilation. The examiner should be aware, however, that the very patients whose pupils are most resistant to dilatation due to plus disease are the ones harboring the most threatening ROP. Other difficulties encountered include residual pupillary membrane strands (tunica vasculosis lentis), transient cataracts of prematurity, hyaloid vascular remnants, and vitreous haze.

A lid speculum is placed after instillation of topical anesthetic, such as proparacaine. A variety of lid speculums are available for the premature infant (Fig. 10-14). As a precaution against viral or chlamydial transfer, the lid speculum should be sterile for each infant. Some NICUs may require gloves as a routine

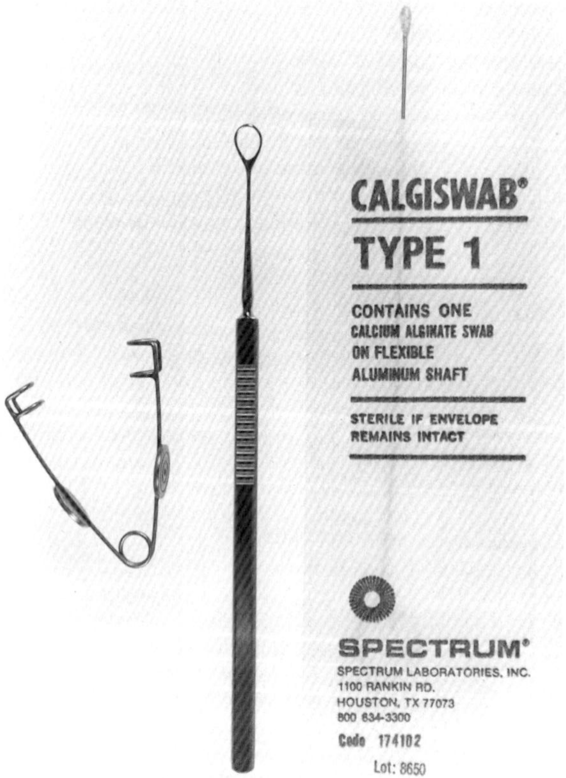

FIGURE 10-14. Alphonso lid speculum used for ROP screening examinations (*left*). Small lens loop (*middle*) or an aluminum wire nasopharyngeal culture swab (*right*) can be used for peripheral scleral depression and rotation of the globe.

policy for infant examinations or they may be worn at the discretion of the examiner. It is advisable to have a nursing staff member present during the entire examination to assist in physically restraining the infant, as well as monitoring the infant's vital signs and airway. Bradycardia, due to the oculocardiac reflex, is a recognized complication of the examination, and may be caused by traction on the extraocular muscles, pressure on the globe, scleral depression, and the use of a lid speculum.[21]

The examination is performed about 30 to 45 min after instillation of dilating drops with a binocular indirect ophthalmoscope and a 28 diopter lens. Gentle scleral depression and ocular rotation can be accomplished with either a sterile small lens loop or an aluminum wire nasopharyngeal culture swab (see Fig. 10-13). If the examiner thinks of these depressors as primarily for rotating the eye, scleral depression can be performed atraumatically and provides information regarding the peripheral retina, such as extent of avascularity, zone III fibrovascular proliferation, and early traction retinal detachment, which will assist the clinician in determining treatment decisions, follow-up examination schedules, and the patient's prognosis. Also, in a teaching institution residents and fellows should be instructed to appreciate the entire spectrum of retinal manifestations in ROP.

The onset of severe ROP often occurs in infants after their systemic medical problems are stable and they are nearing discharge from the NICU, which makes it especially difficult emotionally on the parents or guardians. Discharge should be delayed if progression seems likely. When an infant reaches prethreshold ROP, we recommend that the attending ophthalmologist inform the parents or guardians of the examination results, prognosis, and follow-up schedule. Whenever possible, this should be accomplished in a conference with the participation of an attending neonatologist, primary nurse, and social worker or in writing. The emotional burden on the parents or guardians may be reduced by a thorough discussion of the problems, especially if an infant requires eventual treatment because of progression of ROP or sustains visual loss.

PROPHYLAXIS AND THERAPY

For infants who are born prematurely, it appears that the extrauterine environment must nurture homeostasis and simulate intrauterine conditions as well as possible. Until the factors that are necessary for the healthy maturation of human infants are better understood, the prevention of blinding ROP hinges on preventing prematurity. Indeed, for each week the infant stays in the normal uterine environment, the odds of eventually developing threshold ROP reduce. In the CRYO-ROP study there was a 19% lowering of the odds of reaching threshold for each additional week of gestational age for all natural history patients.[33]

Surfactant

Clinical trials[82] have demonstrated that surfactant therapy can reduce the severity of respiratory distress syndrome and in some cases lead to a reduction in mortality and a decrease in the incidence of chronic lung disease in preterm infants. A deficiency in natural surfactant (a complex mixture of phospholipids, neutral lipids, and proteins synthesized by type II pneumocytes) is the primary cause of the respiratory distress syndrome. A variety of mammalian, human, and synthetic preparations have been demonstrated to reduce the extent of lung disease by reducing surface tension and stabilizing alveoli, which improves aeration of the newborn's lung.

Several studies have evaluated the effect of prophylactic surfactant therapy on the incidence and severity of ROP.[142,143] In a retrospective study, Repka et al.[143] compared control infants with surfactant-treated infants and noted a significantly lower incidence of any stage of ROP. Their data suggested that surfactant may reduce the incidence and severity of ROP in the VLBW population. However, in a later prospective study,[142] the incidence and severity of ROP did not vary between the control and surfactant-treated infants. These investigators predicted that the absolute number of ROP patients will likely increase because of the decrease in mortality of VLBW surfactant-treated infants.

Vitamin E

In 1949, Owens and Owens[118] first investigated the use of vitamin E for the treatment of ROP in a nonrandomized study. Their rationale for treatment was based on the observation that preterm infants were known to be deficient in vitamin E. Interestingly, at that time the antioxidant properties of vitamin E were not known and oxygen had not yet been implicated as a causative factor in ROP. The antioxidant properties of vitamin E are now well established, and there are theoretical reasons why vitamin E may be important in the premature infant and in ROP. Also, animal studies[132] have suggested that vitamin E may prevent oxygen-induced retinopathy.

Vitamin E belongs to a group of compounds found in human tissue and termed *tocopherols*, alpha-tocopherol accounting for 90% of all tocopherols.[110] Vitamin E is one of several antioxidants found in human tissues; these are essential in protecting molecules from oxidative damage by oxygen-derived free radicals. Free radicals are chemical species with an unpaired electron produced as a result of many biological reactions that may produce cell membrane damage if not countered by antioxidants. Vitamin E traps free radicals formed as a result of the oxidation of the unsaturated fatty acids of membrane phospholipids and is important in maintaining the integrity and stability of biological membranes. Because of exposure to increased oxygen concentration in the face of reduced antioxidant defenses, the premature infant is theoretically at risk of retinal damage from oxygen-derived free radicals.

Kretzer et al.[87,88] developed a hypothesis regarding the role of spindle cells in the development of ROP based on ultrastructural observations from preterm infant postmortem retinas. They demonstrated gap junctions in spindle cells and an increase in endoplasmic reticulum, which synthesizes and secretes an angiogenic factor. This may in turn lead to metaplasia to myofibroblasts that invade the vitreous causing membranes to exert tractional forces on the retina. They postulated that vitamin E supplementation stabilizes spindle cells, minimizing gap junction formation, and interrupting the sequence of events leading to neovascularization and retinal detachment.

The role of vitamin E prophylactic supplementation is controversial because numerous clinical trials have been conducted with conflicting results.[43,44,77,110,133,138,146] Some reported no significant effect of vitamin E,[133,138] others a significant decrease in severity but not in incidence,[44,146] whereas others reported a significant decrease in both severity and incidence of ROP.[43,77] A meta-analysis of 1418 infants reported in the literature found a 52% reduction in incidence of stage 3+ ROP in vitamin E-treated infants, but adverse effects could not be evaluated.[140b] The differences in results may be explained by the relatively small numbers of patients in these studies, the problems associated with low-incidence events, and the number of variables involved.[110] The variables include patient selection; dosage of vitamin E in controls; method of administration (oral, intramuscular, or intravenous); the dose, scheduling, and duration of vitamin E treatment; the plasma vitamin E concentrations achieved; and methods of statistical analysis.[110] Law et al.[97] analyzed seven randomized trials of vitamin E supplementation in ROP. They calculated the relative risk of developing ROP from the individual trials and then combined them using standard statistical techniques to give a summary estimate. Their results showed no statistical reduction in risk of ROP following vitamin E treatment either for all infants with ROP or for those with severe ROP.

Despite inconclusive results, prophylactic vitamin E supplementation might be justified if there were no risks involved with the therapy. However, complications have been reported in premature infants that would place a significant number of infants who would not develop severe ROP at risk of developing complications from vitamin E supplementation. A significant increase in the incidence of necrotizing enterocolitis has been reported in infants treated with vitamin E.[43,76] Johnson et al.[76] also reported a significantly increased incidence of sepsis in their treated group. In 1983, E-Ferol, which is an intravenous vitamin E preparation, was recalled following the deaths of 38 infants who received this preparation.[129] The carrier (polysorbate 80) may have been responsible for this syndrome, rather than vitamin E itself.[2]

In summary, the neonatologist must consider the risk–benefit relationship when using vitamin E supplementation; however, the risks appear minimal for premature infants so long as "physiological" serum vitamin E levels (1–3 mg/dl) are maintained. Vitamin E is a component of intravenous multiple vitamin supplements, and "physiological" serum vitamin E levels can be safely achieved even if this preparation is administered on the first day of life in the recommended doses with intravenously supplied maintenance fluids.[40] However, caution should be used when considering high doses, because the American Committee of Fetus and Newborn[23] concluded that "at this time, however, the Committee regards prophylactic use of pharmacologic vitamin E as experimental and cannot recommend that high doses of vitamin E be given routinely to infants weighing less than 1500 g, even if said use is limited to infants who require supplemental oxygen."

Cryotherapy

Transscleral cryotherapy to the avascular retina in infants with ROP was first advocated as a treatment modality in Japan in the 1970s.[145] The treatment rationale for cryotherapy in ROP is based on previous studies that showed successful regression of neovascularization in other ischemic retinopathies using ablative techniques with cryotherapy or photocoagulation. Theories regarding the mechanism of action of cryotherapy have included the belief that ablation of ischemic retina reduces the formation of vasoformative substances and, thus, the stimulus to neovascularization.

The use of cryotherapy also gained acceptance in other parts of the world.[10,69] Ben-Sira et al.[10] treated only the avascular peripheral retina in 18 eyes of 9 infants with active retinopathy. Regression of active retinopathy occurred in all eyes with long-term retention of good vision in 15 eyes. Hindle[69] reported successful results in severe acute ROP treating both the neovascular ridge and the avascular retina anterior to the ridge. However, other reports were more skeptical regarding the outcomes following cryotherapy for acute ROP.[67,80,83] Keith[80] applied cryotherapy to the vascular ridge of 15 eyes in 9 infants with active retinopathy. He observed that infants in the treated group fared considerably worse than in the untreated group, and final outcome was not influenced. Harris and McCormick[67] treated 10 eyes of 10 infants with either photocoagulation and/or cryopexy, and their early observations suggested that treatment was neither harmful nor particularly beneficial. Kingham[83] treated 14 eyes in 12 infants with acute retrolental fibroplasia with cryotherapy. He concluded that for only 1 or possibly 2 eyes was the treatment of value; for the remaining 12 eyes, it was either ineffective or deleterious. He concluded that treatment by cryotherapy was rarely, if ever, indicated or justified. Pilot studies randomizing eyes with severe ROP to either cryotherapy or observation have been performed.[164,165] Palmer and Goodman[122] reported inconclusive results in the management of 15 severe ROP patients. Tasman et al.[164,165] suggested that cryotherapy appears to be preferred over no treatment in the management of 28 patients with bilateral symmetrical stage 3 ROP where one eye was assigned to cryotherapy and the other to control.

These early conflicting reports are probably a result of multiple factors including small groups of patients, variations in the timing of treatment intervention, lack of a common classification system, lack of control eyes, and difference in treatment technique. Two major different treatment techniques included ablation to either the neovascular ridge (arteriovenous shunt) or the avascular retina anterior to the shunt.[109]

CRYO-ROP Study

To resolve the uncertainty about the value of cryotherapy for ROP, a multicenter trial (the CRYO-ROP study) was designed to evaluate its safety and efficacy.[26] In January 1986, 23 participating centers began enrolling eligible infants weighing less than 1251 g. Infants were initially examined between 4 and 6 weeks of age and examinations were recorded every 2 weeks unless the ROP reached a "prethreshold" level (zone I, any stage; zone II, stage 2 with "plus" disease, or zone II, stage 3) (see Table 10-2). Examinations were then repeated at least weekly until the prethreshold disease either regressed or showed progression to threshold disease, which was defined as at least five continuous or eight cumulative 30° sectors (clock hours) of stage 3 ROP in zone I or II in the presence of plus disease (see Table 10-2; Figs. 10-6, 10-15). If both eyes developed threshold ROP, one eye was randomly assigned to receive cryotherapy, while the other eye served as a control. If only one eye developed threshold, only that eye was randomized to either cryotherapy or no treatment. If the less severely affected fellow eye reached threshold and the first eye had been randomized to "no cryotherapy," cryotherapy was offered for the second eye, so that all infants who had two eyes with threshold ROP had the opportunity to receive cryotherapy in one eye. If ROP in either eye reached stage 4, the infant was considered monocular and deemed ineligible for enrollment in the trial.

Treatment Technique

Cryotherapy may be applied transconjunctivally under topical, local, or general anesthesia. In the CRYO-ROP study, 27.5% of all treatments were performed under general anesthesia while the remainder were done with local anesthesia.[27] Cryotherapy can be performed with a standard retinal probe, pediatric probe, or cataract probe. A pediatric T-shaped probe with a reverse curve may be useful because of the small shaft, yet larger area

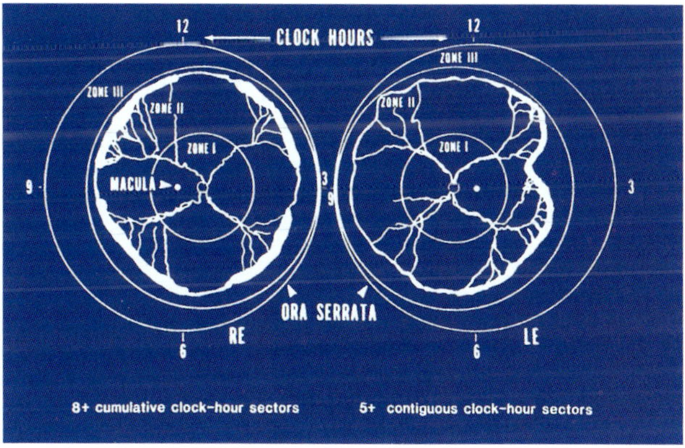

FIGURE 10-15. Diagram of two representative eyes that have reached threshold for randomization. Right eye (*RE*): at least eight cumulative 30° sectors (clock hours) of stage 3. Left eye (*LE*): at least five contiguous 30° sectors of stage 3. *Thin line* of ROP represents stage 1 or 2, and *broader sketched line* signifies stage 3. (From Cryotherapy for Retinopathy of Prematurity Cooperative Group. Multicenter trial of cryotherapy for retinopathy of prematurity: Preliminary results. Arch Ophthalmol 1988;106:471–479, with permission.)

of treatment that can be applied. The smaller (1.5 mm) spherical pediatric probe may also be helpful for treating posteriorly located disease or when retreating between "skipped" areas at a later date. If a disease is located in posterior zone II, or in zone I, one approach is to treat the most posterior avascular retina with laser using an indirect ophthalmoscopic delivery system (see below), and completing the treatment anteriorly with cryotherapy. With increasing experience and the use of pediatric probes, there is less need to open the conjunctiva to treat posteriorly with cryotherapy, but in zone I cases it may be necessary, unless laser is used for the posterior application of the treatment. If necessary, the conjunctiva is opened with a scissors snip in the oblique quadrants between the rectus muscles. Each conjunctival incision is closed with a single 8-0 chromic suture. Whenever the conjunctiva is surgically incised or is inadvertently torn by the cryoprobe, it is an open surgical procedure and should be treated with appropriate sterile technique.

Cryotherapy is begun under direct visualization anteriorly at the ora serrata, followed by more posterior applications. The instant a freeze is noted, the footpedal should be released and thawing begun. A freeze usually takes approximately 2s to appear; however, when insulated by an extraocular muscle it may take much longer. If a freeze is delayed, the probe should be checked for contact with the globe. One then moves to another area of the avascular retina and treats again, constantly being aware of avoiding unnecessary pressure on the globe, and releasing the probe periodically to restore circulation. Approximately 50 treatment applications will be necessary in an average eye, using a standard retinal probe.[26] If a smaller probe is used, more applications will be necessary. Previously treated areas blanch within a few minutes and remain visible during the surgery. Treatment should be contiguous and nonoverlapping, and treatment of the neovascular ridge should be avoided; however, treatment should extend to the anterior edge of the ridge. Treatment can be technically difficult and time-consuming, even to an experienced surgeon. The first-time premie cryosurgeon should be prepared for at least an hour's session and, if the ROP is located in zone I, probably substantially longer.

Following cryotherapy the infant will require reevaluation by a neonatologist. Occasionally, in infants not intubated, the stress of treatment necessitates reintubation and resumption of assisted ventilation. Even in stable infants, close systemic monitoring is necessary after treatment. The eyes are inspected daily for signs of infection. There is no proven necessity for any postoperative topical medication, but a topical antibacterial seems prudent. Posterior synechiae are not often a significant problem in the immediate postoperative period, but a mydriatic or cycloplegic (such as 2% homatropine hydrobromide) to move the pupil for a few days may be beneficial and may decrease pain. Topical steroids may be considered if significant inflammation occurs.

In cases that show a favorable effect from cryotherapy, plus disease subsides within the first few days, and this is followed by regression of extraretinal fibrovascular proliferation in 10 to 21 days. Postoperative examination of the fundus should be performed 5 to 7 days following treatment, to evaluate for untreated (skipped) areas. If these are found near the ridge in association with persistence of plus disease, and if there is either segmental shallow retinal detachment or progression of extraretinal fibrovascular proliferation in this same quadrant, additional treatment of untreated avascular retina is indicated.[26]

In an effort to minimize surgical and visual morbidity, a modification of the standard treatment technique in the CRYO-

ROP study has been proposed.[113,153] Nissenkorn et al.[113] reported successful anatomic results in 23 infants using only one row of cryo applications to the avascular retina anterior to the fibrovascular ridge of stage 3 ROP. Spencer et al.[153] reported regression in 17 of 18 eyes with stage 3+ ROP using cryotherapy applications limited to the avascular retina adjacent to the areas of stage 3 disease. These approaches have not been validated by adequate controlled studies.

Results of the CRYO-ROP Study

The CRYO-ROP study registered 9751 infants with birth weights less than 1251 g at 23 study centers between January 1986 and November 1987.[27] Many of these infants (3929) were excluded from further follow-up for various reasons (death, transfer out of study center, or declined consent), leaving 4099 infants remaining who were followed up sequentially according to the protocol. Of these, 291 eventually reached threshold ROP and were randomized into the cryotherapy trial. At 3 and 12 months after randomization, a detailed fundus examination was performed and stereoscopic photographs of the posterior pole and anterior segment were taken. The primary outcome for eyes in this clinical trial was derived from masked assessment of the photographs. Outcomes were classified as "unfavorable" if the photographs showed (1) a posterior retinal fold involving the macula, (2) a retinal detachment involving zone I of the posterior pole, or (3) a retrolental mass obscuring the posterior pole. All eyes with other fundus appearances were classified as having a "favorable" outcome.

The randomized cohort of 291 infants had a mean birth weight of 800 g and a mean gestational age of 26.3 weeks. Bilateral threshold disease was present in 82.5% of the infants and 22.7% of the infants were from multiple births. The mean chronological age at which randomization occurred was 11.3 weeks and the mean postconception age (gestational age plus chronological age) was 37.7 weeks. Of the 265 treated eyes, 17 required additional cryotherapy. The criteria for retreatment were the persistence of plus disease 3 to 17 days after cryotherapy, with adjacent untreated avascular retina.

Of the 279 infants who survived 3 months following randomization, 273 returned for outcome examination at that time.[27] Of these infants, 260 had fundus photographs that could be graded for anatomic outcome. Although 51.4% of control eyes had an unfavorable outcome, this was significantly less frequent in the eyes that received cryotherapy (31.1%). There was also good correlation between the outcome assessment of the clinician and that of the photograph readings. These data demonstrated the efficacy of cryotherapy in reducing by approximately one-half the risk of unfavorable retinal outcome from threshold ROP.

Of the original cohort of 291 infants who underwent the randomization procedure, 246 returned for the 12-month follow-up examination.[28] Results of masked grading of fundus photographs of the posterior pole were similar to results obtained 3 months after randomization, and indicated an unfavorable outcome in 25.7% of eyes that received cryotherapy compared with 47.4% of the control eyes. Also, masked Teller Acuity Card[39] assessment of grating acuity was performed in this study group and indicated an unfavorable functional outcome in 35.0% of the treated eyes compared with 56.3% of the control eyes.

The overall incidence of an adverse cosmetic outcome (strabismus, corneal opacity, eyelid fissure asymmetry) in a group of survivors in the natural history cohort ($n = 2759$) was 15.1%.[31] In patients with bilateral threshold ROP who underwent randomization to cryotherapy in one eye, more frequent adverse cosmetic outcomes were found in the untreated fellow eyes.[31]

Results were reported at the $3^1/_2$-year follow-up examination on 92% of the 256 survivors from the original cohort of 291 infants in the randomized trial.[32] Functional outcome was evaluated by masked assessment of letter acuity using the HOTV crowded letter test and grating acuity using the Teller Acuity Card procedure. Structural outcome was evaluated by physician's assessment of ROP residua in the posterior pole. All three outcome measures showed a reduction in unfavorable outcomes in treated versus control eyes: 46.6% versus 57.5% for letter acuity, 52.4% versus 65.6% for grating acuity, and 26.1% versus 45.4% for posterior pole status. These results supported the long-term efficacy and safety of cryotherapy in the treatment of severe ROP.

Intraoperative ocular complications during the course of the trial were limited and included conjunctival or subconjunctival hematomas; unintended conjunctival lacerations; retinal, preretinal, or vitreous hemorrhage; transient closure of the central retinal artery; and inadvertent freezing to an area outside of the target zone (Table 10-5).[26,27] Intraoperative systemic complica-

TABLE 10-5. Complications During Cryotherapy.

Complications	*Number*	*%*
Intraoperative ocular complications		
Conjunctival or subconjunctival hematoma	31	11.7
Conjunctival laceration, unintended	14	5.3
Hemorrhage: retinal, preretinal, vitreous	59	22.3
Closure of the central retinal artery (transient)	1	0.4
Inadvertent freeze to area outside of target zone	2	0.8
Other	2	0.8
Systemic complications		
Bradycardia	25	9.4
Acquired or increased cyanosis	3	1.1
Seizure	1	0.4
Other	6	2.3

$n = 265$.

Source: From Cryotherapy for Retinopathy of Prematurity Group. Arch Ophthalmol 1990;108:195–204, with permission.

tions included bradycardia, tachycardia, arrhythmia, apnea, cyanosis, hypoxemia, transient blood pressure changes, temporary respiratory arrest, and seizure (Table 10-5).[26,27] No deaths from treatment occurred. Additional potential complications secondary to cryotherapy that were not reported in the study include occlusion amblyopia, elevation of intraocular pressure, preretinal membrane formation, inadvertent freezing of the optic nerve or macula, perforation of the globe, orbital wall injury, and cardiorespiratory arrest.[13] Greven and Tasman[61] reported retinal tears developing at the junction between treated and untreated retina and resulting in retinal detachment in two patients several months after cryopexy. A 10-year follow-up study of children in the CRYO-ROP study found that peripheral retinal ablation by cryotherapy for advanced ROP produced only a small reduction in visual field (approximately 5% compared to the fellow eye). However, with or without cryotherapy, visual field area was smaller (by approximately 30%) in eyes that had severe ROP than in eyes of preterm children who did not develop ROP.[25a]

Selection of Patients

Zone I disease is a particular problem in management. Because the CRYO-ROP study demonstrated relatively weak benefit of cryotherapy in threshold zone I eyes, some investigators[116,156,162] advocate redefining threshold to allow earlier treatment intervention in zone I disease. Laser photocoagulation treatment for subthreshold eyes[45] or threshold eyes[16] offers promise for zone I eyes. Laser photocoagulation combined with supplementary oxygen for prethreshold ROP has been advocated.[9] A multicenter trial investigating the use of supplemental oxygen at prethreshold did not significantly reduce the number of infants requiring peripheral ablative therapy.[156a]

Laser Photocoagulation

Xenon photocoagulation was first used in Japan for active ROP before the use of cryotherapy.[112] However, due to technical difficulties in delivery, this treatment modality was eventually replaced by cryotherapy. Renewed interest in photocoagulation treatment for active ROP occurred in the 1980s when technological advances made indirect ophthalmoloscopic delivery systems for argon laser photocoagulation available. Landers et al.[95] first reported the application of argon laser with the indirect ophthalmoscope to the entire area of avascular retina in one premature infant with threshold ROP. This study was followed by an additional report[96] in which 15 eyes of 9 infants at or beyond threshold stage 3+ ROP were treated with argon laser photocoagulation and followed for a minimum of 6 months. A favorable outcome was seen in 73% of eyes, which was comparable to the results in the CRYO-ROP study. McNamara et al.[104] compared the efficacy of transcleral cryotherapy versus laser photocoagulation in 22 infants with threshold stage 3+ ROP in a prospective, randomized clinical trial. Fifteen of 16 eyes randomized to laser, and 9 of 12 eyes randomized to cryotherapy in 18 infants followed for at least 3 months showed regression of extraretinal neovascularization. These results also suggested that laser therapy is as effective as cryotherapy in the treatment of ROP. In the same clinical trial, McNamara et al.[105] reported their treatment results with the portable diode laser (emitting light at 810nm) compared with transcleral cryotherapy. Twenty-five of 28 eyes treated with diode laser photocoagulation using indirect ophthalmoscopic delivery and followed up for at least 3 months underwent regression. Of 24 fellow eyes treated with cryotherapy and followed up for at least 3 months, 20 underwent regression. Hunter and Repka[73] reported their results in a prospective randomized study comparing diode laser with cryotherapy in 19 infants (33 eyes) with threshold ROP. Only 1 infant in each group progressed to an unfavorable outcome.

These studies[16,73,105] suggest that diode laser, in addition to argon laser, is as effective as cryotherapy in the treatment of threshold ROP.

Laser treatment to the avascular retina in ROP has several practical advantages over cryotherapy. The laser unit is portable, more convenient, and laser treatment is technically easier to apply. Most importantly, because laser therapy is better tolerated by the patient, it can sometimes be delivered without the need for subconjunctival or general anesthesia. The use of topical anesthesia, with or without sedation, may avoid some of the systemic complications seen with local or general anesthesia.[13] Complications associated with laser therapy include corneal haze, burns of the iris, cornea, and tunica vasculosa lentis, transient lens opacities, and choroidal hemorrhage.[16a,39b,73] Blinding cataracts have also been observed following laser therapy for ROP.[134] Outcomes following surgery for laser-induced cataracts in ROP are usually poor; this appears to be due to hypotony, possibly from damage to the posterior ciliary arteries.[94a] Laser treatment is applied with a dull white laser burn as an end point, usually leaving one-half to one "burn width" between lesions (Fig. 10-16). All avascular retina is treated anterior to the ridge. As in the CRYO-ROP study, retreatment may be necessary if complete regression of extraretinal fibrovascular proliferation is not observed.

Laser photocoagulation may offer significant advantages over cryotherapy for treatment of zone I threshold ROP. This is a critical issue because the CRYO-ROP study reported a 91.7% unfavorable outcome in control eyes and a 75.0% unfavorable outcome in treated eyes with zone I disease.[28] Capone et al.[16] treated 17 (30 eyes) infants with zone I threshold ROP with diode laser photocoagulation. A favorable outcome was attained in 25 eyes (83.3%). Other reports[45,155,156] have recognized that posterior ROP may have an aggressive course and may require earlier treatment intervention instead of waiting for threshold criteria. Fleming et al.[45] used diode laser photocoagulation to treat 18 eyes in 9 infants with prethreshold, posterior ROP. Treatment was commenced as soon as plus disease developed (defined as tortuosity and dilation of posterior vessels) and disease regression was achieved in all eyes. They recommended lowering the threshold criteria for the treatment of posterior ROP because of the extremely poor prognosis of this form of ROP. Other reports[156,162] have recommended the reassessment of present threshold criteria in view of the experience gained from the

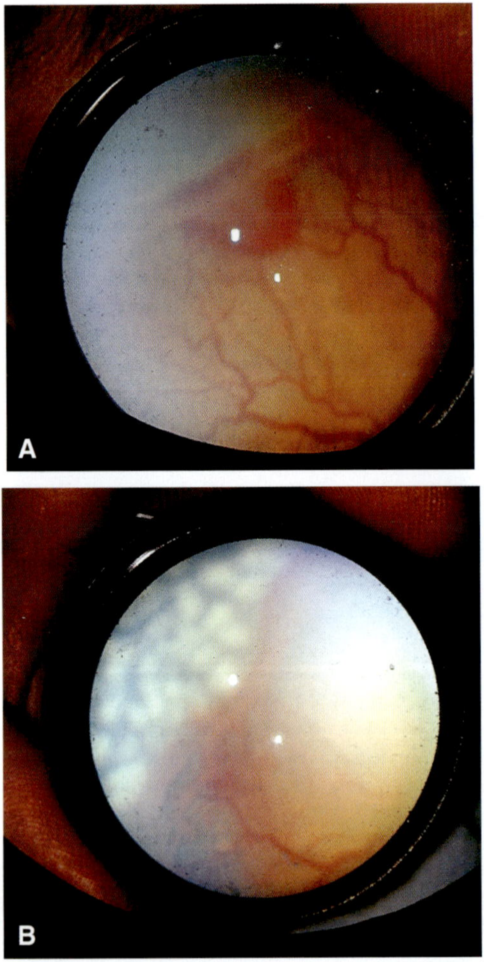

FIGURE 10-16A–C. **(A)** Threshold ROP: ridge of active fibrovascular proliferation between vascular and avascular retina. **(B)** Dull white laser burns seen immediately after laser photocoagulation to avascular retina anterior to fibrovascular ridge. **(C)** Chorioretinal scarring 3 weeks following laser photocoagulation to avascular retina. Note regression of extraretinal fibrovascular proliferation. (Courtesy of Dr. R.R. Ober.)

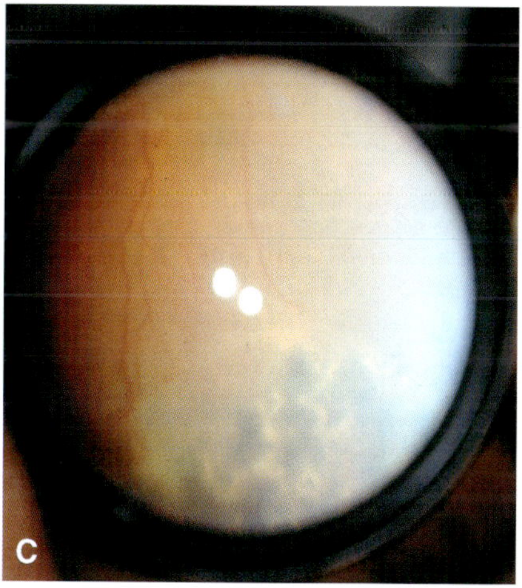

FIGURE 10-16A–C. (continued)

CRYO-ROP study and recent laser studies in the treatment of ROP. This idea is currently being tested in the Early Treatment for ROP study, sponsored by the National Eye Institute.

Several studies[9,16,73,96,104,105] suggest that laser therapy is as effective as cryotherapy for ROP. The Laser ROP Study group,[175] after conducting a meta-analysis of three published, randomized laser ROP trials and one unpublished, nonrandomized ROP trial, came to the same conclusion. The risks of laser versus cryotherapy must be weighed for each individual patient.

MANAGEMENT OF ADVANCED ROP

STOP-ROP Trial

The STOP-ROP multicenter trial studied the use of supplemental therapeutic oxygen late in the hospital course for the treatment of advanced ROP (pre-threshold ROP).[78a,111] The hypothesis stated that increasing the oxygen in patients with Stage 3 ROP would down regulate VEGF and cause regression of the neovascularization. The results from the trial showed no significant decrease in poor outcomes. It is important to note that the supplemental oxygen therapy was given late in the infant's hospital stay. Hyperoxia early in the premature infant's course may be detrimental and increases the risk for severe ROP.[30a,57a,79a]

Scleral Buckling

Despite the significant reduction in the incidence of an unfavorable anatomic outcome (posterior pole macular fold or retinal detachment) noted in the CRYO-ROP study, 31.1% of treated eyes progressed to this outcome.[28] Reports before completion of the CRYO-ROP study utilizing encircling scleral buckling to reattach the retina in advanced ROP indicated encouraging results.[106,107,161,168] However, the optimum timing and modality of surgical intervention for advanced ROP are unclear. A significant advantage of scleral buckling over vitrectomy is in maintaining phakia. Lens-sparing vitrectomy techniques have been developed and may be superior to buckling in some settings.[102] Lens-sparing vitrectomy in stage 4+ eyes may prevent progression to more advanced stages.[16b]

Eyes selected for scleral buckling usually are stage 4B eyes or stage 5 eyes with open funnels and minimal vitreous traction. Because the retinal detachment in stage 4A eyes, in particular, may remain stable or even undergo spontaneous reattachment, surgery may be withheld until progression of the detachment into the fovea.[62] However, visual outcomes are generally poor despite successful macular reattachment, possibly because of retinal abnormalities as a result of detachment and amblyopia.[19a,115] Thus, scleral buckling for stage 4A eyes, before macular detachment, may possibly yield better visual results.[171]

The technique of scleral buckling involves placement of a 2- to 2.5-mm-wide, 360° circumferential silicone band on episclera. Supplemental buckling elements can be placed to support the area of highest ridge elevation. Peripheral cryoablation may be applied to avascular attached retina if neovascular activity is still present and preoperative treatment is absent or inadequate. Subretinal fluid drainage is performed routinely by some surgeons,[62] whereas others[115,171] rarely drain, but instead perform anterior chamber paracentesis. The encircling band usually must be divided or removed several months following surgery to prevent retardation of eye growth and reduce the likelihood of extrusion of the band later in life.[62,171] The retina usually remains attached after buckle removal, and myopia may decrease.[19b]

Scleral buckling for advanced ROP appears to play a role in reducing progression from stage 4 to stage 5 ROP. Greven and Tasman[62] achieved anatomic attachment of the retina in 13 (59%) of 22 eyes with either stages 4B or 5. Of these patients achieving anatomic reattachment with follow-up of 18 months or more, 4 (40%) of 10 had 20/400 or better visual acuity. Noorily et al.[115] used scleral buckling alone to successfully reattach 10 of 15 eyes (67%). However, of these cases only 2 (20%) of 10 were able to achieve fix-and-follow acuities. Trese[171] reported anatomic retinal reattachment in 12 (70%) of 17 stage 4A eyes, 29 (67%) of 43 stage 4B eyes, and 4 (40%) of 10 stage 5 eyes. This study was not designed to tabulate visual results, but isolated cases yielded visual acuities as good as 20/30.[171]

As it was estimated in 1991 that 440 to 770 infants would be affected with low vision due to retinal detachments, the exact role of scleral buckling in the management of advanced ROP is a critical issue.[111] Because spontaneous retinal reattachment in stage 4 ROP can occur (and rarely stage 5 ROP), it is critical to compare current data with the natural history of retinal detachment as it becomes available. Ideally, a randomized, prospective clinical trial of scleral buckling should be performed to define its role in the management of advanced ROP.

Vitreoretinal Surgery

If vitreous traction is severe, especially if the posterior pole is involved, scleral buckling may not be sufficient to reattach the retina, and vitrectomy may be indicated. Eyes considered for vitrectomy are usually stage 5 eyes, although stage 4B eyes with significant posterior vitreous traction may qualify. Refinements in vitrectomy instrumentation and techniques have been developed that allow meticulous removal of proliferative membranes and reattachment of the retina in some ROP eyes that previous were unsalvageable.

The two major surgical approaches to vitrectomy for advanced ROP are the closed- and open-sky techniques. Both techniques offer advantages and disadvantages. Charles[18] and others[20,37,169,170,176] helped to pioneer the closed technique, which is now the technique used most commonly. Charles[18] utilized a two-port technique; one port for right-angle 20-gauge scissors and the other for an infusion needle. He advocated a pars plicata entry site because of the usual marked anterior displacement of the retina and the underdeveloped pars plana in the premature infant eye. After lensectomy, the retrolental tissue and epiretinal membranes are removed by scissors delamination. Air is injected at the completion of the dissection, but subretinal fluid is usually not drained because of the risk of retinal break with forceful posterior expansion of the retina. deJuan and Machemer[37] use a similar technique, but advocate using a limbal entry site and a three-port technique with suturing of the infusion cannula to the globe. This technique allows both true bimanual membrane removal (forceps and scissors) and posterior dissection with the use of an intraocular fiberoptic light pipe. Trese[169,170] reported a two-port system combined with sodium hyaluronate infusion; this allows for a true bimanual technique and the use of a fiberoptic light pipe for posterior dissection.

Hirose et al.[72] advocated an open-sky technique, because of some of the inherent difficulties with closed vitrectomy. With this technique, the cornea is removed and stored in tissue culture fluid during surgery. The lens is then extracted intracapsularly with a cryoprobe. The retrolental membranes are then dissected with a microspatula and Vannas scissors and removed from the detached retina in one piece. Hyaluronic acid is used to expand the funnel detachment to facilitate removal of membranes and fibrous tissue. The corneal button is then replaced and sutured with 10-0 running nylon sutures. The open-sky technique allows direct access to the retrolental membranes, affords an excellent view, and allows a true bimanual technique. The potential disadvantages of the open-sky technique include prolonged hypotony, prolonged operating time, limiting posterior dissection, and induced astigmation.

Indications for surgical intervention are not established, but most surgeons recommend operating when vascular activity is regressing or regressed. In general, surgery is performed between 6 and 12 months of age. However, ambulatory vision has been reported in patients operated between 2 and 3 years of age.[72] Better results have been attained if the configuration of the retinal detachment funnel was wide anteriorly and wide posteriorly.[72,169,170]

The anatomic results following either closed-sky or open-sky vitrectomy are variable. Hirose et al.[72] reported reattachment in 205 (39.2%) of 524 eyes in 338 infants with the open-sky technique during the period 1974 through 1989. Trese[170] achieved anatomic retinal attachment in 48% of eyes with stage

5 ROP. Zilis et al.[176] achieved partial attachment in 9 (64%) of 14 eyes with stage 4 ROP and in 38 (31%) of 121 eyes with stage 5 ROP; complete attachment in stage 5 eyes was achieved in 11 eyes (9%). Quinn et al.[140] reported a reattachment rate of 28% in 20 of 71 eyes (defined as retinal reattachment of some degree). Charles[18] reported a 46% anatomic success rate in 580 patients.

Unfortunately, despite anatomic reattachment following vitrectomy, visual outcome is extremely disappointing.[79] These poor visual outcomes are probably a result of ocular and neurological (amblyopia) causes.[19a,79,170,176] Hirose et al.[72] reported visual results among 82 eyes with attached retinas; vision was 20/200 in 3 eyes, 20/400 in 4 eyes, 20/800 in 9 eyes, 20/1600 in 11 eyes, and 20/3200 in 24 eyes. In 26 eyes, vision was limited to light perception. Trese[170] reported 26 of 85 eyes (31%) exhibiting visual behavior (light reaction, follow objects, identify shapes). Zilis et al.[176] reported final visual acuity of fix and follow or greater in 6 (43%) of 14 eyes with stage 4 and in 13 eyes (11%) with stage 5 ROP. Quinn et al.[140] reported pattern vision (response to low-vision acuity card with 2.2-cm-wide stripes[39]) in only 2 of 20 eyes with retinal reattachment following vitrectomy. A study by Cherry et al. demonstrated that in 5 eyes with reattached retinas after stage 5 ROP, the ERG was nonrecordable. Thus, persistent retinal dysfunction limits vision even after retinal surgery for severe ROP.[19a]

In selected cases, lens-sparing vitreous surgery may be performed in stage 4B or stage 5 eyes[16b,102]; this offers several potential advantages over standard vitrectomy methods, in which lensectomy is performed, regarding development of the visual system following surgery, such as better optical rehabilitation and shorter periods of postoperative visual deprivation. Finally, vitreous surgery may be beneficial in selected eyes of older patients with advanced ROP in eliminating media opacities and for uncovering areas of functional, attached retina.[11] The visual-evoked potential and contact B-scan ultrasound of the globe may be useful in predicting which older patients may benefit from vitreous surgery. A randomized clinical trial is needed.

FUTURE DIRECTIONS IN CLINICAL RESEARCH FOR ROP

Although great strides have been made in treating the active stages of ROP, the cicatricial sequelae, for example, retinal detachment, retinal folds, and retrolental membranes, are best prevented rather than managed after they occur because of severe limitations in successful anatomic and visual outcomes. Therefore, clinical research regarding any of the aspects of prenatal, perinatal, or neonatal care that could result in lower rates of premature birth is vital. In addition, knowledge gained about the basic mechanisms of control of neovascular retinopathies and vitreoretinal disorders may be applied clinically to aid in the reduction or elimination of the cicatricial sequelae of ROP. Some day, perhaps control can be achieved pharmacologically.

References

1. Addison DJ, Font Rl, Manshot WA. Proliferative retinopathy in anencephalic babies. Am J Ophthalmol 1972;74:967–976.
2. Alade SL, Brown RE, Paquet A. Polysorbate 80 and E-ferol toxicity. Pediatrics 1986;77:593–597.
3. American Academy of Pediatrics, American Association for Pediatric Ophthalmology and Strabismus, American Academy of Ophthalmology. Screening examination of premature infants for retinopathy. Pediatrics 2001;108:809–811.
4. Ashton N. Oxygen and the growth and development of retinal vessels. In vivo and in vitro studies. Am J Ophthalmol 1966;62:412–435.
5. Ashton N, Ward B, Serpell G. Effect of oxygen on developing retinal vessels with particular reference to the problem of retrolental fibroplasia. Br J Ophthalmol 1954;38:397–432.
6. Avery GB, Glass P. Light and retinopathy of prematurity: what is prudent for 1986? Pediatrics 1986;78:519–520.
7. Avery ME, Oppenheimer EH. Recent advances in mortality from hyaline membrane disease. J Pediatr 1960;57:553–559.
8. Benner JD, Landers MB. Hyperoxia and transient resolution of vascular vasodilation and tortuosity in threshold retinopathy of prematurity. Am J Ophthalmol 1993;115:258–259.
9. Benner JD, Morse LS, Hay A, Landers MB. A comparison of argon and diode photocoagulation combined with supplemental oxygen for the treatment of retinopathy of prematurity. Retina 1993;13:222–229.
10. Ben-Sira I, Nissenkorn I, Grunwald E, Yassur Y. Treatment of acute retrolental fibroplasia by cryopexy. Br J Ophthalmol 1980;64:758–762.

10a. Berkowitz BA, Berlin ES, Zhang W. Variable supplemental oxygen during recovery does not reduce retinal neovascular severity in experimental ROP. Curr Eye Res 2001;22(6):401–404.

11. Bradford JD, Trese MT. Management of advanced retinopathy of prematurity in the older patient. Ophthalmology 1991;98:1105–1108.

12. Brown DR, Biglan AW, Stretavsky MAM. Screening criteria for the detection of retinopathy of prematurity in patients in a neonatal intensive care unit. J Pediatr Ophthalmol Stabismus 1987;24:212–215.
13. Brown GC, Tasman WS, Naidoff M, et al. Systemic complications associated with retinal cyroablation for retinopathy of prematurity. Ophthalmology 1990;97:855–858.
14. Campbell R. Intensive oxygen therapy as a possible cause of retrolental fibroplasia. Med J Aust 1951;2:48–50.
15. Campbell PB, Bull MJ, Ellis FD, et al. Incidence of retinopathy of prematurity in a tertiary newborn intensive care unit. Arch Ophthalmol 1983;101:1686–1688.
16. Capone A Jr, Diaz-Rohena R, Sternberg P Jr, et al. Diode-laser photocoagulation for zone I threshold retinopathy of prematurity. Am J Ophthalmol 1993;116:444–450.
16a. Capone A Jr, Drack AV. Transient lens changes after diode laser retinal photoablation for retinopathy of prematurity. Am J Ophthalmol 1994;118(4):533–535.
16b. Capone A Jr, Trese MT. Lens-sparing vitreous surgery for tractional 4A ROP retinal detachments. Ophthalmology 2001;108(11):2068–2070.
17. Carpel EF, Kalina RE. Pupillary responses to mydriatic agents in premature infants. Am J Ophthalmol 1973;75:989–991.
18. Charles S. Vitrectomy with ciliary body entry for retrolental fibroplasia. In: McPherson AR, Hittner HM, Kretzer FL (eds) Retionopathy of prematurity—current concepts and controversies. Toronto: Decker, 1986.
19. Charles BJ, Ganthier R, Appiah AA. Incidence and characteristics of retinopathy of prematurity in a low-income inner-city population. Ophthalmology 1991;98:14–17.
19a. Cherry TA, Lambert SR, Capone A Jr. Electroretinogram findings in stage 5 ROP after retinal reattachment. Retina 1995;15(1):21–24.
19b. Choi MY, Yu YS. Efficacy of removal of buckle after scleral buckling surgery for ROP. J Pediatr Ophthalmol Strabismus 2000; 4(6):362–365.
20. Chong LP, Machemer R, de Juan E. Vitrectomy for advanced stages of retinopathy of prematurity. Am J Ophthalmol 1986;102:710–716.
21. Clark WN, Hodges R, Noel LP, et al. The oculocardiac reflex during ophthalmoscopy in premature infants. Am J Ophthalmol 1985;99: 649–651.
22. Clemett RS, Darlow BA, Hidajat RR, Tarr KH. Retinopathy of prematurity: review of a five-year period, examination techniques and recommendations for screening. Aust NZ J Ophthalmol 1986;14: 121–125.
23. Committee on Fetus and Newborn: vitamin E and the prevention of retinopathy of prematurity. Pediatrics 1985;76:315–316.

23a. Connolly BP, McMamara JA, Sharma S, Regillo CD, Tasman W. A comparison of laser photocoagulation with transscleral cryotherapy in the treatment of threshold retinopathy of prematurity. Ophthalmology 1998;105(9):1628–1631.
24. Criswick VG, Schepens CI. Familial exudative vitreoretinopathy. Am J Ophthalmol 1969;68:578–594.
25. Cross KW. Cost of preventing retrolental fibroplasia? Lancet 1973; 2:954–956.
25a. Cryotherapy for Retinopathy of Prematurity Cooperative Group. Effect of retinal ablative therapy for threshold retinopathy of prematurity: results of Goldmann perimetry at the age of 10 years. Arch Ophthalmol 2001;119(8):1120–1125.
26. Cryotherapy for Retinopathy of Prematurity Cooperative Group. Multicenter trial of cryotherapy for retinopathy of prematurity: preliminary results. Arch Ophthalmol 1988;106:471–479.
27. Cryotherapy for Retinopathy of Prematurity Cooperative Group. Multicenter trial of cryotherapy for retinopathy of prematurity: three month outcome. Arch Ophthalmol 1990;108:195–204.
28. Cryotherapy for Retinopathy of Prematurity Cooperative Group. Multicenter trial of cryotherapy for retinopathy of prematurity: one-year outcome. Structure and function. Arch Ophthalmol 1990; 108:1408–1416.
29. Cryotherapy for Retinopathy of Prematurity Cooperative Group. Incidence and early course of retinopathy of prematurity (Palmer EA, Flynn JT, Hardy RJ, et al.: Cryotherapy for Retinopathy of Prematurity Group). Ophthalmology 1991;98:1628–1640.
30. Cryotherapy for Retinopathy of Prematurity Cooperative Group. Development of myopia in infants with birth weights less than 1251 grams (Dobson V, Quinn GE, Repka MX, et al.: Cryotherapy for Retinopathy of Prematurity Group). Ophthalmology 1992;99: 329–340.
30a. Hong PH, Wright KW, et al. Strict oxygen management is associated with decreased incidence of severe retinopathy of prematurity. Association for Research in Vision and Ophthalmology Abstracts. 2002 Abstract #4011.
31. Cryotherapy for Retinopathy of Prematurity Cooperative Group. Ocular cosmesis in retinopathy of prematurity (Summers G, Phelps DL, Tung B, Palmer EA; Cryotherapy for Retinopathy of Prematurity Cooperative Group). Arch Ophthalmol 1992;110:1092–1097.
32. Cryotherapy for Retinopathy of Prematurity Cooperative Group. Multicenter trial of cryotherapy for retinopathy of prematurity: $3^1/_2$-year outcome: structure and function. Arch Ophthalmol 1993; 111:339–344.
33. Cryotherapy for Retinopathy of Prematurity Cooperative Group. Prognostic factors in the natural course of retinopathy of prematurity (Palmer EA, Schaffer DB, Plotsky DF: The Cryotherapy for Retinopathy of Prematurity Cooperative Group). Ophthalmology 1993;100:230–273.

34. Cryotherapy for Retinopathy of Prematurity Group. The natural ocular outcome of premature birth and retinopathy: status at 1 year. Arch Ophthalmol 1994;112:903–912.
35. Cryotherapy for Retinopathy of Prematurity Group. Correlation of retinopathy of prematurity in fellow eyes in the CRYO-ROP study (Quinn GE, Dobson V, Biglan A, Evans J, Plotsky D, Hardy RJ: Cryotherapy for Retinopathy of Prematurity Group). Arch Ophthalmol 1995;113(4):469–473.
36. Darlow BA, Horwood LJ, Clement RS. Retinopathy of prematurity: risk factors in a prospective population-based study. Paediatr Perinatal Epidemiol 1992;6:62–80.
37. deJuan E Jr, Machemer R. Retinopathy of prematurity: surgical technique. Retina 1987;7:63–69.
38. deJuan E Jr, Shields S, Machemer R. The role of ultrasound in the management of retinopathy of prematurity. Ophthalmology 1988; 95:884–888.
39. Dobson V, Quinn GE, Biglan AW, et al. Acuity card assessment of visual function in the cryotherapy for retinopathy of prematurity trial. Investig Ophthalmol Vis Sci 1990;31:1702–1708.
39a. Drack AV. Preventing blindness in premature infants. N Engl J Med 1998;338(22):1620–1621.
39b. Drack AV, Burke JP, Pulido JS, Keech RV. Transient punctate lenticular opacities as a complication of argon laser photoablation in an infant with ROP. Am J Ophthalmol 1992;113(5):583–584.
40. Ehrenkranz RA. Vitamin E and retinopathy of prematurity: still controversial. J Pediatr 1989;114:801–803.
41. Faris BM, Brockhurst RJ. Retrolental fibroplasia in the cicatricial stage: the complication of rhegmatogenous retinal detachment. Arch Ophthalmol 1969;82:60–65.
42. Fielder AR, Shaw DE, Robinson J, Ng YK. Natural history of retinopathy of prematurity: a prospective study. Eye 1992;6:233–242.
43. Finer NN, Peters KL, Hayek Z, Merel CL. Vitamin E and necrotizing enterocolitis. Pediatrics 1984;73:387–393.
44. Finer NN, Schindler RF, Grant F, Hill GB, Peters KL. Effect of intramuscular vitamin E on frequency and severity of retrolental fibroplasia. Lancet 1982;2:1087–1091.
44a. Fivgas GD, Capone A Jr. Pediatric rhegmatogenous retinal detachment. Retina 2001;21(2):101–106.
45. Fleming TN, Rung PE, Charles ST. Diode laser photocoagulation for prethreshold, posterior retinopathy of prematurity. Am J Ophthalmol 1992;114:589–592.
46. Fletcher MC, Brandon S. Myopia of prematurity. Am J Ophthalmol 1955;40:474–481.
47. Flynn JT. Acute proliferative retrolental fibroplasia: multivariate risk analysis. Trans Am Ophthalmol Soc 1983;81:549–591.
48. Flynn JT. Retinopathy of prematurity. Pediatr Clin North Am 1987; 34:1487–1515.

49. Flynn JT. The premature retina: a model for the in vivo study of molecular genetics? Eye 1992;6:161–165.
50. Flynn JT, Bancalari E, Bawol R, et al. Retinopathy of prematurity. A randomized, prospective trial of transcutaneous oxygen monitoring. Ophthalmology 1987;94:630–638.
51. Flynn JT, Bancalari E, Bachynski BN, et al. Retinopathy of prematurity: Diagnosis, severity, and natural history. Ophthalmology 1987;94:620–629.
52. Flynn JT, Bancalari E, Snyder ES, et al. A cohort study of transcutaneous oxygen tension and the incidence and severity of retinopathy of prematurity. N Engl J Med 1992;326:1050–1054.
53. Flynn JT, O'Grady GE, Herrera J, et al. Retrolental fibroplasia. I. Clinical observations. Arch Ophthalmol 1977;95:217–223.
54. Foos RY. Acute retrolental fibroplasia. Albrecht von Graefe's Arch Klin Exp Ophthalmol 1975;195:87–100.
55. Foos RV. Chronic retinopathy of prematurity. Ophthalmology 1985; 92:563–574.
56. Foos RY. Retinopathy of prematurity: pathologic correlation of clinical stages. Retina 1987;7:260–276.
57. Foos RY, Kopelow SM. Development of retinal vasculature in paranatal infants. Surv Ophthalmol 1973;18:117–127.
57a. Pierce EA, Foley ED, Smith LE. Regulation of vascular endothelial growth factor by oxygen in a model of retinopathy of prematurity. Arch Ophthalmol 1996;114:1219–1228.
58. Gallo JE, Holmström G, Kugelberg U, et al. Regressed retinopathy of prematurity and its sequelae in children aged 5–10 years. Br J Ophthalmol 1991;75:527–531.
59. Glass P, Avery GB, Kolinjavadi N, et al. Effect of bright light in the hospital nursery on the incidence of retinopathy of prematurity. N Engl J Med 1985;313:401–404.
60. Graham MV, Gray OP. Refraction of premature babies' eyes. Br Med J 1963;1:1452–1454.
61. Greven CM, Tasman W. Rhegmatogenous retinal detachment following cryotherapy in retinopathy of prematurity. Arch Ophthalmol 1989;107:1017–1018.
62. Greven C, Tasman W. Scleral buckling in stages 4B and 5 retinopathy of prematurity. Ophthalmology 1990;97:817–820.
63. Gunn TR, et al. Risk factors in retrolental fibroplasia. Pediatrics 1980;65(6):1096–1100.
64. Hack M, Fanaroff AA. Outcomes of extremely-low-birth-weight infants between 1982 and 1988. N Engl J Med 1989;321:1642–1647.
65. Hammer ME, Mullen PW, Ferguson JG, et al. Logistic analysis of risk factors in acute retinopathy of prematurity. Am J Ophthalmol 1986;102:1–6.
66. Harris GS. Retinopathy of prematurity and retinal detachment. Can J Ophthalmol 1976;11:21–25.
67. Harris GS, McCormick AQ. The prophylactic treatment of retrolental fibroplasia. Mod Probl Ophthalmol 1977;18:364–367.

68. Hartnett ME, Gilbert MM, Richardson TM, et al. Anterior segment evaluation of infants with retinopathy of prematurity. Ophthalmology 1990;97:122–130.
69. Hindle NW. Cryotherapy for retinopathy of prematurity to prevent retrolental fibroplasia. Can J Ophthalmol 1982;17:207–212.
70. Hindle NW. Cryotherapy for retinopathy of prematurity: timing of intervention. Br J Ophthalmol 1986;70:269–276.
71. Hindle NW. Cryotherapy for retinopathy of prematurity: none, one, or both eyes. Arch Ophthalmol 1990;108:1375.
72. Hirose T, Schepens CL, Katsumi O, Mehta MC. Open-sky vitrectomy for severe retinal detachment caused by advanced retinopathy of prematurity. In: Flynn JT, Tasman W (eds) Retinopathy of prematurity. New York: Springer-Verlag, 1992.
72a. Holmstrom M, el Azazi M, Kugelberg U. Ophthalmological long-term follow-up of preterm infants: a population-based, prospective study of the refraction and its development. Br J Ophthalmol 1998;82(11):1265–1271.
73. Hunter DG, Repka MX. Diode laser photocoagulation for threshold retinopathy of prematurity. A randomized study. Ophthalmology 1993;100:238–244.
74. Ibayashi H, Nishimura M, Yamana T. Avascular zone in the macula in cicatricial retinopathy of prematurity. Am J Ophthalmol 1985;99:235–239.
75. Isenberg SJ. Macular development in the premature infant. Am J Ophthalmol 1986;101:74–80.
76. Johnson L, Bowen FW, Abbasi S, et al. Relationship of prolonged pharmacological serum levels of vitamin E to incidence of sepsis and necrotizing enterocolitis in infants with birth weights 1500 grams or less. Pediatrics 1985;15:619–638.
77. Johnson L, Quinn GE, Abhasi S, et al. Effect of sustained pharmacologic vitamin E levels on incidence and severity of retinopathy of prematurity: a controlled clinical trial. J Pediatr 1989;114:827–838.
78. Kalina RE, Hodson WA, Morgan BC. Retrolental fibroplasia in a cyanotic infant. Pediatrics 1972;50:765–768.
78a. The STOP-ROP Multicenter Study Group. Supplemental therapeutic oxygen for prethreshold retinopathy of prematurity (STOP-ROP), a randomized, controlled trial. I. Primary outcomes. Pediatrics 2000;105:295–310.
79. Kalina RE. Treatment of retinal detachment due to retinopathy of prematurity: documented disappointment [editorial]. Ophthalmology 1991;98:3–4.
79a. Tin W, Milligan DWA, Pennefather P, Hey E. Pulse oximetry, severe retinopathy, and outcome at one year in babies of less than 28 weeks gestation. Arch Dis Child Fetal Neonatal Ed 2001;84:F106–F110.
80. Keith CG. Visual outcome and effect of treatment in stage III developing retrolental fibroplasia. Br J Ophthalmol 1982;66:446–449.

81. Kelly SP, Fielder AR. Microcornea associated with retinopathy of prematurity. Br J Ophthalmol 1987;71:201–203.
82. Kendig JW, Notter RH, Cox C. A comparison of surfactant as immediate prophylaxis and as a rescue therapy in newborns of less than 30 weeks gestation. N Engl J Med 1991;324:865–871.
82a. Kent D, Pennie F, Laws D, et al. The influence of retinopathy of prematurity on ocular growth. Eye 2000;14(1):23–29.
83. Kingham JD. Acute retrolental fibroplasia. II. Treatment by cryosurgery. Arch Ophthalmol 1978;96:2049–2053.
84. Kinsey VE. Retrolental fibroplasia: co-operative study of retrolental fibroplasia and the use of oxygen. Arch Ophthalmol 1956;56: 481–543.
85. Kinsey VE, Arnold HJ, Kalina RE, et al. PaO_2 levels and retrolental fibroplasia: a report of the co-operative study. Pediatrics 1977;60: 655–668.
85a. Knight-Nanan DM, O'Keefe M. Refractive outcome in eyes with retinopathy of prematurity treated with cryotherapy or diode laser: 3 year follow-up. Br J Ophthalmol 1996;80(11):998–1001.
86. Kraushar MF, Harper RG, Sia CG. Retrolental fibroplasia in a full term infant. Am J Ophthalmol 1975;80:106–108.
87. Kretzer FL, Hittner HM. Retinopathy of prematurity: clinical implications of retinal development. Arch Dis Child 1988;63:1151–1167.
88. Kretzer FL, Mehta RS, Johnson AT, et al. Vitamin E protects against retinopathy of prematurity through action on spindle cells. Nature (Lond) 1984;309:793–795.
89. Kushner BJ. Strabismus and amblyopia associated with regressed retinopathy of prematurity. Arch Ophthalmol 1982;100;256–261.
90. Kushner BJ. Ciliary block glaucoma in retinopathy of prematurity. Arch Ophthalmol 1982;100:1978–1079.
91. Kushner BJ. The sequelae of regressed retinopathy of prematurity. In: Silverman WA, Flynn JT (eds) Retinopathy of prematurity. Boston: Blackwell, 1985.
92. Kushner BJ, Gloeckner E. Retrolental fibroplasia in full-term infants without exposure to supplemental oxygen. Am J Ophthalmol 1984;97:148–153.
93. Kushner BJ, Sondheimer S. Medical treatment of glaucoma associated with cicatricial retinopathy of prematurity. Am J Ophthalmol 1982;94:313–317.
94. Kwitko ML. Secondary glaucoma in infancy and childhood. In: Glaucoma in Infants and Children. New York: Appleton-Century-Croft, 1973.
94a. Lambert SR, Capone A Jr, Cingle KA, Drack AV. Cataract and phthisis bulbi after laser photoablation for threshold ROP. Am J Ophthalmol 2000;129(5):585–591.
95. Landers MB III, Semple HC, Ruben JB, Serdahl C. Argon laser photocoagulation for advanced retinopathy of prematurity. Am J Ophthalmol 1990;110:429–431.

96. Landers MB III, Toth CA, Semple HC, Morse LS. Treatment of retinopathy of prematurity with argon laser photocoagulation. Arch Ophthalmol 1992;110:44–47.
97. Law MR, Wijewardene K, Wald NJ. Is routine vitamin E administration justified in very low birth weight infants? Dev Med Child Neurol 1990;32:442–450.
98. Laws D, Shaw DE, Robinson J, et al. Retinopathy of prematurity: a prospective study. Review at six months. Eye 1992;6:477–483.
99. Liberfarb RM, Eavey RO, De Long GR, et al. Norrie's disease: a study of two families. Ophthalmology 1985;92:1445–1451.
100. Lucey JF, Dangman B. A reexamination of the role of oxygen in retrolental fibroplasia. Pediatrics 1984;73:82–96.
101. Machemer R. Description and pathogenesis of late stages of retinopathy of prematurity. Ophthalmology 1985;92:1000–1004.
102. Maguire AM, Trese MT. Lens-sparing vitreoretinal surgery. Arch Ophthalmol 1992;110:284–286.
103. McDonald AD. Cerebral palsy in children of very low birth weight. Arch Dis Child 1963;38:579–588.
104. McNamara JA, Tasman W, Brown GC, Federman JL. Laser photocoagulation for stage 3+ retinopathy of prematurity. Ophthalmology 1991;98:576–580.
105. McNamara JA, Tasman W, Vander JF, Brown GC. Diode laser photocoagulation for retinopathy of prematurity: preliminary results. Arch Ophthalmol 1992;110:1714–1716.
106. McPherson A, Hittner HM. Scleral buckling in $2^1/_2$- to 11-month old premature infants with retinal detachment associated with acute retrolental fibroplasia. Ophthalmology 1979;86:819–836.
107. McPherson AR, Hittner M, Lemos R. Retinal detachment in young premature infants with acute retrolental fibroplasia: thirty-two new cases. Ophthalmology 1982;89:160–169.
108. Michael AJ, Pesin SR, Katz LJ, Tasman WS. Management of late-onset angle-closure glaucoma associated with retinopathy of prematurity. Ophthalmology 1991;98:1093–1098.
109. Mousel D, Hoyt CS. Cryotherapy for retinopathy of prematurity. Ophthalmology 1980;87:1121–1127.
110. Muller DPR. Vitamin E therapy in retinopathy of prematurity. Eye 1992;6:221–225.
111. Manual of Procedures of the Multicenter Trial of Supplemental Therapeutic Oxygenation for Prethreshold Retinopathy of Prematurity (STOP-ROP), May 1993.
112. Nagata M, Kanerari S, Fukuda H, Suekane K. Photocoagulation for the treatment of the retinopathy of prematurity. Jpn J Clin Ophthalmol 1968;24:419–427.
113. Nissenkorn I, Axer-Siegel R, Kremer I, Ben-Sira I. Effect of partial cryoablation on retinopathy of prematurity. Br J Ophthalmol 1991;75:160–162.
114. Nissenorn I, Kremer I, Gilad E, et al. "Rush" type retinopathy of prematurity: report of three cases. Br J Ophthalmol 1987;71:559–562.

115. Noorily SW, Small K, deJuan E Jr, Machemer R. Scleral buckling for stage 4B retinopathy of prematurity. Ophthalmology 1992;99: 263–268.
116. Ober RR. Diode laser photocoagulation for threshold stage 3+ retinopathy of prematurity. Investig Ophthalmol Vis Sci 1993;34: 1448.
117. Ober RR, Bird AC, Hamilton AM, Sehmi K. Autosomal dominant exudative vitreoretinopathy. Br J Ophthalmol 1980;64:112–120.
118. Owens WC, Owens EU. Retrolental fibroplasia in premature infants. II. Studies on the prophylaxis of the disease: the use of alpha-tocopheryl acetate. Am J Ophthalmol 1949;32:1631–1637.
119. Palmer EA. Optimal timing of examination for acute retrolental fibroplasia. Ophthalmology 1981;88:662–668.
120. Palmer EA. Optimal timing for acute retrolental fibroplasia (from discussion by John T. Flynn, 667). Ophthalmology 1981;88:662–668.
121. Palmer EA. Risks of dilating a child's pupils. Trans Pac Coast Oto-Ophthalmol Soc 1982;63:141–145.
122. Palmer EA, Goodman S. A pilot randomized trial of cryotherapy for retinopathy of prematurity. Investig Ophthalmol Vis Sci 1987; 23(3)(suppl):105.
123. Palmer EA, Hardy RJ. Zone 1 retinopathy of prematurity. Arch Ophthalmol 1994;112:156.
124. Patz A. Current concepts of the effects of oxygen on the developing retina. Curr Eye Res 1984;3:159–163.
125. Patz A, Eastham A, Higginbotham DH, Kleh T. Oxygen studies in retrolental fibroplasia. II. The production of the microscopic changes of retrolental fibroplasia in experimental animals. Am J Ophthalmol 1953;36:1511–1522.
126. Patz A, Hoeck LE, De La Cruz E. Studies on the effects of high oxygen administration in retrolental fibroplasia. I. Nursery observations. Am J Ophthalmol 1952;35:1248–1253.
127. Patz A, Payne JW. Retrolental fibroplasia. In: Duane TD, Jaeger (eds) Clinical ophthalmology, vol 3. Philadelphia: Harper and Row, 1983.
128. Phelps DL. Retinopathy of prematurity: an estimate of vision loss in the United States—1979. Pediatrics 1981;67:924–926.
129. Phelps DL. E-Ferol: what happened and what now? Pediatrics 1984; 74:1114–1116.
130. Phelps DL. Reduced severity of oxygen-induced retinopathy in kittens recovered in 28% oxygen. Pediatr Res 1988;24:106–109.
131. Phelps DL, Brown DR, Tung B, et al. 28-Day survival rates of 6676 neonates with birth weights of 1250 grams or less. Pediatrics 1991;87:7–17.
132. Phelps DL, Rosenbaum AL. Vitamin E in kitten oxygen-induced retinopathy. II. Blockage of vitreal neovascularization. Arch Ophthalmol 1979;97:1522–1526.
133. Phelps DL, Rosenbaum AL, Isenberg SJ, et al. Tocopherol efficacy and safety for preventing retinopathy of prematurity:

a randomized, controlled, double-masked trial. Pediatrics 1987;79: 489–500.

134. Pogrebniak AE, Bolling JP, Stewart MW. Argon laser-induced cataract in an infant with retinopathy of prematurity. Am J Ophthalmol 1994;117:261–262.
135. Pollard ZF. Secondary angle-closure glaucoma in cicatricial retrolental fibroplasia. Am J Ophthalmol 1980;89:651–653.
136. Pollard ZF. Lensectomy for secondary angle-closure glaucoma in advanced cicatricial retrolental fibroplasia. Ophthalmology 1984; 91:395–398.
137. Pulido JS, Byrne SF, Clarkson JG, et al. Evaluation of eyes with advanced stages of retinopathy of prematurity using standardized echography. Ophthalmology 1991;98:1099–1104.
138. Puklin JE, Simon RM, Ehrenkranz RA. Influence on retrolental fibroplasia of intramuscular vitamin E administration during respiratory distress syndrome. Ophthalmology 1982;89:96–102.
139. Pruett RC, Schepens CL. Posterior hyperplastic primary vitreous. Am J Ophthalmol 1970;69:535–543.
140. Quinn GE, Dobson V, Barr CC, et al. Visual acuity in infants after vitrectomy for severe retinopathy of prematurity. Ophthalmology 1991;98:5–13.
140a. Quinn GE, Dobson V, Kivlin J, et al. Prevalence of myopia between 3 months and $5^1/_2$ years in preterm infants with and without ROP. CRYO-ROP Cooperative Group. Ophthalmology 1998;105(7):1292–1300.
140b. Raju TN, Langenberg P, Bhutani V, Quinn GE. Vitamin E prophylaxis to reduce retinopathy of prematurity: a reappraisal of published trials. J Pediatr 1997;131(6):844–850.
140c. Reddy VM, Capone A Jr, Drack AV. The role of light toxicity in retinopathy of prematurity and congenital cataract. Am J Ophthalmol 1994;117(2):262–264.
141. Reese AB, King MJ, Owens WC. A classification of retrolental fibroplasia. Am J Ophthalmol 1953;36:1333–1335.
142. Repka MX, Hardy RJ, Phelps DL, Summers CG. Surfactant prophylaxis and retinopathy of prematurity. Arch Ophthalmol 1993; 111:618–620.
142a. Repka MX, Palmer EA, Tung B for the Cryotherapy for Retinopathy of Prematurity Group. Involution of retinopathy of prematurity. Arch Ophthalmol 2000;118:645–649.
143. Repka MX, Hudak ML, Parsa CF, Tielsch JM. Calf lung surfactant extract prophylaxis and retinopathy of prematurity. Ophthalmology 1992;99:531–536.
143a. Reynolds JD, Hardy RJ, Kennedy KA, et al. Lack of efficacy of light reduction in preventing retinopathy of prematurity. Light-ROP Cooperative Group. N Engl J Med 1998;338(22):1572–1576.
144. Robinson J, Fielder AR. Light and the immature visual system. Eye 1992;6:166–172.

144a. Saito V, Omoto T, Cho Y, et al. The progression of retinopathy of prematurity and fluctuation in blood gas tension. Graefés Arch Clin Exp Ophthalmol 1993;231(3):151–156.

145. Sasaki K, Yamashita Y, Maekawa T, Adachi T. Treatment of retinopathy of prematurity in active stage by cryocautery. Jpn J Ophthalmol 1976;20:384–395.

146. Schaffer DB, Johnson L, Quinn GE, et al. Vitamin E and retinopathy of prematurity: follow-up at one year. Ophthalmology 1985;92: 1005–1011.

147. Schaffer DB, Quinn GE, Johnson C. Sequelae of arrested mild retinopathy of prematurity. Arch Ophthalmol 1984;102:373–376.

147a. Seiberth V, Linderkamp O. Risk factors in retinopathy of prematurity: a multivariate statistical analysis. Ophthalmologica 2000; 214(2):131–135.

147b. Shastry BS, Hejtmancik JF, Hiraoka M, et al. Linkage and candidate gene analysis of autosomal-dominant familial exudative vitreoretinopathy. Clin Genet 2000;58(4):329–332.

147c. Shastry BS, Pendergast SD, Hartzer MK, Liu X, Trese MT. Identification of missense mutations in the Norrie disease gene associated with advanced ROP. Arch Ophthalmol 1997;115(5):651–655.

148. Shohat M, Reisner SH, Krikler R, et al. Retinopathy of prematurity: Incidence and risk factors. Pediatrics 1983;72:159–163.

149. Shulman J, Jampol LM, Schwartz H. Peripheral proliferative retinopathy without oxygen therapy in a full-term infant. Am J Ophthalmol 1980;90:509–514.

150. Silverman W. Retrolental fibroplasia: a modern parable. New York: Grune & Stratton, 1980.

151. Smith J, Shivitz I. Angle-closure glaucoma in adults with cicatricial retinopathy of prematurity. Arch Ophthalmol 1984;102:371–372.

152. Sneed Sr, Pulido JS, Blodi CF, et al. Surgical management of late-onset retinal detachments associated with regressed retinopathy of prematurity. Ophthalmology 1990;97:179–183.

153. Spencer R, Hutton WG, Snyder WB, et al. Limited applications of cryotherapy for severe retinopathy of prematurity. Ophthalmic Surg 1992;23:766–769.

154. Stannard KP, Mushin AS, Gamsu HR. Screening for retinopathy of prematurity in a regional neonatal intensive care unit. Eye 1989; 3:371–378.

155. Sternberg P Jr, Lopez PF, Capone A, et al. Management of threshold retinopathy of prematurity. Retina 1992;12:S60–S63.

156. Sternberg P Jr, Lopez PF, Lambert HM, et al. Controversies in the management of retinopathy of prematurity. Am J Ophthalmol 1992;113:198–202.

156a. Supplemental therapeutic oxygen for prethreshold retinopathy of prematurity (STOP-ROP), a randomized, controlled trial. Pediatrics 2000;105(2):295–310.

157. Szewczyk TS. Retrolental fibroplasia. Etiology and prophylaxis. Am J Ophthalmol 1952;35:301–311.
158. Tasman W. Vitreoretinal changes in cicatricial retrolental fibroplasia. Trans Am Ophthalmol Soc 1970;68:548–594.
159. Tasman W. Retinal detachment in retrolental fibroplasia. Albrecht von Graefe's Klin Ophthalmol 1975;195:129–139.
160. Tasman W. Late complications of retrolental fibroplasia. Ophthalmology 1979;86:1724–1740.
161. Tasman W. Management of retinopathy of prematurity. Ophthalmology 1985;92:995–999.
162. Tasman W. Threshold retinopathy of prematurity revisited (Editorial). Arch Ophthalmol 1992;110:623–624.
163. Tasman W, Annesley W Jr. Retinal detachment in the retinopathy of prematurity. Arch Ophthalmol 1966;75:608–614.
164. Tasman W, Brown GC, Schaffer DB, et al. Cryotherapy for active retinopathy of prematurity. Ophthalmology 1986;93:580–585.
165. Tasman W, Brown GC, Schaffer DB, et al. Cryotherapy for active retinopathy of prematurity (from discussion by Earl A. Palmer, pp 584–585). Ophthalmology 1986;93:580–585.
166. Terry TI. Extreme prematurity and fibroblastic overgrowth of persistent vascular sheath behind each crystalline lens. I. Preliminary report. Am J Ophthalmol 1942;25:203–204.
167. Terry TL. Fibroblastic overgrowth of persistent tunica vasculosa lentis in premature infants. II. Report of cases. Arch Ophthalmol 1943;29:36–53.
168. Topilow HW, Ackerman AL, Wang FM. The treatment of advanced retinopathy of prematurity by cryotherapy and scleral buckling surgery. Ophthalmology 1985;92:379–387.
169. Trese MT. Surgical results of stage V retrolental fibroplasia and timing of surgical repair. Ophthalmology 1984;91:461–466.
170. Trese MT. Visual results and prognostic factors for vision following surgery for stage V retinopathy of prematurity. Ophthalmology 1986;93:574–579.
171. Trese MT. Scleral buckling for retinopathy of prematurity. Ophthalmology 1994;101:23–26.
172. Trese MT, Batton DG. Ocular examination schedule for infants with fetal hydrops. Am J Ophthalmol 1989;108:459.
173. The Committee for the Classification of Retinopathy of Prematurity: an international classification of retinopathy of prematurity. Arch Ophthalmol 1984;102:1130–1134.
174. The Committee for the Classification of Retinopathy of Prematurity. An international classification of prematurity: the classification of retinal detachment. Arch Ophthalmol 1987;105:906–913.
175. The Laser ROP Study Group. Laser therapy for retinopathy of prematurity. Arch Ophthalmol 1994;112:154–156.
176. Zilis JD, de Juan E, Machemer R. Advanced retinopathy of prematurity: the anatomic and visual results of vitreous surgery. Ophthalmology 1990;97:821–826.

11

Infectious, Inflammatory, and Toxic Diseases of the Retina and Vitreous

William L. Haynes, Jose S. Pulido, and Peter H. Spiegel

The first portion of this chapter discusses inflammatory and infectious disorders that affect the posterior segment of the eye. Some of the disorders that are discussed are much more common in children than in adults (e.g., pars planitis). Although others are more common in adults, the ability to recognize their appearance is important because they can occur in pediatric patients (e.g., the presumed ocular histoplasmosis syndrome). In the last portion of the chapter, nutritional and toxic disorders of the retina are presented. Table 11-1 lists various infectious, inflammatory, toxic, and nutritional disorders of the retina and vitreous in the approximate order of their prevalence in children. Disorders that occur primarily in children are marked with a "c"; disorders that occur primarily in adults are marked with an "a"; conditions that occur in both groups are marked "a,c."

PARS PLANITIS

Pars planitis is a chronic inflammatory disorder of the retina and vitreous that commonly occurs in children and young adults. The etiology of the disease is not known. However, pars planitis has been associated with HLA-DR2 suballele-DR1501.[27a] Pars planitis is characterized by vitreous inflammation, commonly associated with *"snowball" opacities* of the vitreous and *"snowbank" opacities* along the pars plana (Fig. 11-1A). *Retinal periphlebitis* may also be seen. Patients usually present with

TABLE 11-1. Infectious, Inflammatory, Toxic, and Nutritional Disorders of the Retina and Vitreous.

I. Infectious and inflammatory disorders
   A. Primarily vitreitis
      1. Pars plantis (a,c)
      2. Juvenile rheumatoid arthritis (c)
      3. Toxocariasis (a,c)
      4. Sarcoidosis (a,c)
      5. Lyme disease (a,c)
      6. Inflammatory bowel disease (a)
      7. Whipple's disease (a)
   B. Primarily retinitis
      1. Toxoplasmosis (a,c)
      2. Acute retinal necrosis (a,c)
      3. AIDS (CMV retinitis) (a,c)
      4. Rubella (a,c)
      5. Syphilis (a,c)
      6. DUSN (a,c)
      7. Candida (a,c)
      8. Wegener's (a,c)
      9. SSPE (c)
      10. Leptospirosis (Leber's stellate neuroretinitis) (a,c)
      11. Behcet's (a)
      12. Lupus erythematosis (a)
      13. Cat-scratch neuroretinitis (a,c)
   C. Primarily choroiditis
      1. Onchocerchiasis (a,c)
      2. Ophthalmomyiasis (a,c)
      3. POHS (a,c)
      4. APMPPE (a)
      5. Sympathetic ophthalmia (a,c)
      6. Tuberculosis (a)
      7. VKH (a)
      8. MEWDS (a)
      9. Vitiliginous chorioretinitis (birdshot) (a)
      10. Serpiginous chorioretinitis (a)
      11. PIC (a)
      12. Multifocal choroiditis (a)
   D. Other
      1. Scleritis (a,c)
      2. Bacterial endophthalmitis (a,c)

II. Toxic and nutritional retinal disorders
   A. Vitamin A deficiency (Uyemura's syndrome) (a,c)
   B. Chalcosis (a,c)
   C. Siderosis (a,c)
   D. Oxalosis (a,c)
   E. Desferoxamine toxicity (a,c)
   F. Carbon monoxide toxicity (a)
   G. Methoxyflurane toxicity (a)
   H. Chloroquine toxicity (a)
   I. Canthaxanthine toxicity (a)
   J. Talc retinopathy (a)
   K. Plaquenil toxicity (a)
   L. Thioridazine toxicity (a)
   M. Nicotinic acid toxicity (a)
   N. Quinine toxicity (a)
   O. Tamoxifen toxicity (a)

CMV, cytomegalovirus; DUSN, diffuse unilateral subacute neuroretinitis; SSPE, subacute sclerosing panencephalitis; POHS, presumed ocular histoplasmosis syndrome; APMPPE, acute posterior multifocal placoid pigment epitheliopathy; VKH, Vogt–Koyanagi–Harada syndrome; MEWD, multifocal evanescent white dot syndrome; PIC, punctate inner choroidopathy.

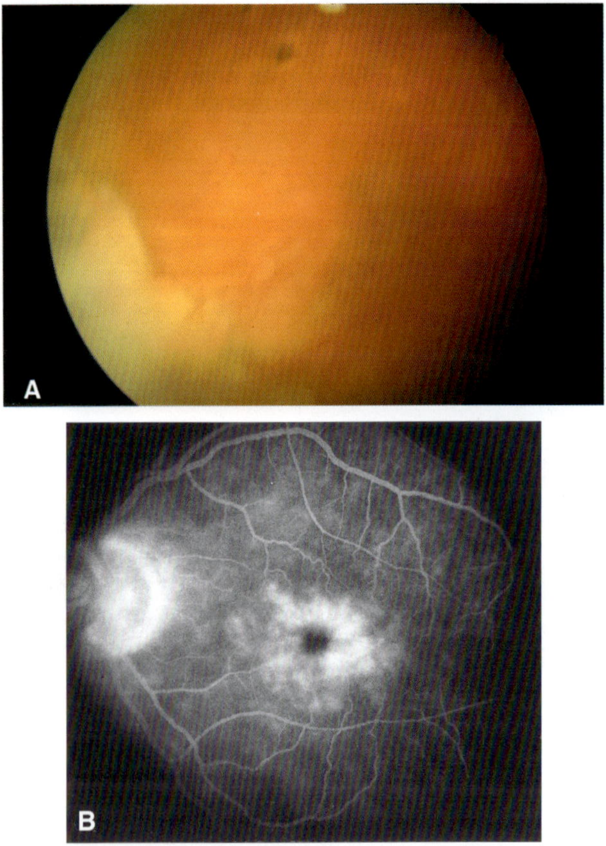

FIGURE 11-1A,B. (A) Peripheral "snowbanking" is the hallmark of pars planitis. **(B)** Angiographic appearance of cystoid macular edema, the most common cause of visual loss in patients with pars planitis.

blurred vision and floaters but do not usually complain of pain or photophobia. Up to 80% of cases are eventually bilateral. Anterior chamber inflammation is usually mild or absent although children seem to have more anterior chamber inflammation than adults. The snowbank opacities along the pars plana are characteristic of the disease but are sometimes present in only one eye of a patient with bilateral inflammation. The snowbanks represent fibroglial masses and are most commonly seen inferiorly. Peripheral neovascularization may occur along an area of snowbanking and vitreous hemorrhage can occur. Optic disc edema may be seen, more commonly in children, in whom it occurs in up to 50% of cases. In cases of severe vitritis, children may present with decreased red reflexes.

The course of pars planitis is variable. Inflammation is usually chronic but may not result in severe visual loss. The amount of visual loss is usually related to the presence of *cystoid macular edema* (CME) (Fig. 11-1B). CME is typically worse in patients having more inflammation. Cataracts, glaucoma, and retinal detachments may also cause visual loss in these patients. Vitreous hemorrhage is an important cause of visual loss in children with pars planitis. In addition, about 16% of patients with pars planitis develop optic neuritis or multiple sclerosis. There are no characteristic laboratory abnormalities. The differential diagnosis of pars planitis includes sarcoidosis, tuberculosis, syphilis, toxocariasis, and toxoplasmosis. Conversely, a pars planitis-like inflammation may also be seen in patients with multiple sclerosis.[4]

Treatment of pars planitis with corticosteroids is often effective. Corticosteroids can have significant ocular and systemic side effects and should be used with caution. Aggressive treatment is indicated in cases of visual loss from 20/20 or severe floaters that cause visual impairment. Periocular steriods (20–40 mg triamcinolone diacetate per injection) are the first line of treatment, especially for unilateral cases. More than one injection may be necessary to achieve a decrease in inflammation or resolution of CME. Intraocular corticosteroids may also be considered and appear to be of significant value. Cryotherapy or laser photocoagulation to areas of snowbanking or to the retina behind the snowbanking may be effective in decreasing inflammation in some cases and can decrease peripheral neovascularization. Oral corticosteroids (1–2 mg/kg per day, tapering 5–10 mg/wk), may be effective, although significant side effects are common with prolonged treatment, and treatment for longer than 3 weeks should be avoided. Methotrexate, cyclosporine, or chlorambucil may be effective and can decrease peripheral neovascularization, but should be reserved for severe cases.[21,31a,35] These agents, particularly cyclosporine, should be used with great caution. Peripheral scatter photoaocagulation[41] is also useful in treating vitreous base neovascularization. Pars plana vitrectomy also has a role in cases with severe vitreitis, macular edema, vitreous hemorrhage, and epiretinal membrane.

SARCOIDOSIS

Sarcoidosis is an inflammatory systemic disease characterized by the formation of noncaseating granulomas. The disease is most common in adults, although children may be affected. Posterior segment manifestations are seen in approximately 20% of patients with ocular sarcoidosis. Vitreous inflammation classically presents as clumps of vitreous debris ("snowballs"). Perivascular sheathing is common, and severe forms of periphlebitis can occur. Vascular occlusion (most commonly branch vein occlusion) may be seen. Multifocal, deep, white, choroidal lesions are characteristic but similar lesions are seen in other inflammatory ocular disorders (Fig. 11-2). Granulomatous infiltration of the optic nerve may lead to severe visual loss.

The diagnosis may be made presumptively (e.g., in a patient with uveitis and bilateral hilar adenopathy) or by biopsy of conjunctival, skin, or lung lesions. Laboratory testing may be of some use in making the diagnosis. Serum *angiotensin-converting enzyme* (ACE) is often elevated in patients, and an

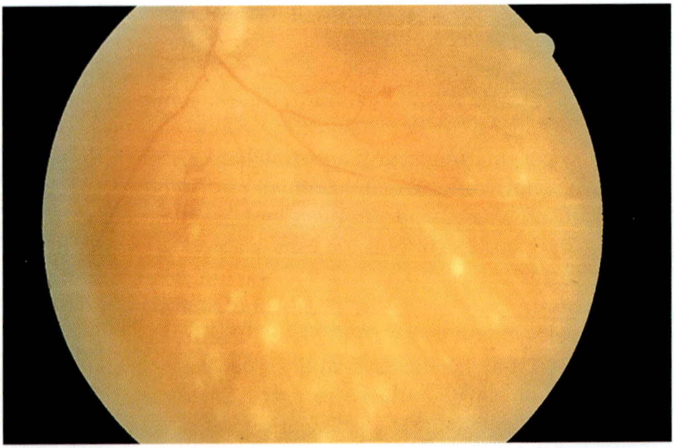

FIGURE 11-2. Peripheral "punched-out" chorioretinal lesions in the presence of active posterior uveitis in a patient with sarcoidosis.

elevated serum ACE supports the diagnosis of sarcoidosis. Random conjunctival biopsy (when no nodules are seen) has been advocated by some and may be useful in some cases.[33]

The differential diagnosis of ocular sarcoidosis includes many entities. In children, one must consider juvenile rheumatoid arthritis and pars planitis. Other diseases that may have a similar presentation include sympathetic ophthalmia, Behcet's disease, and the "white-dot" syndromes.[37]

Corticosteroids are effective in treating ocular (and systemic) manifestations of sarcoidosis. Acute iridocyclitis responds well to topical corticosteroids. Chronic granulomatous uveitis may require periocular, intraocular, or systemic steroids. In treating children, one must remember the severe side effects of chronic systemic corticosteroids and limit their use when possible. Choroidal lesions are associated with CNS sarcoidosis and appropriate evaluation is required.

OCULAR TOXOCARIASIS

Ocular toxocariasis is caused by invasion of the eye by larval forms of the dog roundworm, *Toxocara canis* or, rarely, by the cat roundworm, *Toxocara cati*. The first cases of ocular toxocariasis to be described were patients who had undergone enucleation for suspicion of retinoblastoma.[57] Most of these patients had dense vitreous inflammation (vitreous abscess) and retinal detachment. The more common presentation is a gray to white mass in the posterior pole or retinal periphery (a focal granuloma) with variable amounts of vitreous inflammation (Fig. 11-3). The inflammation may resolve over time. Vitreoretinal *traction bands* may be seen extending from the mass. Pathologically, the mass lesion represents a choroidal granuloma. Peripheral inflammation similar to that seen in pars planitis has also been described, but only one eye is usually afffected.[20] Ultrasound biomicroscopy may identify characteristic pseudocysts in the peripheral vitreous of affected eyes.[54] In some cases, there are no overt signs of inflammation and a child may present with strabismus or poor vision on screening tests. The disease is usually unilateral and almost always occurs in children. The diagnosis is usually made clinically, but serum antibody titers determined by enzyme-linked immunosorbent assay (ELISA) may be helpful in some cases. Titers are often lower in patients with ocular toxocariasis than in those with visceral larva migrans. Serum titers of 1:8 have been suggested to be supportive of the diagnosis, but titers of this level may be seen in up to 30% of young children with no evidence of ocular disease.[13]

Severe infections or those that threaten vision by proximity to the macula or optic nerve should be treated with periocular or systemic corticosteroids in an attempt to quiet the inflammation. The antihelminthics *thiabendazole* and *albendazole* have been used with some success, but corticosteroids should be given concomitantly to blunt the intense inflammatory reaction that occurs following the death of intraocular organisms.[38] Cryotherapy and photocoagulation may be used in some cases.[1a] Cycloplegic agents should also be used. In cases with less inflammation, topical steroids may be of some benefit. Cases that develop epiretinal membranes, traction retinal detachment, and combined traction-rhegmatogenous retinal detachment may be treated with modern vitreoretinal surgery techniques including vitrectomy, scleral buckling, endolaser, and fluid–gas exchange.[1] The optimum timing of surgery and how aggressive the surgeon should be in attempting to remove posterior granulomas in undetermined.[1]

Partly because of the similarity of their names, ocular toxocariasis is sometimes confused with ocular toxoplasmosis (see

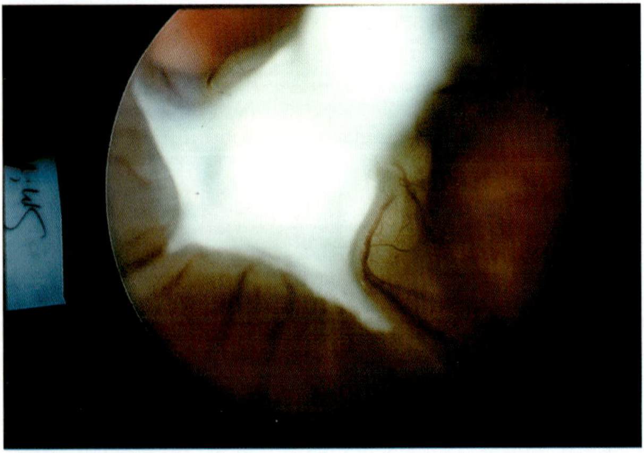

FIGURE 11-3. Fundus photograph shows the typical posterior pole granuloma of toxocariasis. (From Pollard ZF, Jarrett WH, Hagler WS, et al: ELISA for diagnosis of ocular toxocariasis. Ophthalmology 1979;86:743–752, with permission.)

TABLE 11-2. Clinical Features of Ocular Toxoplasmosis and Ocular Toxocariasis.

	Toxoplasmosis	*Toxocariasis*
Age of onset	Children or adults; may be congenital	Almost always children, usually over age 3
Associated ocular conditions	Microphthalmos in congenital cases; may present with strabismus or poor vision 2° to macular scarring	May present with strabismus or poor vision 2° to macular scarring
Associated systemic conditions	Microcephaly, convulsions, cerebral calcifications, organomegaly in congenital cases	None
Vitritis	Common	Common
Retinal lesions	Fluffy retinitis, often in an area of chorioretinal scarring	Retinochoroidal mass lesion (granuloma)
Serological testing	ELISA for antibodies to *Toxoplasma gondii* usually positive. PCR of vitreous can also be performed in some centers.	ELISA for antibodies to *Toxocara canis* may be positive

following). Table 11-2 summarizes the distinguishing features of these two entities.

JUVENILE RHEUMATOID ARTHRITIS

Juvenile rheumatoid arthritis (JRA) is a group of disorders characterized by persistent arthritis with an onset before 16 years of age. Certain types of JRA are associated with a high incidence of uveitis. The predominant ocular manifestation of the disorder is chronic iridocyclitis. A few patients may have significant vitritis, but the posterior vitreous is usually clear. The uveitis may initially be asymptomatic but can cause severe visual disability in some patients. Glaucoma, band keratopathy, anterior and posterior synechiae, cataracts, and cystoid macular edema may occur (Fig. 11-4). The uveitis is most commonly seen in young girls under age 5 with pauciarticular arthritis (four or fewer joints involved at onset of disease) and positive antinuclear antibodies (ANA).[7]

Treatment of chronic uveitis in patients with JRA is often difficult. Topical, periocular, or possibly intraocular corticosteroids are the treatment of choice. Oral corticosteroids should be avoided if possible because of the chronic course of the

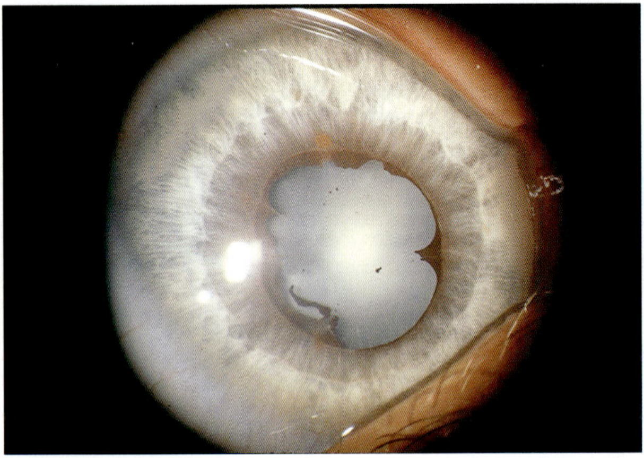

FIGURE 11-4. Patient with juvenile rheumatoid arthritis, showing the sequelae of chronic anterior uveitis that include posterior synechiae and cataract formation. Band keratopathy is also seen in many of these patients.

disease and many side effects of the treatment, but aggressive treatment is required. It may not be possible to clear the anterior chamber of cells, and the flare often persists after adequate treatment, but aggressive treatment is required.[34] Many children will be on systemic *methotrexate*, which may have a steroid-sparing effect. Systemic cyclosporin A is effective in many refractory cases.[21] *Etanercept*, which neutralizes tumor necrosis factor-α, may also be effective in certain cases of treatment-resistant cases; however, further research is needed regarding its effectiveness in ocular disease.[46]

OCULAR TOXOPLASMOSIS

Ocular toxoplasmosis results from infection with the protozoan parasite *Toxoplasma gondii*. Congenital toxoplasmosis is classically described as a triad of convulsions, cerebral calcifications, and retinochoroiditis. If the fetus is infected in the first trimester, the resulting illness may be severe, with microcephaly, seizures, intracranial calcification, hydocephalus, jaundice, and organomegaly. Retinochoroiditis is present in 75% to 80% of cases.[8,48] Microphthalmos, optic atrophy, anterior and posterior uveitis, strabismus, and nystagmus may also be seen. Histopathologic features include retinitis, retinal necrosis, RPE disruption, choroidal inflammation and congestion, and optic neuritis.[47] Infections acquired later in gestation are typically less severe and may initially be asymptomatic. Some patients present with strabismus or poor vision on screening examinations due to macular scarring. Some cases of "acquired" toxoplasma retinochoroiditis are probably the result of reactivation of congenitally acquired infection.[42]

Older patients with active ocular toxoplasmosis often present with complaints of decreased vision and floaters. A focal area of retinitis is often seen adjacent to an old scar (Fig. 11-5A). The active area is fluffy and white and has an overlying vitritis. When vitreous inflammation is intense, the classic "headlight-in-a-fog" presentation is seen, representing an area of retinitis seen through vitreous haze (Fig. 11-5B). A typical attack may last a week to several months despite treatment. The visual prognosis depends mainly on the presence or absence of macular involvement. Papillitis is rarely seen but is a cause of permanent visual loss in some patients. Punctate retinal lesions have also been described.[14] One study found a 6% incidence of retinal detachment and an additional 5% incidence of retinal breaks in 150 patients with ocular toxoplasmosis.[6] Patients with severe inflammation and myopia were at greatest risk. The diagnosis is made when a typical fundus lesion is found in a patient with positive serological testing. The presence of IgG or IgM antibodies in serum can be detected by indirect immunofluorescence or ELISA. Neonates with congenital infections may demonstrate IgM antibodies in the cerebrospinal fluid (CSF). Because many patients without active toxoplasmosis may have positive antibody titers, the diagnosis is mainly a clinical one, with serology playing a supportive role. More recent work has shown that polymerase chain reaction of blood, aqueous, and vitreous can identify *T. gondii* DNA.[18,32]

Congenital infections should be treated agressively for a duration of 1 year. Triple drug therapy with pyramethamine, sulfadiazine, and leukovorin (folinic acid) is clearly superior to treatment for 1 month or no treatment.[29,30,48] Prednisone is added for elevation of CSF protein and for vision-threatening chorioretinitis. Prolonged triple-agent treatment has been shown to lead to quite favorable neurological and ophthalmologic outcomes, despite severe disease at presentation.[29,30,48] Therefore, early, accurate diagnosis and prompt referral are imperative.

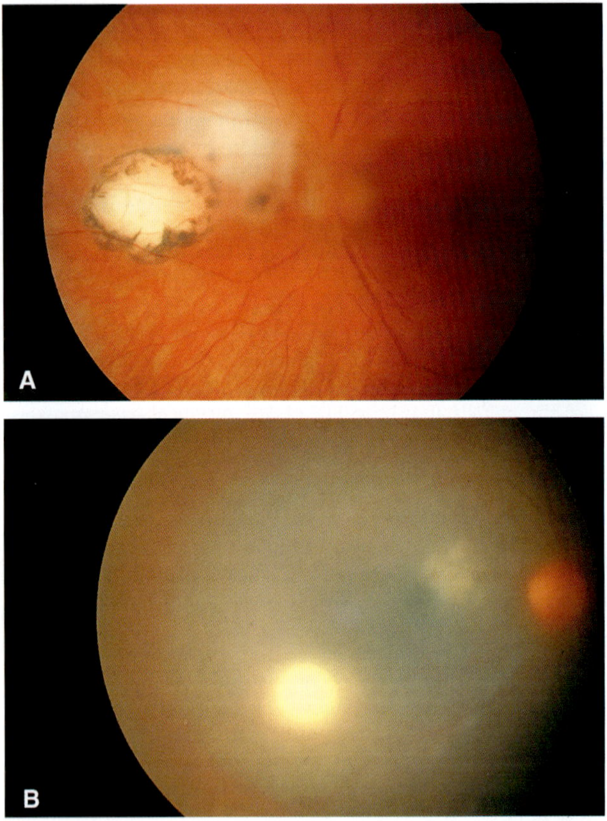

FIGURE 11-5A,B. **(A)** Active inflammation at the edge of an old chorioretinal scar in a patient with toxoplasmosis. **(B)** Classic "headlight-in-the-fog" appearance of active toxoplasmosis represents a posterior pole inflammatory mass seen through the haze caused by posterior uveitis.

In older patients, treatment should be considered if the macula or optic nerve is threatened or if the patient is immunodeficient. Triple-drug therapy also is commonly used in older patients [pyrimethamine (50 mg loading dose, then 25 mg orally twice a day), sulfadiazine (1g orally four times a day), and prednisone (20–40 mg or more daily usually starting 1–2 days after the other drugs)]. Folinic acid (3–5 mg orally three times per week) is also given to counteract the toxic side effects of pyrimethamine (mainly bone marrow toxicity). Prednisone should not be used alone to treat ocular toxoplasmosis.[50] Clindamycin and azithromycin has been used as an alternative or additional drug to treat ocular toxoplasmosis and may have some efficacy.[24] Preventative measures such as adequate cooking of meats and the avoidance of cats and cat feces by pregnant women and high-risk individuals are recommended.

LYMPHOCYTIC CHORIOMENINGITIS VIRUS CHORIORETINITIS AND HTLV-1

Lymphocytic choriomeningitis virus (LCMV) is an arena virus harbored by the common house mouse and other rodents. Transmission to humans may occur through the air and through consumption of food infected by urine, feces, and saliva. Bites may also transmit the virus. Only a few dozen cases of disease attributable to LCMV have been published, but this entity is probably more common than previously believed.[31]

Vertical transmission may lead to a congenital syndrome of chorioretinal scarring and retinal pigment epithelium (RPE) migration, with consequent visual impairment. Central nervous system sequelae include microcephaly, cerebral atrophy, hydrocephalus and periventricular calcification. Infections causing only ocular disease have been documented. Infections acquired by older children and adults are less severe and may be subclinical. Diagnosis is made through immunofluorescent antibody testing and ELISA testing. The differential diagnosis of LCMV chorioretinitis includes the constituents of the *TORCH* cluster; however, the appearance of congential LCMV most closely resembles toxoplasmosis.[5] Exposure to rodents during pregnancy should be avoided.[31] HTLV-1 can cause uveitis. This has been noted most commonly in Asia and the Caribbean.[30a]

ACUTE RETINAL NECROSIS

The acute retinal necrosis syndrome (ARN) is characterized by necrotizing retinitis and vitritis in immunocompetent patients. Although it is most common in the 20- to 50-year-old age group, it can occur in children. The disease is most commonly unilateral, but up to one-third of cases are bilateral. The second eye is usually affected within a few weeks of the first but occasionally this occurs much later.

Patients often initially present with a painful red eye secondary to a granulomatous anterior uveitis (Fig. 11-6A). Patchy

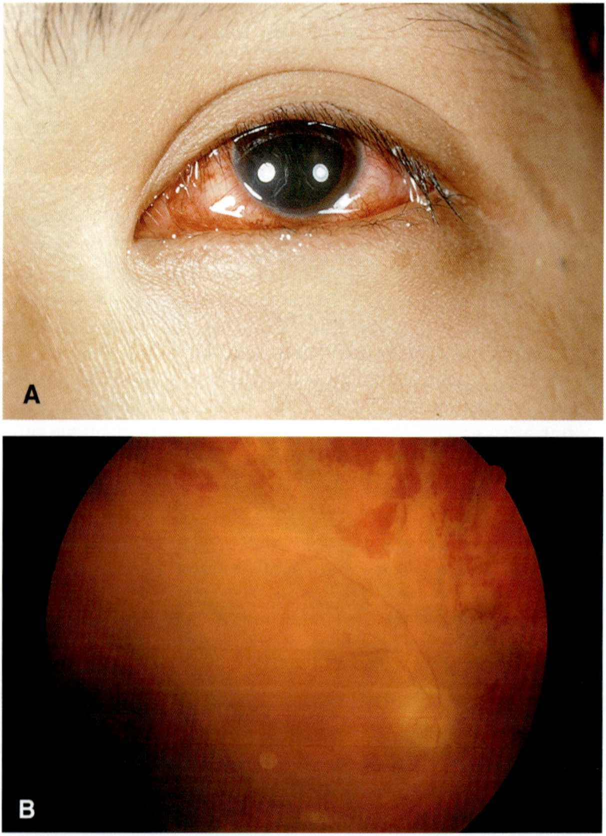

FIGURE 11-6A,B. Common features of the acute retinal necrosis syndrome. The affected eye is usually red and painful. Diffuse whitening of the retina is seen on ophthalmoscopy. Retinal hemorrhage may also be seen.

whitening of the peripheral retina and vitreous inflammation may be present initially or may develop over days to weeks. Arterial sheathing is common. The white areas may coalesce and spread posteriorly (Fig. 11-6B). The active phase of retinitis lasts 4 to 6 weeks. When lesions clear, they leave atrophic scars with RPE stippling. Three-fourths of these patients develop retinal detachment in the involved eye within 1 to 2 months, often complicated by large breaks and tractional components. Visual loss secondary to optic nerve involvement may also occur.

Herpesvirus particles have been identified within necrotic retina from eyes with ARN. Varicella zoster virus (VZV) and herpes simplex type 1 and 2, demonstrated by polymerase chain reaction (PCR) and antibody testing, have been shown to be the most common causes.[9,23,53,55]

The treatment of ARN is difficult, and no randomized clinical trials have been performed. However, the retinitis responds to acyclovir. Retinal tears often occur despite treatment, commonly leading to retinal detachment. Prophylactic laser at the edge of the involved retina and i.v. acyclovir therapy may improve the prognosis.[19] Poor visualization may preclude laser therapy, and early vitrectomy may be required in patients with ARN and hazy vitreous. The role of corticosteroids in this disorder is controversial.

RUBELLA

Expectant mothers who are infected with the rubella (*German measles*) virus during pregnancy may give birth to infants with a variety of congenital anomalies affecting the eyes, ears, heart, and other organs. Depending on the stage of gestation at the time of infection, a wide variety of clinical features may be seen. The most common ocular findings of the congenital rubella syndrome are nuclear cataract (often eccentric), microphthalmos, and a salt-and-pepper retinopathy. Other findings include congenital glaucoma, strabismus, and iris hypoplasia. Nonocular findings include sensorineural hearing loss and congenital heart disease.

Rubella retinopathy is classically described as a "salt and pepper" mottling of the retinal pigment epithelium (RPE) (Fig. 11-7A,B) that is often most prominent in the posterior fundus. Eighty percent of cases are bilateral. The abnormal fundus

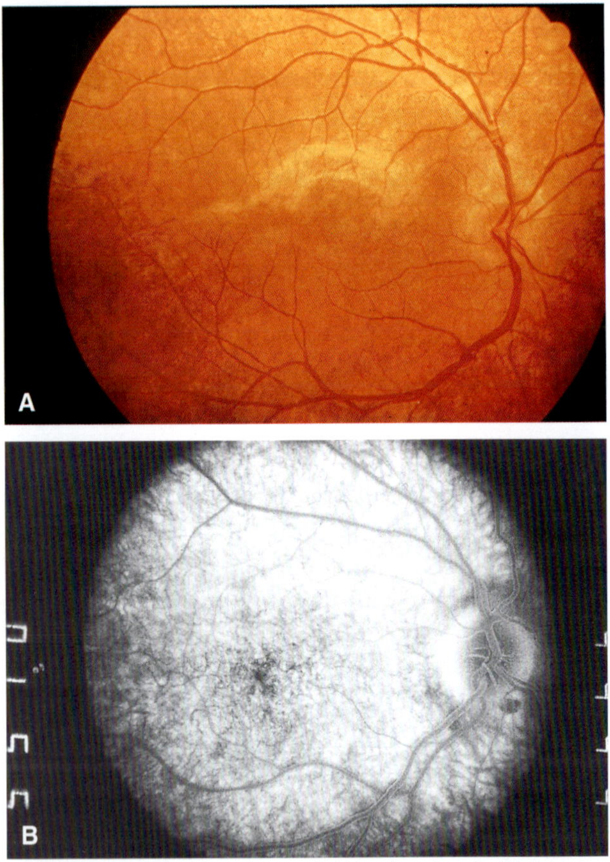

FIGURE 11-7A,B. Fundus photograph (**A**) and angiogram (**B**) from two different patients with congenital rubella show the characteristic "salt-and-pepper" retinopathy.

appearance may be seen alone or may be accompanied by other ocular abnormalities such as cataract and microphthalmos. When seen alone, the abnormal fundus appearance does not usually result in a decrease in visual acuity. Visual fields, color vision, electroretinography, and electro-oculography are usually normal. Fundus changes may progress throughout childhood, and choroidal neovascularization has been described. The fundus picture is not specific for rubella. A similar appearance may occur in patients with congenital syphilis as well as toxic or inherited diseases of the RPE and the carrier state of X-linked ocular albinism.[16] Positive serum titers of antibody against the rubella virus are indicative of prior infection and may aid in making the diagnosis. However, negative antibody titers do not rule out the diagnosis of congenital rubella because antibodies may disappear with time. Treatment for the choroidal neovascularization can be performed with conventional laser photocoagulation or photodynamic therapy.

SYPHILIS

Syphilis is a sexually transmitted disease caused by the spirochete *Treponema pallidum*. Syphilitic eye disease may be congenital or acquired. Congenital syphilis is associated with a pigmentary retinopathy that is classically described as a "salt-and-pepper" mottling of the fundus (Fig. 11-8A). The retinal pigment epithelial clumping may mimic retinitis pigmentosa. Optic atrophy is also commonly seen. Infants with congenital syphilis acquire the disease transplacentally. Affected infants may have failure to thrive, hepatosplenomegaly, and anemia. Classic nonocular physical signs include *saddle nose, sabre shins*, and *Hutchinson's teeth*. Some cases are asymptomatic and are recognized later in life (e.g., after an episode of interstitial keratitis). Acquired syphilis commonly produces a patchy neuroretinitis that may result in profound visual field loss. Uveitis (Fig. 11-8B) or optic disc edema may also occur with or without chorioretinitis.

The diagnosis of syphilitic eye disease is made with a combination of clinical and laboratory examinations. In congenital cases, the serum VDRL and FTA-ABS tests may be negative early in the course of the disease. However, in cases of congenital syphilis that present late, as well as in cases of acquired syphilis, these tests are usually useful. Because the serum VDRL may be falsely negative in some patients, the FTA-ABS is a more reliable test. However, false-positive results occur with both tests. VDRL testing of the CSF should be performed in patients with suspected secondary or tertiary syphilis.

Treating affected mothers is the best preventative treatment for congenital syphilis. Infants with congenital syphilis should

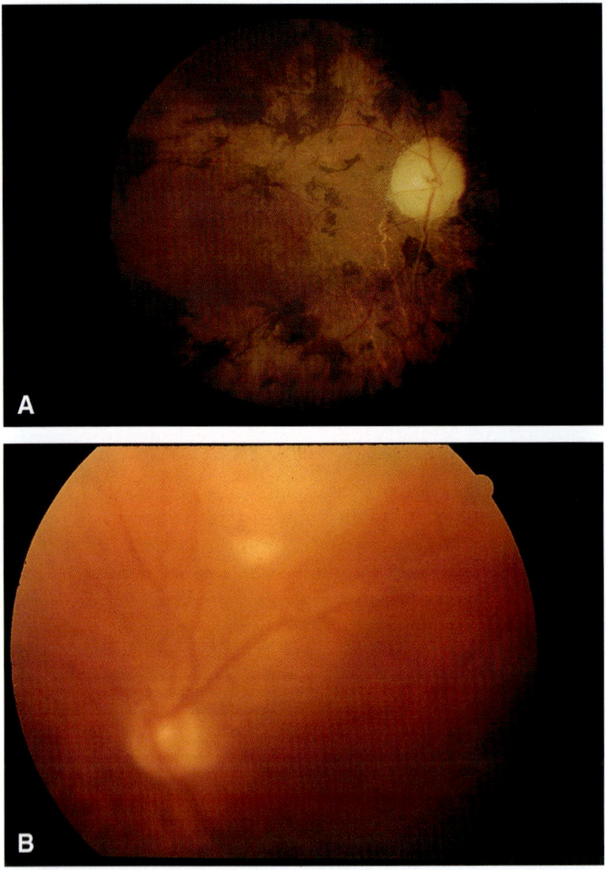

FIGURE 11-8A,B. **(A)** Fundus photograph from patient with congenital syphilis. Note the pigmentary abnormalities and pale optic disc. **(B)** Anterior or posterior uveitis may be seen in patients with secondary syphilis. This patient presented with posterior uveitis and a chorioretinal inflammatory mass.

be treated similarly regardless of CSF serologies.[17] Treatment of acquired cases depends on CSF serologies. The latest recommendations from the Centers for Disease Control should be consulted before starting therapy. Ocular syphilis should be treated as if it were neurosyphilis. Cycloplegics and topical or periocular steroids may be helpful adjuncts in patients with uveitis.

AIDS AND OPPORTUNISTIC OCULAR INFECTIONS

Acquired immunodeficiency syndrome (AIDS) is caused by infection with HIV-1, a retrovirus. Infection with the virus may occur in any age group and most commonly occurs through sexual intercourse or shared intravenous needles. Infants can acquire the disease in utero from an infected mother (vertical transmission) or from breast milk. Patients who are infected with the virus develop a profound depression in cell-mediated immunity. The disease may manifest itself many years after the initial infection with the virus. Patients are prone to develop opportunistic infections such as *Pneumocystis carinii* pneumonia and unusual neoplasms such as Kaposi's sarcoma.

Ocular involvement is quite common in affected patients and ranges from scattered cotton wool spots to potentially blinding *cytomegalovirus (CMV) retinitis*.[2] Cotton wool spots are commonly seen in affected patients. Clinically, these nerve fiber layer infarcts appear as whitish fluffy lesions of the inner retina (Fig. 11-9A) that may be up to 0.5 disc diameters in size. They do not enlarge with time (as do the lesions of CMV retinitis) and rarely cause any visual disturbance. Cytomegalovirus is a herpesvirus that can cause a severe retinitis. The disease occurs almost exclusively in immunocompromised hosts (e.g., organ and bone marrow transplant patients, cancer patients, patients with AIDS). Approximately 1.6% to 6% of children with AIDS develop CMV retinitis, which is significantly less frequent than in adults.[2,12] CMV retinitis may appear as fluffy whitish retinal lesions with hemorrhage that enlarge over time (Fig. 11-9B). Alternatively, the lesions may be granular centrally with hemorrhage and retinal whitening at the periphery. The edges of the lesions are areas of active viral infection whereas the central areas represent necrotic retina. Lesions often start peripherally, and visual acuity may be normal until the macula or optic nerve are involved.

The diagnosis of CMV retinitis in children may be delayed because of their inability to report visual loss. Therefore, screening examinations on a more frequent schedule than in adults may be desirable. Retinal examinations should also be

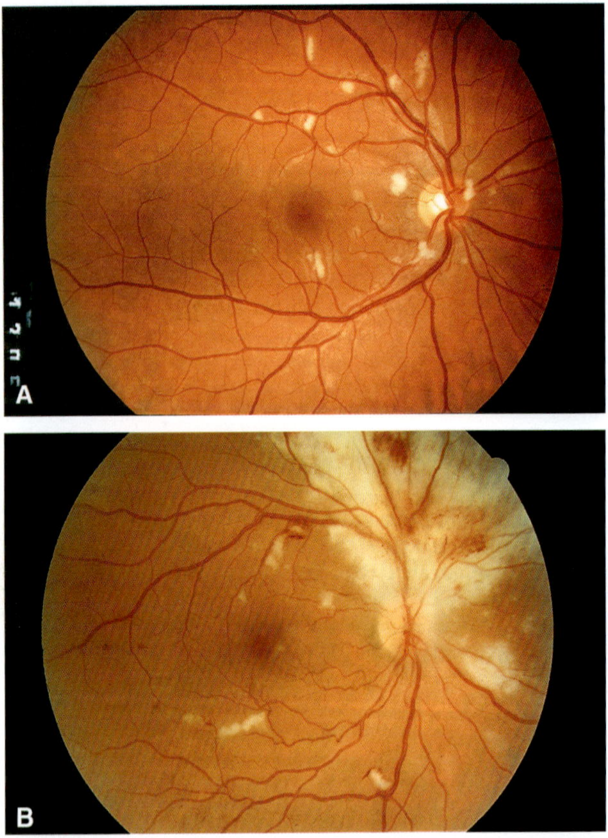

FIGURE 11-9A,B. **(A)** Cotton wool spots are commonly seen in patients with the acquired immunodeficiency syndrome (AIDS) but do not seem to be predictive of other ocular complications. **(B)** Cytomegalovirus retinitis encroaching upon the optic disc in patient with AIDS.

performed when systemic CMV infections are detected. Du et al.[12] found that children with HIV and a CD4 lymphocyte count less than 20 were at greater risk for retinitis whereas those with higher counts did not develop retinitis. Optimal treatment of CMV retinitis in children has not yet been established. Treatment with intravenous *foscarnet* or *ganciclovir* often results in a clinical response.[51,56] These drugs are virostatic, and maintenance therapy is required. If ganciclovir alone fails to control the retinitis, the addition of foscarnet may control the disease.[51] The use of ganciclovir and foscarnet together decreases the incidence of reactivation. For severe infections or for patients who cannot tolerate systemic medication, intravitreal ganciclovir (1 mg in 0.1 ml) or placement of sustained-release ganciclovir implants may be tried in conjunction with oral valganciclovir.[10,28] Other opportunistic infections may occur in AIDS patients and may be difficult to differentiate from CMV retinitis. Both herpes simplex and herpes zoster may produce a retinitis in immunocompromised patients.[36] If the patient has AIDS, HAART (highly active anti-retroviral therapy) may help cause resolution of the CMV retinitis, but a secondary iridocyclitis may develop (immune reconstitution uveitis). This iridocyclitis is responsive to topical corticosteroids.

OPHTHALMOMYIASIS AND DIFFUSE UNILATERAL SUBACUTE NEURORETINITIS

The term ophthalmomyiasis applies to cases of ocular infestation with the larval forms of flies. The larval forms may be transmitted by adult flies through bites or by touching the ocular area with hands contaminated with larvae.[57]

Characteristically, ocular findings consist of subretinal tracks with or without an encysted or moving organism within the subretinal space (Fig. 11-10A). The amount of inflammatory response is variable. Patients may complain of photopsias. Loss of vision may occur if the macula or optic nerve is involved.

Treatment of affected patients depends on the amount of inflammation present and whether the organism can be localized. Severe inflammatory reactions should be treated with periocular or oral corticosteroids. If the organism can be localized, photocoagulation of the organism has been recommended.[44] Organisms may also be removed with vitrectomy.

Diffuse unilateral subacute neuroretinitis (DUSN) is caused by ocular infestation with nematode larvae other than *Toxocara canis*.[15] These larvae are not found within granulomatous masses, as are *T. canis* organisms, but may be seen moving through the subretinal space. Patients typically present with scotomata and/or visual blurring. Diffuse patchy pigment epithelial atrophy and/or deep gray-white retinal lesions may be

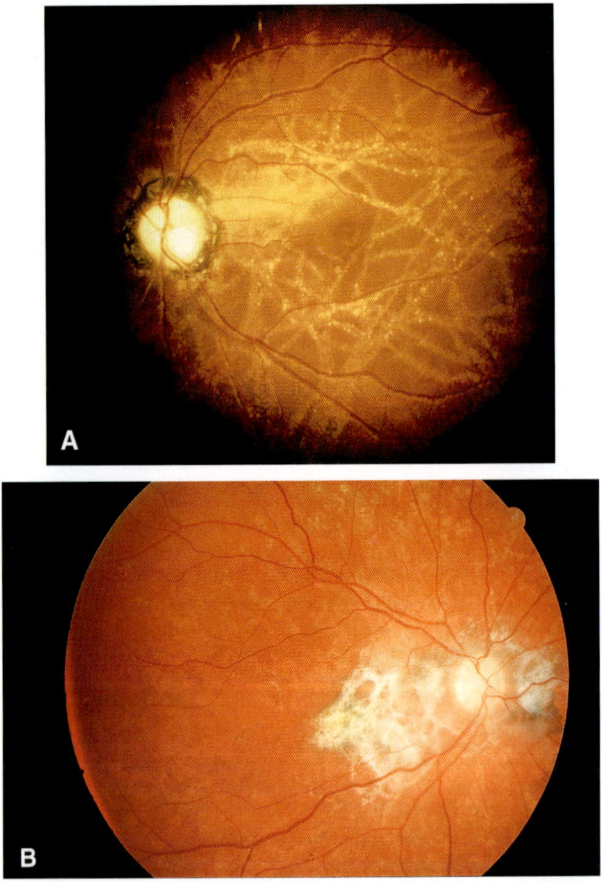

FIGURE 11-10A,B. (A) Young patient with ophthalmomyiasis who presented with complaints of flashing lights in this eye. Note the numerous tracks made by the motile nematode. (Courtesy of Dr. W. Johnson.) **(B)** Note the pale optic disc, narrowed vessels, peripapillary scarring, and diffuse pigmentary abnormality in this photograph of an eye with the late stage of diffuse unilateral subacute neuroretinitis (DUSN).

seen. Optic nerve swelling is common, and visual field loss may be severe. In the late stages, optic atrophy, pigmentary retinal changes, and narrowing of the retinal vessels may be seen (Fig. 11-10B). Motile organisms may be seen at any stage of the disease. *Toxocara* ELISA titers are typically low. Electroretinogram (ERG) abnormalities are present in all stages of the disease, with the b-wave being affected more than the a-wave. Many entities are in the differential diagnosis of DUSN, depending on the stage of the disease. Early in the course, DUSN may mimic various "white-dot" syndromes or presumed ocular histoplasmosis syndrome (POHS) whereas late in the course it may mimic retinitis pigmentosa. It should be remembered that DUSN occurs most often in children and young adults who are otherwise healthy. This condition is almost always unilateral. A case of living nematodes in both eyes was referred to as diffuse *bilateral subacute neuroretinitis*.[11]

Treatment is similar to that for ophthalmomyiasis. Laser photocoagulation of the organism is the definitive treatment.

PRESUMED OCULAR HISTOPLASMOSIS SYNDROME

The presumed ocular histoplasmosis syndrome (POHS) is characterized by peripheral "punched-out" chorioretinal scars, pe ripapillary scarring, disciform macular scarring, and a lack of inflammation (Fig. 11-11A). The disease is thought to be related to infection with *Histoplasma capsulatum*, a fungus that is a common soil contaminant in the Mississippi and Ohio river valleys of the United States. Initial infection with the organism occurs by respiratory contact and may result in a mild upper respiratory syndrome but is more commonly asymptomatic. An active choroiditis may occur at this early stage. In immunocompetent individuals, the syndrome (including ocular lesions) resolves spontaneously, resulting in multifocal areas of chorioretinal scarring. The disease is most commonly recognized in adults but may be seen in older children. Many patients are asymptomatic and the syndrome is recognized by noting the multifocal chorioretinal scars during routine ophthalmoscopy. However, choroidal neovascular membranes may occur adjacent to these scars, and these may cause hemorrhage and serous detachment of the retina (Fig. 11-11B,C). If this occurs in the macular area, visual acuity can be seriously affected. If left

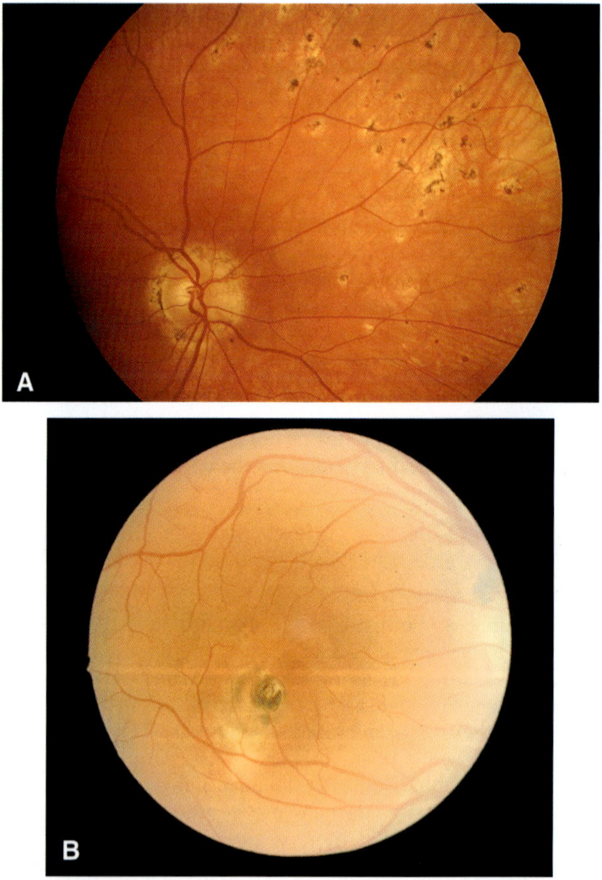

FIGURE 11-11A–C. (**A**) Peripapillary atrophic changes and peripheral pigmented "punched-out" chorioretinal lesions without uveitis are the most common manifestations of the presumed ocular histoplasmosis syndrome (POHS). Photograph (**B**) and angiographic view. (**C**) show a perifoveal neovascular membrane secondary to POHS.

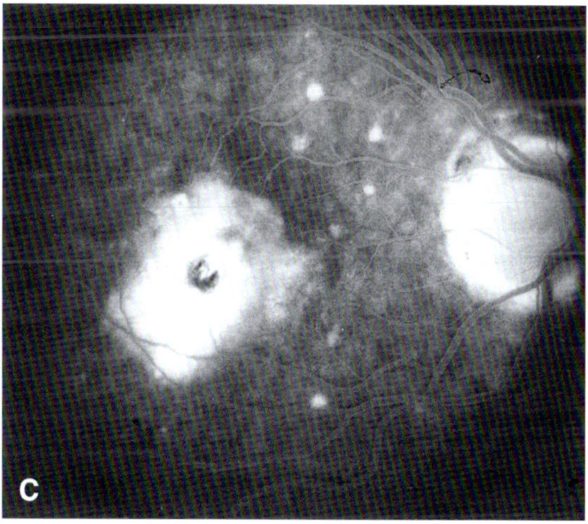

FIGURE 11-11A–C. (continued)

untreated, these lesions may progress to disciform scarring, although some resolve spontaneously with maintenance of good visual acuity. Submacular surgery to remove peripapillary and subfoveal choroidal neovascular membranes is sometimes used. Ablation of these neovascular membranes with argon laser has been shown to reduce the risk of severe visual loss in some patients.[39] Photodynamic therapy is helpful in cases of subfoveal or juxtafoveal neurovascular memory.

SYMPATHETIC OPHTHALMIA

Sympathetic ophthalmia is an uncommon but potentially devastating ocular disease of unknown etiology. It is a bilateral granulomatous uveitis that occurs after penetrating trauma or, less commonly, after intraocular surgery. The disease is thought to represent an autoimmune response to an unidentified antigen. The inflammatory response occurs not only in the traumatized eye (*exciting eye*) but also in the fellow eye (*sympathizing eye*). The disease is more common in males. Children and young adults are most commonly affected, probably reflecting the higher incidence of trauma in these age groups. Sympathetic ophthalmia is uncommon (<1% of trauma cases and <0.05% of surgical cases).[26] The incidence of sympathetic ophthalmia has apparently decreased over time, possibly because of advances in surgical technique.

The clinical course of sympathetic ophthalmia is variable. The onset may occur days or many years after the initial injury. Typically, there is a mild inflammatory response in the sympathizing eye with a worsening of inflammation in the exciting eye.[43] The anterior chamber inflammation may be intense, with formation of keratic precipitates. Anterior chamber inflammation is accompanied by injection, pain, and photophobia. Vitritis and retinal changes typically follow. Yellow-white peripheral choroidal lesions are known as *Dalen–Fuchs nodules*, which are classic but not pathognomonic of the disease. Optic disc swelling is often seen (Fig. 11-12A). Pathologically, there is diffuse infiltration of the choroid with lymphocytes, epithelioid cells, and scattered giant cells (Fig. 11-12B). Dalen–Fuchs nodules represent focal accumulations of inflammatory cells beneath the RPE. The choriocapillaris is classically not involved in the inflammation.

The diagnosis of sympathetic ophthalmia is made clinically. Ultrasound demonstrates a thickened choroid. There are no laboratory tests that aid in the diagnosis. Fluorescein angiography shows multiple enlarging hyperfluorescent spots at the level of the RPE. Indocyanine green shows hypofluorescence.[7a]

Untreated, the disease tends to run a chronic destructive course. Before the the use of corticosteroids, less than 50% of patients retained any useful vision. The prognosis has improved with corticosteroid treatment, although many patients require long-term steroid treatment and the disease tends to recur when steroids are withdrawn.[27] Enucleation of the injured eye before the development of inflammation in the fellow eye may prevent sympathetic ophthalmia. If an eye has no useful vision and is traumatically disorganized, it should probably be enucleated within 2 weeks of the injury to minimize the likelihood of sensitization to the antigen to which the inflammatory response occurs. It is unknown whether enucleation of the injured eye is beneficial after inflammation has begun in the sympathizing eye. Large doses of systemic corticosteroids are advisable in treating sympathetic ophthalmia in most cases. These doses may be necessary for many weeks. Once the inflammation has been controlled, one should attempt to taper the steroids slowly,

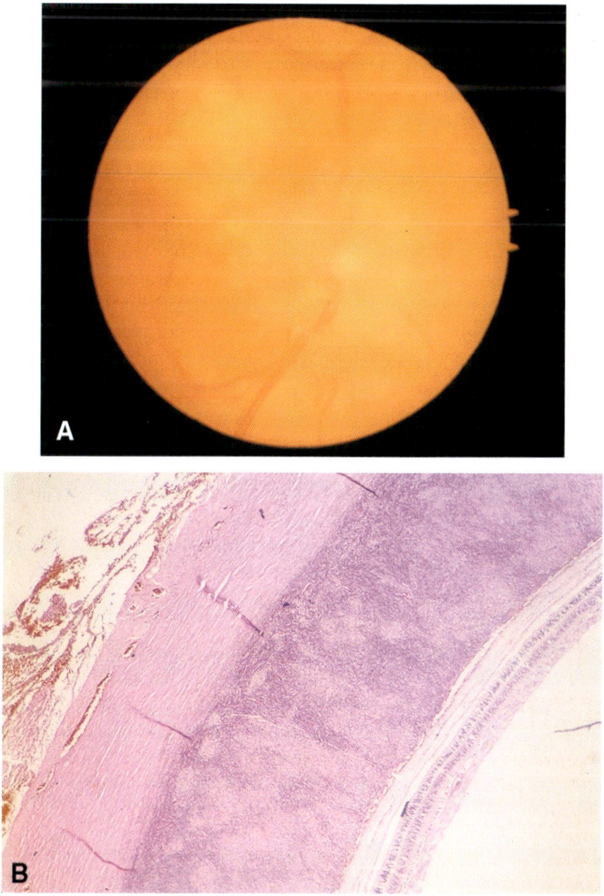

FIGURE 11-12A,B. **(A)** Fundus appearance of the sympathizing eye in a patient with sympathetic ophthalmia. Both anterior and posterior uveitis were present, as were optic disc edema and choriodal infiltrates. There was a history of penetrating trauma to the other eye. **(B)** Histological section demonstrates marked granulomatous inflammation of the choroid in a patient with sympathetic ophthalmia.

eventually using an alternate-day regimen with the lowest possible dose. *Cyclosporine, methotrexate* and alkylating agents such as *chlorambucil* are alternatives to steroids in refractory cases or in patients unable to tolerate corticosteroids.[7a,43]

VOGT–KOYANAGI–HARADA SYNDROME

The Vogt–Koyanagi–Harada syndrome (VKH) is a multisystem disorder with a predilection for darkly pigmented individuals and those of Asian ancestry. In the United States, it is most common in patients with Native American heritage. VKH occurs most commonly in the second to fifth decades of life. The disease has been termed the uveomeningitic syndrome because it classically presents with uveitis and a meningeal prodrome with headache, fever, neck stiffness, and CSF pleocytosis. *Vitiligo, poliosis, alopecia,* tinnitus, and neurosensory hearing loss may occur later in the course of the disease.

Ocular involvement usually begins as a posterior uveitis. Optic disc swelling and retinal edema occur early and, as the disease evolves, exudative retinal detachment may occur (Fig. 11-13A,B). Additional complications include cataract, glaucoma, choroidal neovascular membrane, and subretinal fibrosis.[22,45]

Fluorescein angiography will show characteristic leakage of fluorescein from the choroid (and not from the retinal vessels) at this stage. An anterior uveitis with keratic precipitates and iris nodules usually occurs later. Pathologically, there is invasion of the choroid with inflammatory cells similar to that seen in sympathetic ophthalmia. In contrast to sympathetic ophthalmia where the choriocapillaris is usually spared, the choriocapillaris is often involved in the inflammatory response in VKH.

The etiology of VKH is unknown. T-lymphocyte-mediated autoimmunity probably plays a role. The HLA-DR4 antigen is associated with VKH in Native American, Italian, Japanese, Chinese, and Hispanic patients.[40]

Corticosteroids are the drugs of choice in the treatment of VKH. High-dose oral or intravenous steroids may be necessary for severe cases with exudative retinal detachment. As a therapeutic response is obtained, the steroid dose may be tapered. The response to therapy is variable, and inflammation may recur

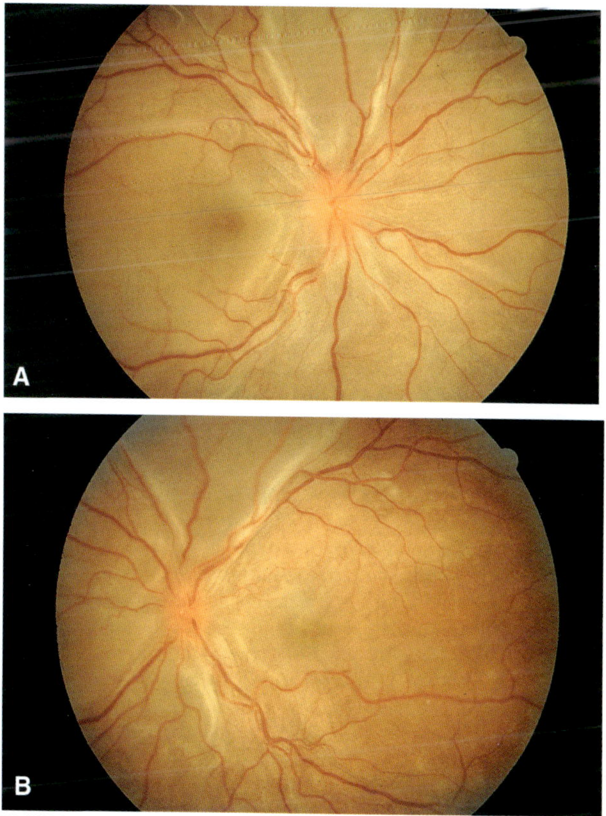

FIGURE 11-13A,B. Bilateral exudative retinal detachments in patient with Vogt–Koyanagi–Harada syndrome.

after steroids are stopped. Cyclosporine may be used in refractory cases or in patients who do not tolerate corticosteroids. Table 11-3 compares the clinical features of sympathetic ophthalmia and VKH syndrome.

TABLE 11-3. Comparison of Sympathetic Ophthalmia and Vogt–Koyanagi–Harada Syndrome.

	Sympathetic ophthalmia	*Vogt–Koyanagi–Harada syndrome*
Age	All ages	20–50 years
Racial predisposition	None	Asian and black
Penetrating trauma	Always present	Usually absent
Skin changes	Uncommon	Common (63%–90%)
Central nervous system findings	Uncommon	Common (84%)
Hearing dysfunction	Uncommon	Common (75%)
Choriocapillaris involvement	Usually spared	Frequently involved

Source: Power WJ, Foster CS. Update on Sympathetic Ophthalmia. Int Ophthalmol Clin 1995;35:127–137, with permission.[43]

VITAMIN A DEFICIENCY

Depletion of tissue stores of vitamin A leads to an ocular syndrome characterized by night blindness and *xerophthalmia*. Vitamin A is a fat-soluble vitamin found in meat, eggs, and milk. Carotenes can be metabolized to vitamin A in humans, and thus yellow fruits and green leafy vegetables are also important sources of Vitamin A. Hypovitaminosis A is an important problem in Third World countries. It is uncommon in the United States but can occur in malnourished patients, those with malabsorption disorders, and patients on abnormal diets.

Nyctalopia (night blindness) is the earliest and most common manifestation of vitamin A deficiency. In untreated cases, the conjunctiva becomes dry (xerosis) and *Bitot's spots* (plaques of keratinizing debris at the limbus) appear (Fig. 11-14). Corneal drying occurs and may progress to ulceration with resultant blindness. Fundus changes consisting of peripheral yellow-white dots may occur, but this is uncommon.

The diagnosis is usually made clinically. Dark adaptation is characteristically prolonged. Serum vitamin A levels may be abnormal, but this is a late occurrence because serum levels may be normal in the face of severe tissue depletion of the vitamin. Treatment of the condition is systemic replacement of vitamin A. The prognosis for vision depends on the state of the ocular tissues at the time therapy is instituted. Healing of corneal and conjunctival lesions will occur, but in cases where perforation has occurred, vision may not be restored. Artificial tears, topical

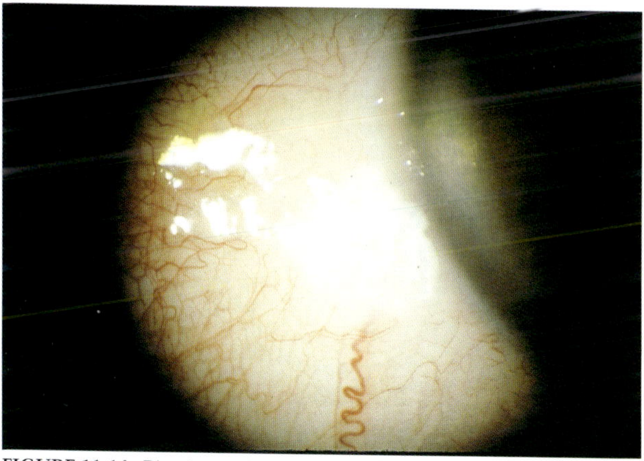

FIGURE 11-14. Bitot's spot in a patient with vitamin A deficiency. These whitish, poorly wetting patches are seen early in the course of the disease. Progression to severe xerosis may occur in untreated cases.

antibiotics, and topical retinoic acid may be of some adjunctive use in therapy.[52] Bitot's spots do not respond to systemic therapy and may require excision.

SIDEROSIS AND CHALCOSIS (RETAINED METALLIC FOREIGN BODIES)

Intraocular foreign bodies containing iron or copper may not cause an immediate severe inflammatory reaction and may not be recognized by the patient or a physician at the time of initial trauma. However, their presence may lead to severe consequences at a later time.

Siderosis is produced by oxidation of iron to ferrous (Fe^{2+}) ions with absorption of these toxic ions by various ocular tissues. Iron may accumulate in the iris causing heterochromia and pupillary sphincter palsy. Rust spots may appear on the lens, and a cataract may form (Fig. 11-15A,B). Glaucoma may result from accumulation of iron in the trabecular meshwork. Retinal toxicity results in ERG changes beginning with an increase in the height of the a-wave followed by a decrease in the height of both the a-wave and the b-wave. The ERG may eventually

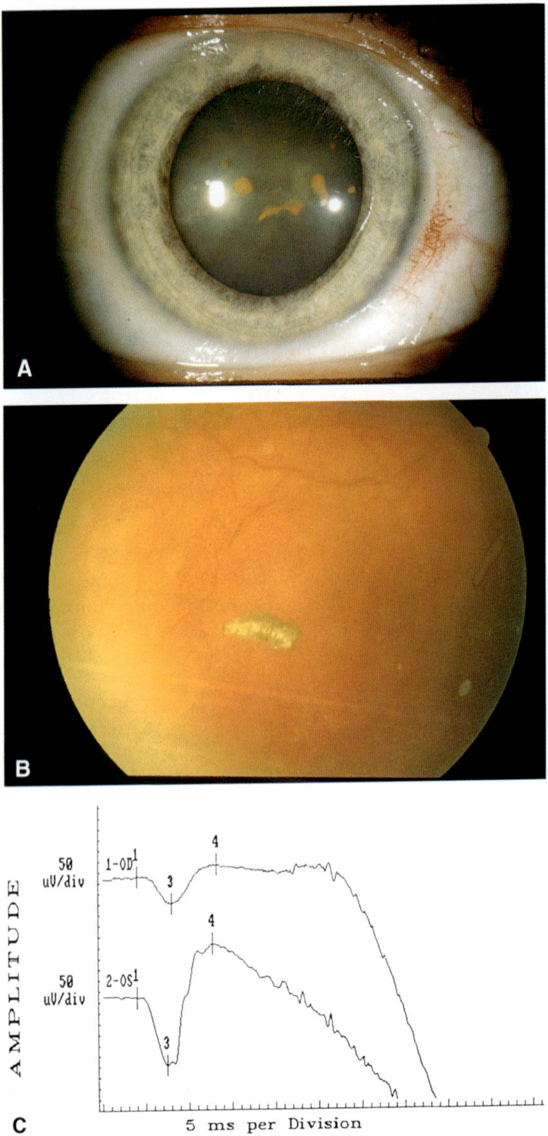
A
B
C
AMPLITUDE
50 uV/div
1-OD
50 uV/div
2-OS
1
3
4
5 ms per Division

become flat (Fig. 11-15C). Even at this point, removal of the foreign body may be indicated as useful vision may remain.

Pure copper is extremely toxic to the eye, and a pure copper intraocular foreign body may cause an acute suppurative endophthalmitis. Foreign bodies containing small amounts of copper typically will not cause such an acute inflammatory response. However, copper ions may, over time, be disseminated throughout the eye, leading to a syndrome known as *chalcosis*. Copper ions have an affinity for basement membranes. Deposits of copper in the lens capsule may lead to a *"sunflower" cataract*. Deposits in Descemet's membrane lead to the formation of the characteristic *Kayser–Fleischer ring*, a golden-colored corneal ring at the limbus. There may be *iris heterochromia* with a greenish tint to the iris in the involved eye. Retinal toxicity is much less severe than that seen in *siderosis*. A small decrease in the height of the b-wave may be seen. Macular pigmentary changes have been described. Visual loss may result from cataract formation or vitreous changes.[49] The decision as to whether a copper-containing foreign body should be removed in patients with chalcosis should be individualized.

All patients with a history consistent with the possibility of an intraocular foreign body should have appropriate radiologic studies at the time of their presentation.

ACUTE POSTERIOR MULTIFOCAL PLACOID PIGMENT EPITHELIOPATHY

In 1968, Gass described a syndrome of temporary loss of vision associated with large plaquelike lesions at the level of the retinal pigment epithelium and termed this disorder acute posterior multifocal placoid pigment epitheliopathy (APMPPE). This disorder is typically bilateral but may not affect both eyes at the

FIGURE 11-15A–C. (**A**) "Rust spots" beneath the anterior capsule of the lens are a typical feature of siderosis in a patient with a retained iron-containing foreign body. (**B**) Retained metallic foreign body seen in the same patient. Note the hazy vitreous and pigmentary retinal abnormalities. (**C**) Electroretinogram (ERG) shows somewhat selective loss of the b-wave amplitude in the right eye (*top tracing*) in a patient with a metal foreign body and signs of siderosis.

same time. Patients are typically less than 30 years of age. Flashing lights commonly precede the onset of visual acuity loss. Mild vitreous inflammation is common; there may also be mild anterior chamber inflammation. A history of preexisting viral upper respiratory infection is commonly reported.

The characteristic lesions of APMPPE are cream-colored plaques at the level of the retinal pigment epithelium that tend to be oval or round with irregular edges. There are usually multiple lesions randomly distributed over the posterior pole. The presenting visual acuity is usually 20/200 or better. Central and pericentral scotomata are common. Fluorescein angiography and indocyanine green angiography (ICG) may be helpful in making the diagnosis. The cream-colored lesions seen on fundus examination tend to block fluorescence early in the angiogram and stain late. Usually, over a period of a few weeks, the lesions begin to resolve and the vision begins to improve. In most patients, the vision returns to near-normal levels. The disease has been reported to recur, but this is uncommon.

Acute posterior multifocal placoid pigment epitheliopathy may occur as a consequence of a prior viral infection. A 40-year-old man developed APMPPE following an acute group A streptococcal infection.[25] Other causes probably exist. The lesions appear to be related to acute focal decreases in choroidal blood flow.[58] Most cases resolve without treatment over a period of several weeks. The role of corticosteroids in treatment is controversial.

Acknowledgments. The preparation of this chapter was supported in part by an unrestricted grant from Research to Prevent Blindness, Inc.

References

1. Amin HI, McDonald HR, Han DP, et al. Vitrectomy update for macular traction in ocular toxocariasis. Retina 2000;20:80–85.

1a. Barisani-Asenbauer T, Maca SM, Hauff W, et al. Treatment of ocular toxocariasis with albendazole. J Ocul Pharmacol Ther 2001;17:287–294.

2. Baumal CR, Levin AV, Read SE. Cytomegalovirus retinitis in immunosuppressed children. Am J Ophthalmol 1999;127:550–558.

3. Boyer K, Roizen N, Stein L, et al. The child with congenital toxoplasmosis. Curr Clin Top Infect Dis 2000;20:189–208.

4. Breger BC, Leopold IH. The incidence of uveitis in multiple sclerosis. Am J Ophthalmol 1966;62:540–545.

5. Brezin AP, Thulliez P, Cisneros B, et al. Lymphocytic choriomeningitis virus chorioretinitis mimicking ocular toxoplasmosis in two otherwise normal children. Am J Ophthalmol 2000;130:245–247.
6. Bosch-Driessen LH, Karimi S, Stilma JS, Rothova A. Retinal detachment in ocular toxoplasmosis. Ophthalmology 2000;107:36–40.
7. Cassidy JT, Levinson JE, Bass JC, et al. A study of classification criteria for a diagnosis of JRA. Arthritis Rheum 1986;29:274–281.
7a. Chu D, Foster S. Sympathetic Ophthalmia 2002;42(3):179–185.
8. Couvreur J, Desmonts G. Congenital and maternal toxoplasmosis: a review of 300 congenital cases. Dev Med Child Neurol 1962;4:519–530.
9. Culbertson WW, Blumenkranz MS, Pepose JS, et al. Varicella zoster virus is a cause of the acute retinal necrosis syndrome. Ophthalmology 1986;93:559–569.
10. Dalton R, Aylward GW, Sharland M. Use of ganciclovir implants for CMV retinitis in an 18-month-old child with AIDS. Eye 1999;13(pt 1):110–112.
11. DeSouza EC, Abujamra S, Nakashima Y, Gass JDM: Diffuse bilateral subacute neuroretinitis. Arch Ophthalmol 1999;117:1349–1351.
12. Du LT, Coats DK, Kline MW, et al. Incidence of presumed cytomegalovirus retinitis in HIV-infected pediatric patients. POJAAPOS 1999;3:245–249.
13. Ellis GS, Pakalnis VA, Worley G, et al. *Toxocara canis* infection: clinical and epidemiological associations with seropositivity in kindergarten children. Ophthalmology 1986;93:1032–1037.
14. Friedmann CT, Knox DL. Variations in recurrent active toxoplasmic retinochoroiditis. Arch Ophthalmol 1969;81:481–493.
15. Gass JDM, Braunstein RA. Further observations concerning the diffuse unilateral subacute neuroretinitis syndrome. Arch Ophthalmol 1983;101:1689–1697.
16. Gass JDM. Viral retinochoroiditis. In: Stereoscopic atlas of macular diseases. Philadelphia: Mosby, 1987:498–499.
17. Goldman JN. Congenital syphilis. In: Fraunfelder FT, Roy FH (eds) Current ocular therapy, vol 3. Philadelphia: Sauders, 1990:13–14.
18. Figueroa MS, Bou G, Marti-Belda P, et al. Diagnostic value of polymerase chain reaction in blood and aqueous humor in immunocompetent patients with ocular toxoplasmosis. Retina 2000;20:614–619.
19. Han DP, Lewis H, Williams GA, et al. Laser photocoagulation in the acute retinal necrosis syndrome. Arch Ophthalmol 1987;105:1051–1054.
20. Hogan MJ, Kimura SJ, Spencer WH. Visceral larva migrans and peripheral retinitis. JAMA 1965;194:1345–1347.
21. Kilmartin DJ, Forrester JV, Dick AD. Cyclosporin A therapy in refractory noninfectious childhood uveitis. Br J Ophthalmol 1998;82:737–742.
22. Kuo IC, Rechodouni A, Rao NA, et al. Subretinal fibrosis in patients with Vogt–Koyanagi–Harada disease. Ophthalmlology 2000;107:1721–1728.

23. Kychenthal A, Coombes A, Greenwood J, et al. Bilateral acute retinal necrosis and herpes simplex type 2 encephalitis in a neonate. Br J Ophthalmol 2001;85:629–630.
24. Lakhanpal V, Schocket SS, Nirankari VS. Clindamycin in the treatment of toxoplasmoic retinochoroiditis. Am J Ophthalmol 1983;95: 605–613.
25. Lowder CY, Foster RE, Gutman FA. Acute posterior multifocal placoid pigment epitheliopathy after acute group A streptococcal infection. Am J Ophthalmol 1996;122:115–117.
26. Liddy BSL, Stuart J. Sympathetic ophthalmia in Canada. Can J Ophthalmol 1972;7:157–159.
27. Makley TA, Azar A. Sympathetic ophthalmia: a long-term follow-up. Arch Ophthalmol 1978;96:257–262.
27a. Malinowski SM, Pulido JS, Folk JC. Long-term visual outcome and complications associated with pars planitis. Ophthalmology 1993: 100(6):818–824.
28. Malley DS, Barone R, Heinemann MH. Treatment of bilateral cytomegalovirus retinitis with sustained-release ganciclovir implants in a child. Am J Ophthalmol 1996;122:731–732.
29. McAuley J, Boyer KM, Patel D, et al. Early and longitudinal evaluations of treated infants and children and untreated historical patients with congenital toxoplasmosis: the Chicago Collaborative Treatment Trial. Clin Infect Dis 1994;18:38–72.
30. McLeod R, Boyer K, Roizen N, et al. The child with congenital toxoplasmosis. Curr Clin Top Infect Dis 2000;20:189–208.
30a. Merle H, Cabre P, Olindo S, Merle S, Smadja D. Ocular lesions in 200 patients infected by the human T-cell lymphotropic virus type 1 in martinique (French West Indies). Am J Ophthalmol. 2002;134(2): 190–195.
31. Mets MB, Barton LL, Khan AS, Ksiazek TG. Lymphocytic choriomeningitis virus: an underdiagnosed cause of congenital chorioretinitis. Am J Ophthalmol 2000;130:209–215.
31a. Miserochi E, Baltatzis S, Ekong A, et al. Efficacy and safety of chlorambucil in intractable noninfectious uveitis: the Massachusetts Eye and Ear Infirmary experience. Ophthalmology 2002;109:137–142.
32. Montoya JG, Parmley S, Lissenfeld O, et al. Use of the polymerase chain reaction for diagnosis of ocular toxoplasmosis. Ophthalmology 1999;106:1554–1563.
33. Nichols CW, Eagle RC, Yanoff M, et al. Conjunctival biopsy as an aid in the evaluation of a patient with suspected sarcoidosis. Ophthalmology 1980;87:287–291.
34. Nussenblatt RB, Palestine AG. Anterior uveitis. In: Uveitis: fundamentals and clinical practice. Chicago: Yearbook Medical, 1989:175–176.
35. Nussenblatt RB, Palestine AG. Intermediate uveitis and pars planitis. In: Uveitis: fundamentals and clinical practice. Chicago: Yearbook Medical, 1989:194–196.

36. Nussenblatt RB, Palestine AG. Viral diseases. In: Uveitis: fundamentals and clinical practice. Chicago: Yearbook Medical, 1989:424–426.
37. Nussenblatt RB, Palestine AG. White dot syndromes. In: Uveitis: fundamentals and clinical practice. Chicago: Yearbook Medical, 1989:291–308.
38. O'Connor GR. Chemotherapy of toxoplasmosis and toxocariasis. In: Srinivasan BD (ed) Ocular therapeutics. New York: Masson, 1980: 51–57.
39. Ocular histoplasmosis study group. Argon laser photocoagulation for ocular histoplasmosis. Results of a randomized clinical trial. Arch Ophthalmol 1983;101:1347–1357.
40. Ohno S. Immunological aspects of Behcet's disease and VKH. Trans Ophthalmol Soc UK 1981;101:335–341.
41. Park SE, Mieler WF, Pulido JS. Peripheral scatter photocoagulation for neovascularization associated with pars planitis. Arch Ophthalmol 1995;113:1277–1280.
42. Perkins ES. Ocular toxoplasmosis. Br J Ophthalmol 1973;57:1–17.
43. Power WJ, Foster CS. Update on sympathetic ophthalmia. Int Ophthalmol Clin 1995;35:127–137.
44. Raymond LA, Strong LE, Wander AA, et al. Living retinal nematode destroyed with photocoagulation. Ophthalmology 1978;85:944–949.
45. Read RW, Rechodouni A, Butani N, et al. Complications and prognostic factors in Vogt–Koyanagi–Harada disease. Am J Ophthalmol 2001;131:599–606.
46. Reiff A, Takei S, Sadeghi S, et al. Etanercept therapy in children with treatment-resistant uveitis. Arthritis Rheum 2001;44:1411–1415.
47. Roberts F, Mets MB, Ferguson DJP, et al. Histopathological features of ocular toxoplasmosis in the fetus and infant. Arch Ophthalmol 2001;119:51–58.
48. Roizen N, Swisher CN, Stein MA, et al. Neurological and developmental outcome in treated congenital toxoplasmosis. Pediatrics 1995;95:11–20.
49. Rosenthal AR, Marmor MF, Leuenberger P, Hopkins JL. Chalcosis: a study of the natural history. Ophthalmology 1979;86:1956–1972.
50. Sabates R, Pruett RC, Brockhurst RJ. Fulminant ocular toxoplasmosis. Am J Ophthalmol 1981;92:497–503.
51. Sastry SM, Epps CH, Walton RC, et al. Combined ganciclovir and foscarnet in pediatric cytomegalovirus retinitis. J Natl Med Assoc 1996;88:661–662.
52. Sommer A, Emran N. Topical retinoic acid in the treatment of corneal xerophthalmia. Am J Ophthalmol 1978;86:615–617.
53. Tan JCH, Byles D, Stanford MR, et al. Acute retinal necrosis in children caused by herpes simpex virus. Retina 2001;21:344–347.
54. Tran VT, Lumbroso L, LeHoang P, Herbort CP. Ultrasound biomicroscopy in peripheral retinovitreal toxocariasis. Am J Ophthalmol 1999;127:607–609.

55. Van Gelder RN, Willig JL, Holland G, Kaplan HJ. Herpes simplex virus type 2 as a cause of acute retinal necrosis syndrome in young patients. Ophthalmology 2001;108:869–876.
56. Walton RC, Whitcup SM, Mueller BU, et al. Combined intravenous ganciclovir and foscarnet for children with recurrent cytomegalovirus retinitis. Ophthalmology 1995;102:1865–1870.
57. Wilder HC. Nematode endophthalmitis. Trans Am Acad Ophthalmol Otolaryngol 1950;55:99–109.
58. Young NJA, Bird AC, Sehmi K. Pigment epithelial diseases with abnormal choroidal perfusion. Am J Ophthalmol 1980;90:607–618.

12

Myopia

Arlene V. Drack

The term *myopia* refers to a spectrum of ocular disorders in which the far point of the eye is closer to the retina than infinity. The resultant disparity between good vision at "near" (i.e., at a distance from the eye that is at or within the far point plane) and "distance" (any point beyond the far point plane for that particular eye) may be caused by a number of factors. Because most cases of myopia have a benign etiology and course, the importance of this disorder as a predisposing factor for serious retinal pathology is often overlooked.

INCIDENCE AND PREVALENCE

The prevalence of myopia varies greatly between different populations and different ethnic groups. In the United States and western Europe, the prevalence is approximately 25% of the population, but only about 2% of the population has myopia of greater than or equal to 5 diopters.[7] In a Danish study the prevalence of any myopia in 13- and 14-year-olds was 9.5%, whereas the prevalence of high myopia (−6.00 diopters or more) was 0.45%.[15,19] In Asia, the prevalence of myopia is much higher, in some studies up to 75% of the population. In a study done in Hong Kong, the prevalence in kindergarten pupils was 3.3%, in primary school students 36.1%, and among university students 91.7%.[30] The greatest rate of progression of myopia occurred between the ages of 6 and 10 years, at a younger age than most European studies.[29] In mainland China the prevalence was found to be 39% and in Japan it was 55%. The prevalence appears to be increasing over time in Hong Kong and some other Asian countries, as opposed to Denmark and Norway, where a stable percentage of medical school students (50%) were found to have myopia over time.[13] As can be surmised from these prevalence data, the incidence of myopia increases with increasing age. A study from the United Kingdom that analyzed refractive data from patients examined annually between the ages of 7 and 13 years found annual myopia incidence values of 3.5% to 12%, resulting in a rise in prevalence from 5% to 40% over the 6 years of the study.[47]

In a 1975 study, it was estimated that 5.6% of blindness in school children in the United States was secondary to myopia.[21] Myopia is second only to diabetes mellitis as the most common cause of blindness in the working-age population.[7,67] Lower grades of myopia, although not sight threatening, are a cause of significant morbidity.

ETIOLOGY

Myopia can be classified into three broad groups based on clinical findings and prognosis.[7] The first type is *physiological,* or *correlation*, myopia. In these eyes all the components of refraction are within normal limits, but there is a lack of correlation between the refractive powers of the cornea, lens, and axial length, rendering the far point nearer than infinity. Although decreased distance vision results, these eyes are otherwise normal and there are no fundus abnormalities. The degree of myopia is usually low, but there is no "magic number" because a borderline steep cornea, a lens at the upper limit of normal, and an axial length also in the upper normal range, would be expected to yield high amounts of myopia in some cases. This form of myopia generally begins in childhood or adolescence, with a second peak of onset at the end of the second decade or beginning of the third. It usually progresses for several years, then becomes stable or increases very slowly. Some myopes experience another myopic shift in young adulthood.[68]

The second type is *intermediate* myopia.[7] This form of myopia appears to be very similar to *physiological* myopia, although the age of onset may be slightly younger and the final amount of myopia tends to be higher. The main difference is that in these eyes the components of refraction do not fall all of within the normal range; the axial length is notably longer. Over time, fundus changes appear, often beginning in childhood. These eyes are at increased risk of developing open-angle glaucoma, retinal detachment, early cataract, and other disorders.

The third major type, and the most devastating, is *pathological* myopia. In this form, a highly myopic refractive error is often present from early childhood and is usually progressive.[7] Increased axial length and fundus changes are evident at the earliest examination. Prognosis is poor, with legal blindness resulting from maculopathy or retinal detachment in almost 50% of eyes.[8]

High myopia is a term that generally refers to myopia greater than 6 diopters (D). Clinically, eyes may fit into either the intermediate or pathological category because the cause is usually at least partly axial.

The average progression in eyes with *physiological* or *intermediate* myopia in childhood is about −0.50 diopters per year.[23,29,44,54] Factors associated with increased risk for progression to high degrees of myopia include fundus changes, intraocular pressure greater than 16 mm Hg, and myopia greater than −3.00 diopters by 11 years of age.[23] A study of children in Hong Kong found that at age 6 and 7 years, children with at least one myopic parent tended to have higher intraocular pressures than children with two non-myopic parents.[11] A large study of school children in the United States found that the best predictor of juvenile-onset myopia was a cycloplegic refractive error of less than +0.75 diopters of hyperopia in the third grade (usually 8 years of age).[74] Parental history of myopia also plays a role.[73]

There is evidence from both animal and human studies that accommodation plays a role in the development of myopia.[5,51] European and North American studies have repeatedly demonstrated a higher prevalence of myopia in persons with more years of schooling; however, an Asian study failed to find a correlation between type of academic activity and myopia in children.[16] A study done in Newfoundland found that near work and years of education were aspects of a common familial environment that could inflate resemblances of refraction among family members thought to be caused by genetics.[4]

A dramatic increase in the prevalence of myopia in Alaskan Eskimos was noted when compulsory education became mandatory, suggesting that near work was a factor.[69] However, other influences, such as artificial lighting and diet changes, could also be influential.

Use of a night light in infants' bedrooms was found to correlate with development of myopia in one study; however, these data were collected by survey and parental refractive error was not ascertained.[50] A study of infant monkeys reared in continuous ambient lighting,[58] as well as human studies in the United States[20,75] and Asia,[56] failed to find a correlation in other patient populations but did find that myopic parents were more likely to use a night light, suggesting a possible heritability bias.

Although isolated myopia is the most common, it is important to remember that there are other etiologies of myopia that are less benign. Myopia may be secondary to congenital glaucoma, or systemic or ocular syndromes, as is discussed later in this chapter. Most myopia is axial, but other types of "component" myopia should always be considered, such as conditions that cause steep corneas (e.g., keratoconus, microcornea, persistent hyperplastic primary vitreous), or round or misshapen lenses (e.g., microspherophakia, ectopia lentis, posterior lenticonus). Conditions that cause deprivation in infancy may also cause myopia, such as complete congenital ptosis or dense vitreous hemorrhage. In animals such as chicks, tree shrews, and monkeys, deprivation by eyelid suture or occluder contact lens induces axial myopia.[52]

Ciliary spasm and night myopia may coexist with other forms. Ciliary or accommodative spasm may be caused by trauma, central nervous system abnormalities, or psychological issues. Variable esotropia and miosis are usually present. Night myopia is a small myopic shift caused by accommodation that occurs in dim illumination and may neccessitate extra correction for driving. People who have had refractive surgery may also experience decreased night vision; however, this type may be related to larger pupil size, allowing more peripheral, less-corrected cornea to defocus the image.

CLINICAL FEATURES

Vitreous

Vitreous syneresis occurs at a younger age in myopic eyes than emmetropic eyes. The protein, hyaluronic acid, and collagen concentrations are different,[6] and posterior vitreous detachment may occur up to 20 years earlier than in emmetropic eyes.[14] Because onset of liquefaction is related to both the age of the patient and the degree of myopia, it may be present in childhood if the amount of myopia is very high. Examination of the vitreous with the slit lamp, 90 D lens, or direct ophthalmoscope reveals linear filaments with nodules or thickenings. In early liquefaction, there are pockets of fluid within the vitreous gel; later, the fluid portion moves posteriorly, pushing the filaments anteriorly. If there is a posterior vitreous detachment a white ring (Vogt's) corresponding to the vitreous condensation around the disc may be seen floating in the fluid. Patients perceive these filaments as "floaters"; on occasion dense floating particles may obscure vision.

Several systemic syndromes with vitreoretinopathies have pathognomonic vitreous abnormalities that are different than syneresis (see Chapter 6). The vitreous veils in an otherwise optically empty media seen in these disorders should not be confused with the liquefaction and filaments of isolated myopia.

Fundus

In eyes with *physiological* (correlation) myopia, the fundus examination is normal. There may be a tiny crescent of 1/10 diameter of the optic disc.[7] The cardinal fundus findings in *intermediate* myopia (Fig. 12-1A–C) are optic nerve crescent formation, tessellation, and "supertraction."[7] The crescent is usually temporal to the disc and may be white, pigmented, or both[7], and increases in size as myopia progresses.[42] "Supertraction" appears as a rim of heaped choroid and retina slightly overhanging the disc nasally; this may occur with real or apparent tilting of the disc. Because of thinning of the retinal pigment epithelium (RPE) with axial elongation, a tigroid appearance of the fundus may be present; this is most marked in the posterior pole and is referred to as tessellation. It may not be apparent in lightly pigmented individuals. Eyes with crescents, by definition, cannot be considered to have *physiological* myopia.[7] Although the risk of other ocular disorders is higher in these eyes than in normals, most retain good vision throughout life with optical correction.

Peripheral retinal changes such as white without pressure, lattice degeneration (Fig. 12-2), and pavingstone degeneration are found with increased frequency and at a younger age in patients with *intermediate* and *pathological* myopia.[7,24] Retinal holes or tears may be associated with lattice, and this may explain the increased risk of retinal detachment in myopic eyes.

Pathological myopia is an entity distinct from the physiological and intermediate types already described; it is actually a progressive retinal dystrophy with a relatively poor prognosis for retention of good vision throughout life. The earliest signs occur in infancy or childhood, with a variable amount of myopia associated with a localized area of RPE attenuation (tessellation) in

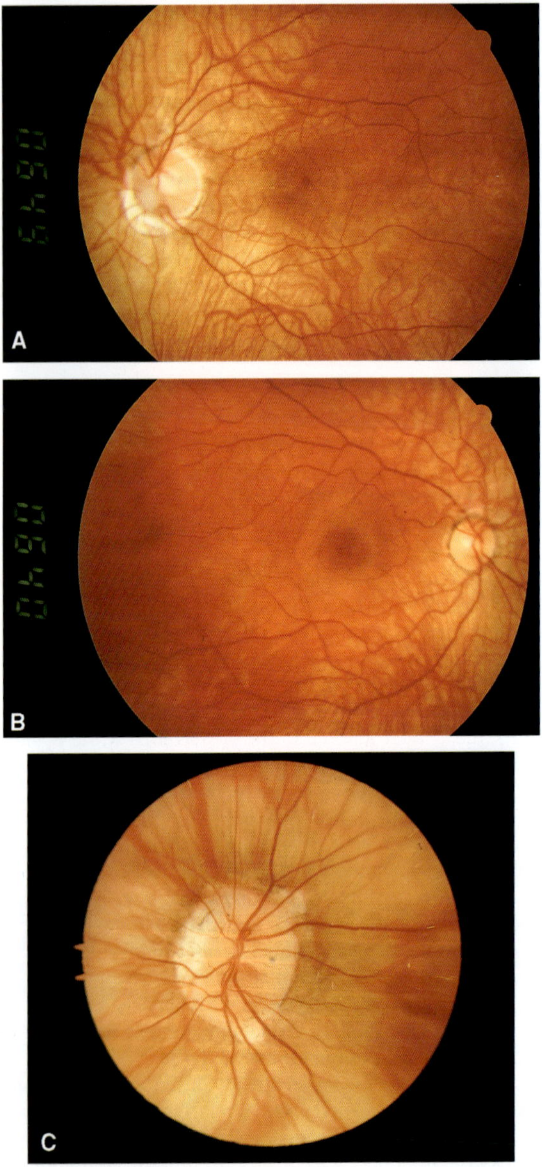
A
B
C

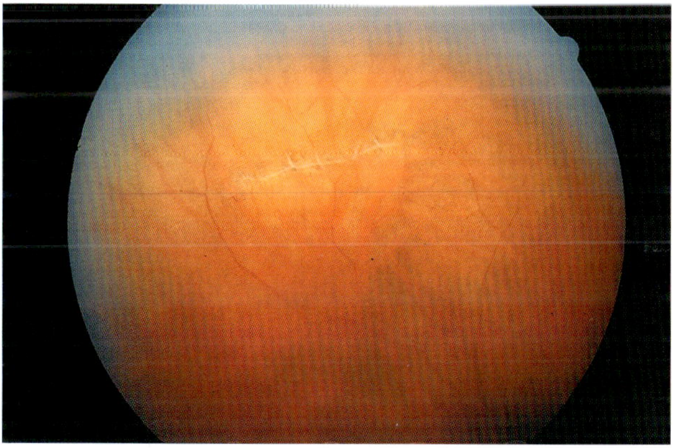

FIGURE 12-2. Typical peripheral lattice degeneration may demonstrate linear white lesions as well as hyperpigmentation. Atrophic holes or flap tears may be associated with lattice.

the posterior pole and an optic nerve crescent. The crescent and tessellation are usually seen on the same side of the nerve. Although these findings in an adult are often secondary to intermediate myopia, in a child they are often the harbinger of a staphyloma, an area of ectasia with thinning of the retina, choroid, and sclera. As pathological myopia progresses, the tessellated area becomes thinned, and eventually excavated (Fig. 12-3). There may be pigment clumping around the edges or within the otherwise hypopigmented area of the staphyloma.

Many types of staphylomas have been described, depending on their location. The most visually significant are those affecting the macula. The presence of a staphyloma is a poor prog-

FIGURE 12-1A–C. **(A)** Left fundus of a 13-year-old girl. The spherical equivalent is −14.00 D. Note that the scleral cresent is most prominent in a somewhat atypical inferonasal location. Tessellation of the posterior pole and a decreased foveal reflex are also present. There is a Bergmeister's papilla on the disc. **(B)** Right fundus of the same patient, with a spherical equivalent −8.00 D. Note the correlation of the size of the crescent with the refraction. **(C)** Myopic disc demonstrates a crescent on one side, with "supertraction" on the other. The *small black dot* seen on the disc is an artifact caused by visualization of the "Allen dot" of the fundus camera that occurs when a highly myopic eye is photographed.

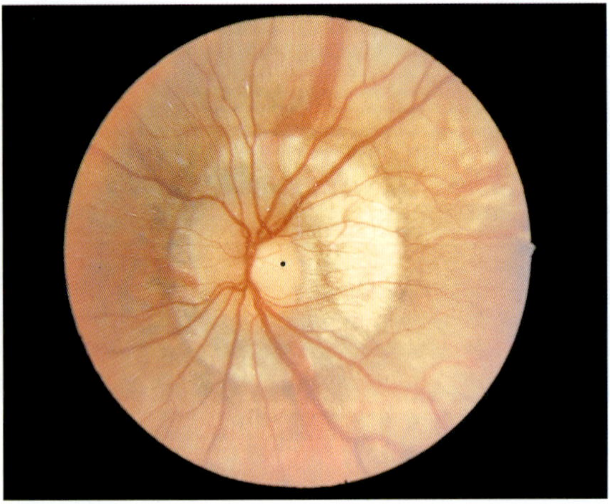

FIGURE 12-3. A peripapillary staphyloma. Note the choroidal vessels diving into the excavation of the staphyloma. The ectasia may occur around the nerve, nasal to the disc, or temporal to the disc. It may also involve the macula, and, because it may increase over time, the prognosis for central vision is poor.

nostic sign. Most of these eyes have best corrected acuities of less than 20/20 early in life and continued loss of vision with increasing age. Almost 50% of eyes with staphylomas are legally blind by the fifth decade of life.[8] "Lacquer cracks" (Fig. 12-4A,B) may develop in or near the macula. These linear, whitish lesions represent breaks in Bruch's membrane. In one study, 4.3% of eyes with an axial length greater than or equal to 26.5 mm exhibited lacquer cracks; the youngest patients seen to have this abnormality were in their late teens.[9] Lacquer cracks themselves usually do not affect acuity; however, they are a poor prognostic sign for the retention of good vision and may be associated with an acquired blue-yellow color deficit.[27] Focal retinal degeneration, hemorrhages, and subretinal neovascular membranes associated with the lacquer cracks are probably responsible for the poor prognosis.

Retinal hemorrhages, particularly in the macula, are not uncommon in pathological myopia and are of two main types. In the first, an acute hemorrhage occurs, unrelated to a subretinal net, causing a severe reduction in acuity but resolving over weeks with vision returning to its previous level. These spontaneous bleeds may recur and may be idiopathic, or related to Valsalva maneuvers, weight lifting, or other activities. The second type of hemorrhage has a much more grave prognosis. These are hemorrhages associated with subretinal neovascular membranes that lead to scarring and chorioretinal clumping called Fuch's spots

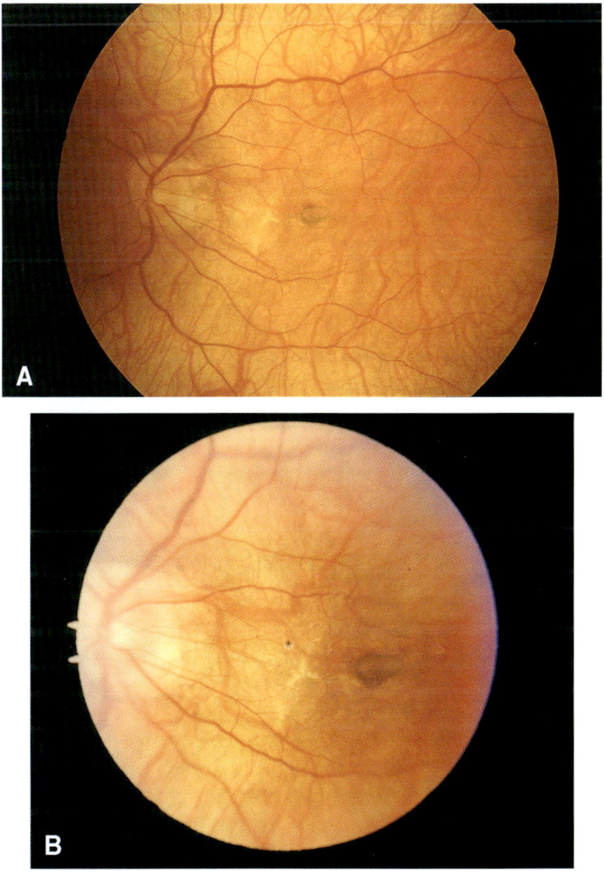

FIGURE 12-4A,B. (**A**) Lacquer crack between the nerve and macula in a highly myopic eye. (**B**) Close-up of the lesion seen in (**A**). Note Fuch's spot near the macula.

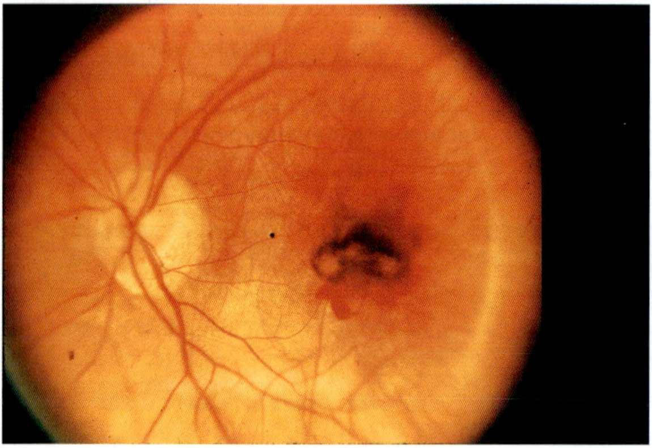

FIGURE 12-5. Multiple Fuch's spots in the macula with a recent hemorrhage as well. The prognosis for good vision in this eye is very poor. (Courtesy of G.F. Judisch, Iowa City, IA.)

(Fig. 12-5); this may be followed by atrophy. Visual loss is severe and may be irreversible in these cases.[63]

Large and small areas of chorioretinal atrophy are seen in some eyes (Fig. 12-6). These areas may coalesce as patients

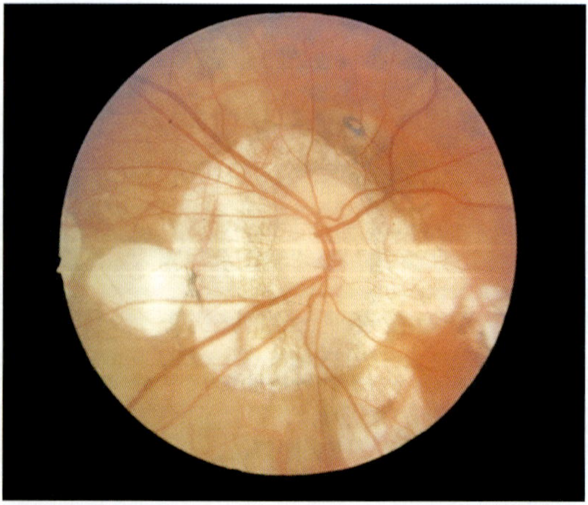

FIGURE 12-6. Geographic atrophy around the optic nerve and in the posterior pole.

become older resulting in large areas of atrophy with somewhat scalloped edges. Even in eyes without macular hemorrhage, the macula may show hyperpigmentation and pigment mottling that is already apparent in childhood.[7]

In later life, eyes with pathological myopia may show marked thinning of all layers of the eye, especially in areas of staphyloma. The choroid in particular becomes thin and sclerotic.

CLINICAL ASSESSMENT

It is of the utmost importance to do a cycloplegic refraction as part of the evaluation of myopia, certainly in all children, and even in adult myopes. Many patients have been over-minussed over years of manifest refractions. Children can accommodate up to 15 diopters with ease, but by the age of 40 years, only about 3 diopters can be easily performed. Overcorrection in adulthood may cause asthenopia and even accommodative esotropia or the breakdown of esophorias because of greater difficulty in accommodating over the extra minus with advancing age.[37]

In older children and adults, a cycloplegic subjective refraction can be done, with or without the duochrome test; 1% cyclopentolate hydrochloride should be used. In younger children, the results of cycloplegic retinoscopy should be prescribed. On subsequent visits, cycloplegic retinoscopy while the child is wearing the glasses can be done to refine the prescription and eliminate vertex distance errors. In patients of all ages with moderate to high levels of myopia, refraction over the patient's existing glasses may give a more accurate final prescription than using a phoropter or trial frames. Because accommodation may play a role in the development of myopia, at the very least, myopic patients should not be "over-minussed" as this induces extra accommodative effort at all distances.

A careful family history should be taken with special emphasis on presence or absence of early-onset refractive errors, retinal detachment, hyperextensibility, cleft palate or bifid uvula, arthritis, best corrected vision below the level necessary to obtain a driver's license, or ectopia lentis. Answers to these questions may point to a more serious ocular or systemic syndrome than isolated simple myopia.

It is important to remember the natural history of physiological myopia when evaluating a new patient. Children are rarely highly myopic before the age of 9 years (although there is evidence that Asian children may develop higher degrees of myopia at younger ages than other ethnic groups). High myopia in children younger than this should prompt a detailed review of systems, birth history asking specifically about prematurity, retinopathy of prematurity either treated or untreated, or other risk factors, and a systemic evaluation for associated syndromes. Intraocular pressure should always be measured at least once, because myopia in infancy can be a presenting sign of congenital glaucoma. Hearing testing should be done in young children presenting with myopia, because several syndromes have deafness as a feature.

SYSTEMIC ASSOCIATIONS

In addition to the types of myopia listed earlier, which are usually isolated, there are special subsets of myopia that fit imperfectly into one of the groups. Unilateral high myopia with increased axial length may occur as a part of a hemihypertrophy syndrome, with myelinated nerve fibers, or as an isolated finding. Myopia related to retinopathy of prematurity (ROP) may be caused by an abnormally spherical lens, increased axial length, or both. Premature infants who develop ROP have a much higher risk of developing myopia than those who did not have ROP, in both Asian and western populations.[60] The prevalence has been found to increase between 3 and 12 months of age on cycloplegic refraction but to remain stable thereafter.[49] A higher prevalence of eyes with more than −8.00 diopters of myopia was found in those treated with cryotherapy versus those who were not treated. Whether this is attributable to the cryotherapy itself or to the opportunity to measure refraction in eyes that otherwise would have developed retinal detachments because of worse, more myopiogenic ROP is unknown.[49]

Myopia may be the presenting sign of several systemic syndromes. Stickler's syndrome, a defect in collagen synthesis caused by mutations in the COL2A1 gene (type 1)[1] and COL11A1 gene (type 2),[53] may present with nystagmus in early childhood as a result of defocus severe enough to cause deprivation, at times in the −15.00 to −20.00 diopter range. In patients with lower degrees of myopia, presentation may be later, when it is noted that the child holds near objects excessively close. Other associated features are early-onset arthritis, hearing loss, flat midface, and cleft palate or bifid uvula. The vitreous is optically empty, with broad veils visible on indirect ophthalmoscopy. It is autosomal dominant.

Kneist dysplasia and spondyloepiphyseal dysplasia (SED) congenita are more severe autosomal dominant manifestations of Col2A1 mutations.[66] Some forms are lethal in the neonatal period. Kneist dysplasia patients resemble Stickler patients, but in addition suffer from dwarfism and scoliosis. Patients with SED congenita have dwarfism with barrel chests, hearing loss, joint disease, and high myopia with a predisposition to retinal detachment. Knobloch syndrome is autosomal recessive and may be associated with an unusual posterior scalp lesion that can overlay an occipital encephalocele. It has been mapped to chromosome 21q22.3.[57] Myopia is also more prevalent in certain ocular disorders such as retinitis pigmentosa, congenital stationary night blindness, Aland eye disease, and gyrate atrophy.

INHERITANCE

The inheritance of myopia is complex, probably because there are many "myopias" with different etiologies. Autosomal dominant, recessive, and sporadic cases of isolated myopia have been reported.[7,33,59] Many pedigrees give the appearance of a complex trait, that is, the frequency is increased within a family relative to the general population, but the inheritance does not follow simple Mendelian laws; this may occur when more than one gene is involved, and/or when there are environmental factors necessary for the expression of the trait.

Some studies have demonstrated that children who have two myopic parents are more likely to become myopic than those with only one, or neither.[38] Axial length is longer in children of myopic parents, even before they develop myopia.[72] In a study of children 6 to 12 years old, the rates of myopia were 12.2% of the children with two myopic parents, 8.2% of those with one myopic parent, and 2.7% of those without myopic parents.[72] Another study found that children with two myopic parents were 6.42 times more likely to become myopic than children without myopic parents.[43] Such studies support the idea that a predisposition is inherited. A similar study done in Hong Kong did not find a correlation with parental myopia, however.[12] Even a U.S. study that sought to find a strong predictor of juvenile myopia found that neither refraction at school entry, refraction in infancy, nor parental myopia had both high sensitivity and specificity.[38] The genetic contribution may be difficult to elucidate because environmental factors, such as nearwork and accommodation, may also play a role and may be similar in members of the same family.[4,73] In addition, it is likely that several different genes for corneal shape, axial length, lens shape, and perhaps eye growth are inherited from each parent, making inheritance of even emmetropia complex to understand. Sorsby found that in refractively normal families there is a mild correlation (0.30) between the midparent refraction (average of the two parents' refractions) and that of offspring.[59] A reevaluation of Goldschmidt's data by Guggenheim et al.[19] found a much higher correlation (0.65) for the midparent/offspring refractions in children with high myopia than in those with refraction near emmetropia, which may suggest autosomal dominant transmission in some cases. Sorsby also found that the concordance in refraction between monozygotic twins was high, 0.71, but not perfect.

Some pedigrees have been reported that appear to represent autosomal dominant inheritance of isolated high myopia. At least two genetic loci have been found, demonstrating genetic heterogeneity.[70,71] Genetic heterogeneity between high and low myopia has also been reported.[46]

TREATMENT AND PREVENTION

The treatment of myopia consists of managing both the visual acuity loss and the complications that may arise. Treatment of the blurred vision in myopia has had a long and checkered history. Everything from physical exercise to palming the eyes to having myopic students study in green rooms has been advocated at one time or another.[31,65] These trials have been uniformly unimpressive in improving acuity.

Prevention

Sight-saving classes, exercises, undercorrection, cycloplegic therapy, contact lenses, pinhole glasses, and many other therapies have been aimed at preventing or slowing the progression of myopia. Surgery has been advocated to retard the progression of staphylomas in pathological myopia. A few of these therapies deserve mention.

There is evidence from several studies that atropinization during childhood slows or prevents an increase in myopia[5,26]; however the effects may not be long lasting.[55] One study that standardized final refractions of atropine and control groups at 20 years of age did find a long-term benefit, with those in the atropine group having a mean refraction of −2.79 diopters whereas those in the control group averaged −3.78.[26] The long-term effects of chronic dilation, including the effect of increased ultraviolet exposure, are not known. Also, the need for bifocals to read during atropine therapy is inconvenient, and patient and parent acceptance is often a problem.[55] The muscarinic antagonist pirenzipine retards axial myopia in nonhuman primates[61] and is currently being tested in clinical trials for use in human children. The rationale for use is that, in animal studies, atropine blocks myopia development even when the optic nerve is severed, meaning the mechanism cannot be lack of accommodation alone. Pirenzipine acts on the same receptors as atropine, yet the mydriasis and cycloplegia are minimal, theoretically producing the same pharmacological or transmitter effect without the side effects.

Undercorrection and near adds have had mixed results, but overall there is little evidence that the chance for benefit warrants the increased expense and effort for most myopes. One study showed no difference in myopic progression over 3 years between children who wore their correction full time, part time, or not at all.[41]

A trial of timolol maleate eyedrops in children with physiological and intermediate myopia showed that there was no significant difference in progression of myopia between the control and timolol groups; some children on topical timolol maleate actually had greater increases in myopia, although axial lengths did not increase more than the control group.[23] The author concluded that timolol maleate has no role in the treatment of these children.

In patients with pathological myopia, however, timolol or other ocular antihypertensives may be beneficial.[7] Scleral reinforcement with various materials also has good results in some hands, and given the poor prognosis in young patients with increasing staphylomas, may be indicated in certain patients.[7,62] Scleral shortening may be useful in cases of detachment secondary to macular hole formation.[39] Activities such as weight lifting, deep sea diving, and sports or hobbies that involve straining or raising intrathoracic pressure should be avoided.

Patients of all ages with high myopia often read better without their myopic correction, and some may prefer under-correction even for distance; this is often related to minification with high minus lenses, and contact lenses may improve the situation. Myopes reading without glasses may be bothered by phorias or tropias causing asthenopia. Low-vision aids should be recommended when appropriate. Highly myopic eyes may develop strabismus later in life, often esotropia, and surgery of the extraocular muscles may be required.[7] In addition, highly myopic eyes may require scleral buckling procedures for retinal detachment, and the buckles themselves may induce strabismus which requires surgical correction. Various vitamin and dietary regimens have been recommended, but scientific evidence of their efficacy is lacking.

TREATMENT

In preverbal children, correction should generally be given for myopia greater than −6.00 diopters, or if they demonstrate symptoms. Older children should be prescribed their full cycloplegic refraction for constant wear once the uncorrected visual acuity drops below the 20/40 range. In children, adolescents, or patients in their late teens or early twenties who develop an increase in myopia during periods of intense study or close work, a case can be made for doing close work without the myopic correction, or with a near plus add.[36,54] Although several studies have failed to find significant benefit from this,[18,23,44] there is a tendency for "high-risk" children (see above) to have less progression of myopia when bifocals are worn.[23] Contact lenses offer improved quality of vision for patients with higher levels of myopia (especially those with anisometropia); they also afford benefits for those who participate in contact sports or other activities in which glasses cannot be worn, and for patients who do not want to wear glasses. The age at which contact lenses should be considered depends on the magnitude of the refractive error, the maturity of the child, and the wishes of the parents. Despite reports that contact lenses halt the progression of myopia, there is evidence that axial length continues to increase.[3] The CLAMP study (Contact Lens and Myopia Progression) will revisit whether rigid contact lenses slow myopic progression, using a different study design that attempts to circumvent limitations of previous trials. At the start of the study,

78.4% of eligible children were able to tolerate rigid contact lens wear.[64] Use of night-time wear contact lenses to temporarily reshape the cornea is also being studied.

Keratorefractive surgery of various types can be performed in an attempt to improve visual acuity without prosthetic devices. The long-term effects of these procedures in children with myopia is not known. Because childhood myopia is a progressive condition, one refractive surgery procedure is unlikely to be sufficient, and reoperation carries a higher risk of complications. Several small studies have examined the role of pediatric refractive surgery for unilateral high myopia with amblyopia. This condition often results in very poor vision in the amblyopic eye because of noncompliance with unilateral contact lens wear or refusal to wear very asymmetrical spectacles. Also, this type of myopia tends to be nonprogressive. Adult nomograms appear to provide good myopic correction in these eyes for children 9 years and older; however, the correction may regress over time.[2,10] Corneal haze following photorefractive keratectomy (PRK) may exacerbate amblyopia, and the possibility of the corneal flap dehiscing with eye rubbing in uncooperative children who have laser in situ keratomileusis (LASIK) could cause serious complications. Also, in children old enough to cooperate with topical anesthesia for the procedure, amblyopia is already well established and best corrected visual acuity is only modestly improved or unchanged in most patients.[40] Clear lens extraction or anterior chamber minus intraocular lenses are also used by some practitioners to correct high myopia. Because these eyes are already at increased risk of retinal detachment and glaucoma and the long-term results are not known, these procedures are not usually recommended for children.

Myopic patients should have yearly examinations to screen for the associated complications of cataracts, glaucoma, and retinal detachment. In young children with physiological myopia, intraocular pressure determinations are not usually necessary unless there are signs of glaucoma. In any infant or young child presenting with myopia, particularly under the age of 3 or 4 years when the sclera is still very distensible, congenital or developmental glaucoma must be excluded as an etiology. Corneal diameters and clarity should be evaluated, and intraocular pressure measurement and/or axial eye length determinations should be made and followed. Sedation may be necessary for some of these tests. Other causes of myopia such as diabetes mellitis and various medications should be considered.

The retinal complications of myopia are the most common and are potentially sight threatening. Approximately 40% of retinal detachments occur in myopic eyes. The risk of retinal detachment following intracapsular cataract surgery is elevated, especially if there is vitreous loss.[22,24] According to a study by Perkins,[45] the risk of retinal detachment increases gradually from eyes with high hyperopia, to low hyperopia, to low myopia, and finally high myopia. Another study showed that retinal detachment is correlated with increased equatorial diameter rather than just with refraction or axial length.[35]

Children and young adults with high myopia may present with complaints of new floaters and flashes of light. Posterior vitreous detachment (PVD) must be looked for in these patients with indirect ophthalmoscopy and (when possible) slit lamp biomicroscopy. Approximately 10% to 15% of eyes with a new PVD develop a retinal tear.[24] Because tears may develop weeks after the PVD, another retinal examination should be performed 4 to 6 weeks after a new PVD is diagnosed. Some children with high myopia complain of bothersome floaters even in the absence of a PVD. If the retinal and vitreous examination are stable, reassurance is all that is required.

Symptomatic retinal tears, large horseshoe tears, and tears in the fellow eye of an eye that has had a detachment should be treated in children just as in adults. If the child is old enough and is cooperative, laser treatment can be done. In younger children general anesthesia and cryotherapy, or laser therapy with an indirect ophthalmoscope delivery system, may be required. In young children with vitreoretinal syndromes such as Stickler's, prophylactic peripheral retinal laser treatment performed under general anesthesia may be indicated. Prophylactic peripheral laser treatment of the fellow eye should be considered, especially if one eye suffers a retinal detachment. All highly myopic children and their parents should know the symptoms of retinal tears and detachments and who to call if they occur. The risk of retinal detachment in children with physiological and low grades of intermediate myopia is very low.

Myopic children or young adults with retinal detachments should be treated with scleral buckling or vitrectomy. If encircling bands are used in the repair of detachments in infants and children, they may need to be divided or removed as the child grows. Encircling bands may induce additional myopia. In premature infants with retinopathy of prematurity in whom large retinal detachments occur within the first year of life, the prog-

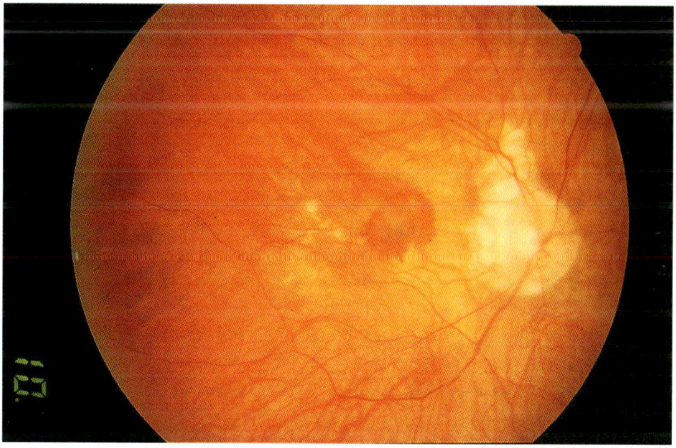

FIGURE 12-7. A choroidal neovascular membrane in a myopic eye. Note the adjacent lacquer crack.

nosis for useful vision is poor, even in many of those with a good anatomic result[48]; this may occur because the retina quickly degenerates after detachment in very young infants.[28] In uncomplicated myopic detachments occurring later in childhood, however, results may be good, unless coexisting myopic macular degeneration, sequelae from ROP, or an associated condition such as Stickler syndrome is present.

Subretinal neovascular membranes may form in the macula (Fig. 12-7). The results of laser treatment have not been as good as for membranes with other etiologies but should be considered if fluorescein angiography demonstrates a discrete membrane in a juxtafoveal or extrafoveal location.

Acknowledgments. Revision of this chapter was supported in part by the Georgia Lions Children's Eyecare Center. This chapter is dedicated to Bill and Elise Emerson.

References

1. Ahmad NN, Ala-Kokko L, Knowlton RG, et al. Stop codon in the procollagen II gene (Col2A1) in a family with Stickler syndrome. Proc Natl Acad Sci USA 1991;88:6624–6627.
2. Alio JL, Artola A, Claramonte P, et al. Photorefractive keratectomy for pediatric myopic anisometropia. J Cataract Refract Surg 1998;24: 327–330.

3. Baldwin WR, West D, Jolley J, et al. Effects of contact lenses on refractive corneal and axial length changes in young myopes. Am J Optom 1969;46:903–911.
4. Bear JC, Richler A, Burke G. Nearwork and familial resemblances in ocular refraction: a population study in Newfoundland. Clin Genet 1981;19(6):462–472.
5. Bedrossian RH. The effect of atropine on myopia. Ophthalmology 1979;86:713–717.
6. Berman ER, Michealson IC. The chemical composition of the human vitreous body as related to age and myopia. Exp Eye Res 1964;3:9–15.
7. Curtin BJ. The myopias: Basic science and clinical management. New York: Harper and Row, 1985.
8. Curtin BJ. The posterior staphyloma of pathologic myopia. Trans Am Ophthalmol Soc 1977;75:67–84.
9. Curtin BJ, Karlin DB. Axial length measurements and fundus changes of the myopic eye. Am J Ophthalmol 1971;71:42–53.
10. Drack A, Nucci P. Refractive surgery in children. Ophthalmol Clin North Am 2001;14(3):457–466.
11. Edwards MH, Chun CY, Leung SS. Intraocular pressure in an unselected sample of 6- to 7-year-old Chinese children. Optom Vision Sci 1993;70(3):198–200.
12. Edwards MH. Effect of parental myopia on the development of myopia in Hong Kong Chinese. Ophthalmic Physiol Optics 1998; 18(6):477–483.
13. Fledelius HC. Myopia profile in Copenhagen medical students 1996–98. Refractive stability over a century is suggested. Acta Ophthalmol Scand 2000;78(5):501–505.
14. Goldmann H. The diagnostic value of biomicroscopy of the posterior parts of the eye. Br J Ophthalmol 1961;45:449–460.
15. Goldschmidt E. On the etiology of myopia. Acta Ophthalmol 1968; 98(suppl):1.
16. Goldschmidt E, Lam CS, Opper S. The development of myopia in Hong Kong children. Acta Ophthalmol Scand 2001;79(3):228–232.
17. Goss DA, Jackson TW. Clinical findings before the onset of myopia in youth. 4. Parental history of myopia. Optom Vision Sci 1996; 73(4):279–282.
18. Grosvenor T, Goss DA. The role of bifocal and contact lenses in myopia control. Acta Ophthalmol (Suppl) 1988;185:162–166.
19. Guggenheim JA, Kirov G, Hodson SA. The heritability of high myopia: a reeanalysis of Goldschmidt's data. J Med Genet 2000;37(3): 227–231.
20. Gwiazda J, Ong E, Held R, Thorn F. Myopia and ambient night-time lighting. Nature (Lond) 2000;404(6774):144.
21. Hatfield EM. Why are they blind? Sight Sav Rev 1975;45:3–22.
22. Hilton GF, McLean EB, Chuang EL. Retinal detachment. Rochester, MN: American Academy of Ophthalmology and Otolarynology, 1989.
23. Jensen H. Myopia progression in young school children: a prospective study of myopia progression and the effect of a trial with bifocal

lenses and beta blocker eye drops. Acta Ophthalmol (Suppl) 1991; 200:69.
24. Kanski JJ. Retinal detachment: a colour manual of diagnosis and treatment. Stoneham: Butterworth, 1986.
25. Kelly TSB, Chatfield C, Tustin G. Clinical assessment of the arrest of myopia. Br J Ophthalmol 1975;59:531–538.
26. Kennedy RH, Dyer JA, Kennedy MA, et al. Reducing the progression of myopia with atropine: a long-term cohort study of Olmstead County students. Binoc Vision Strabismus Q 2000;15(suppl 3):281–304.
27. Klein RM, Curtin BJ. Lacquer crack lesions in pathologic myopia. Am J Ophthalmol 1975;79:386–392.
28. Kretzer FL, Mintz-Hittner HA. The "documented disappointment" of vitrectomy for ROP can be explained histologically. Presented at the 95th Annual Meeting of the American Academy of Ophthalmology, October 13–17, 1991.
29. Lam CS, Edwards M, Millodot M, Goh WS. A 2 year longitudinal study of myopia progression and optical component changes among Hong Kong schoolchildren. Optom Vision Sci 1999;76(6):370–380.
30. Lam DSC. Myopia in the young generation in Hong Kong. Hongkong.com; 2001.
31. Lin LLK, Ko LS. The effect of distance gazing and eye ball exercise on the prevention of myopia progression. Acta Ophthalmol (Suppl) 1988;185:139–140.
32. Lin LLK, Jan JH, Shih YF, Hung PT, Hou PK. Longitudinal study on the ocular refraction and its optical components among children in primary schools. In: Proceedings of the Fourth International Conference on Myopia. Sinapore: Myopia International Research Foundation, 1990:160–168.
33. Mantyjarvi M. High myopia in a family. In: Proceedings of the Fourth International Conference on Myopia. Singapore: Myopia International Research Foundation, 1990:89–98.
34. Mantyjarvi MI. Predicting of myopia progression in school children. J Pediatr Ophthalmol Strabismus 1985;22:71–75.
35. Meyer-Schwickerath G, Gerke E. Biometric studies on the eyeball and retinal detachment. Br J Ophthalmol 1984;68:29–31.
36. Miles PW. A study of heterophoria and myopia in children. Am J Ophthalmol 1962;54:111–114.
37. Moore C, Drack AV. Prism adaptation in decompensated monofixation syndrome. Am Orthopt J 2000;50:80–84.
38. Mutti DO, Zadnik K. The utility of three predictors of childhood myopia: a Bayesian analysis. Vision Res 1995;35(9):1345–1352.
39. Nakagawa N, Parel JM, Murray TG, Oshima K. Effect of scleral shortening on axial length. Arch Ophthalmol 2000;118(7):965–968.
40. Nucci P, Drack A. Refractive surgery for unilateral high myopia in children. J Am Assoc Pediatr Ophthalmol Strabismus 2001;5:348–351.

41. Ong E, Grice K, Held R, Thorn F, Gwiazda J. Effects of spectacle intervention on the progression of myopia in children. Optom Vision Sci 1999;76(6):363–369.
42. Otsuka J. Research on the etiology and treatment of myopia. Acta Soc Ophthalmol Jpn 1967;71:1–212.
43. Pacella R, McLellan J, Grice K, Del Bono EA, Wiggs JL, Gwiazda JE. Role of genetic factors in the etioloty of juvenile onset myopia based on a longitudinal study of refractive error. Optom Vision Sci 1999;76(6):381–386.
44. Parssinen O, Hemminki E. Spectacle use, bifocals and prevention of myopic progression. The two year results of a randomized trial among schoolchildren. Acta Ophthalmol 1988(Suppl)185:156–161.
45. Perkins ES. Morbidity from myopia. Sight Sav Rev 1979;49:11–19.
46. Pintado MH, Olmedo MV, Munoz JI, et al. Genetic differences between low and high myopia. Investig Ophthalmol Vis Sci 1992;33:712.
47. Pointer JS. A 6-year longitudinal optometric study of the refractive trend in school-aged children. Ophthalmic Physiol Optics 2001;21(5):361–367.
48. Quinn GE, Dobson V, Barr CC, et al. Visual acuity in infants after vitrectomy for severe retinopathy of prematurity. Ophthalmology 1991;98(1):5–13.
49. Quinn GE, Dobson V, Siatkowski R, et al. Does cryotherapy affect refractive error? Results from treated versus control eyes in the cryotherapy for retinopathy of prematurity trial. Ophthalmology 2001;108(2):343–347.
50. Quinn GE, Shin CH, Maguire MG, Stone RA. Myopia and ambient lighting at night. Nature (Lond) 1999;399(6732):113–114.
51. Raviola E, Weisel TN. Effect of dark-rearing on experimental myopia in monkeys. Investig Ophthalmol Vis Sci 1978;17:485–488.
52. Raviola E, Weisel TN. An animal model of myopia. N Engl J Med 1985;312(25):1615.
53. Richards AJ, Yates JRW, Williams R, et al. A family with Stickler syndrome type 2 has a mutation in the Col11A1 gene resulting in the substitution of glycine 97 by valine in alpha 1(XI) collagen. Hum Mol Genet 1996;5:1339–1343.
54. Roberts WL, Banford RD. Evaluation of bifocal correction technique in juvenile myopia. Optom Wkly 1967;58(38):25–31; 58(39),21–30; 58(40):23–28; 58(41):27–34; 58(43):19–26.
55. Sampson WG. Role of cycloplegia in the management of functional myopia. Ophthalmology 1979;86:695–697.
56. Saw SM, Wu HM, Hong CY, Chua WH, Chia KS, Tan D. Myopia and night lighting in children in Singapore. Br J Ophthalmol 2001;85(5):527–528.
57. Sertie AL, Quimby M, Moreira ES, et al. A gene which causes severe ocular alterations and occipital encephalocele (Knobloch syndrome) is mapped to 21q22.3. Hum Mol Genet 1996;5:843–847.

58. Smith EL III, Bradley DV, Fernandes A, Hung LF, Boothe RG. Continuous ambient lighting and eye growth in primates. Investig Ophthalmol Vis Sci 2001;42(6):1146–1152.
59. Sorsby A. Refraction. In: Ophthalmic genetics, 2nd edn. London: Butterworths, 1970:38–51.
60. Theng JT, Wong TY, Ling Y. Refractive errors and strabismus in premature Asian infrants with and without retinopathy of prematurity. Singapore Med J 2000;41(8):393–397.
61. Tigges M, Iuvone PM, Fernandes A, et al. Effects of muscarinic cholinergic receptor antagonists on postnatal eye growth of rhesus monkeys. Optom Vision Sci 1999;76(6):397–407.
62. Thompson FB. A re-evaluation of scleral reinforcement surgery. In: Proceedings of the Fourth International Conference on Myopia. Singapore: Myopia International Research Foundation, 1990:427–438.
63. Tokoro T, Mutamatsu T. Macular hemorrhage associated with high myopia. In: Proceedings of the Fourth International Conference on Myopia. New York: Myopia International Research Foundation, 1990:103–108.
64. Walline JJ, Mutti DO, Jones LA, et al. The contact lens and myopia progression study (CLAMP): design and baseline data. Optom Vision Sci 2001;78(4):223–233.
65. Wang AH, Lin LLK, Shi YF, Ko LS. The effect of green classroom on the prevention of myopia progression. Acta Ophthalmol (Suppl) 1988;185:147.
66. Weis MA, Wilkin DJ, Kim HJ, et al. Structurally abnormal type II collagen in a severe form of Kniest dysplasia caused by an exon 24 skipping mutation. J Biol Chem 1998;273(8):4761–4768.
67. Weymouth FW, Hirsch MJ. Theories, definitions and classifications of refractive errors. In: Grosvenor T, Flom MC (eds) *Refractive anomalies: research and clinical applications.* Stoneham, MA: Butterworth-Heinemann, 1991.
68. Working Group on Myopia Prevalence and Progression (WGMPP). Myopia: prevalence and progression. Committee on Vision, National Research Council. Washington, DC: National Academy Press, 1989.
69. Young FA, Baldwin WR, Box RA, Harris E, Johnson C. The transmission of refractive error within Eskimo families. Am J Optom 1969;46:676–685.
70. Young TL, Ronan SM, Drahozal LA, et al. Evidence that a locus for familial high myopia maps to chromosome 18p. Am J Hum Genet 1998;63:109–119.
71. Young TL, Ronan SM, Alvear AB, et al. A second locus for familial high myopia maps to chromosome 12q. Am J Hum Genet 1998;63:1419–1424.
72. Zadnik K, Satariano WA, Mutti DO, Sholtz RI, Adams AJ. The effect of parental history of myopia on children's eye size. JAMA 1994;271(17):1323–1327.
73. Zadnik K. Myopia development in childhood. Optom Vision Sci 1997;74(8).603–608.

74. Zadnik K, Mutti DO, Friedman NE, et al. Ocular predictors of the onset of juvenile myopia. Investig Ophthalmol Vis Sci 1999;40(9): 1936–1943.
75. Zadnik K, Jones L, Irvin B, et al. Myopia and ambient night-time lighting. Nature (Lond) 2000;404(6774):143–144.

13

Patterns of Retinal Disease in Children

Arlene V. Drack

Chapter 30 in this volume stresses that not all diseases that look alike have the same etiology. Very different causes may produce identical clinical pictures, and disorders with similar ophthalmoscopic findings may have widely disparate clinical courses and modes of inheritance. Traditionally, eye disease nomenclature has been based upon underlying etiologies and on which structures in the eye harbor the initial or inciting defect. However, the reality of clinical practice is that when patients present to an ophthalmologist, one of the most important clues the physician has about the disorder is the appearance of the fundus. Therefore, in this chapter, many of the retinal disorders that have been discussed earlier in the retina section are briefly reviewed from two new perspectives: ophthalmoscopic appearance and systemic associations.

The ophthalmoscopic appearance section presents diseases based upon similar fundus findings. A brief explanation of the anatomic basis for the fundus appearance is given, as well as why unrelated disorders are thought to share a common appearance. Differentiating features of some of the entities are discussed. This portion of the chapter can be used to develop a differential diagnosis for patients who present with a well-defined pattern of retinal disease that is known to exist in several different disorders. In most cases, the specific entities can then be studied in more detail elsewhere in this volume. This portion of the chapter is not all inclusive. For example, flecks and dots of the retinal pigment epithelium (RPE), and diffuse pigmentary retinopathies are not listed, because entire Chapters (4, 5) are devoted to the differential diagnosis of these disorders. Uveitis and inflammatory conditions are also readily differentiated from most other entities and are discussed at length in Chapter 11.

The second half of the chapter reviews some of the same disorders from another point of view. Many of the retinal diseases seen in children are part of a larger metabolic or morphological syndrome with physical stigmata. The second section presents categories of disease or dysmorphism commonly associated with retinal disease. Any child presenting with a retinal disorder should have an evaluation by a pediatrician who has been appraised of the most likely associated findings; however, ophthalmologists, after all, are medical doctors and a brief preliminary physical examination in the office can evaluate skin, teeth, palate, fingers and toes. Similarly, a careful, directed history should be taken. Extra digits may have been removed at birth, and parents may not mention the hearing, renal, or neurological problems in other family members unless they are asked about them specifically. Recognition of these syndromes is important for appropriate counseling and general medical care. In several of these disorders, ophthalmologists, not pediatricians, are usually the first physicians with an opportunity to make the diagnosis. Some of these diseases are treatable if detected at an early stage. Even in those for which no treatment is available, prompt recognition may prevent parents from unknowingly having another affected child and, at the very least, may be useful in planning school and other activities for the child. In addition, most parents and children are much better able to accept and live with their disease if they have some knowledge and understanding of why things have occurred and what to expect.

In this chapter, categories and diseases are listed in the tables. All these lists are organized according to the incidence of the diseases in children; that is, the most common causes of a given clinical picture in children are listed first, whereas the least common or very rare causes are last. In some cases, disorders that are extremely common in adults are rare in children. These diseases are marked with an asterisk to indicate that in adolescents or older persons, the differential is notably different. A list of treatable disorders is also given, with a brief discussion in the text of some of the treatment options. Because new treatments may have become available after the writing of this chapter, this list should not be considered all inclusive.

CHARACTERISTIC FUNDUS PATTERNS

Cherry-Red Spot

The ophthalmoscopic appearance of a cherry-red spot is caused by loss of transparency of the extrafoveal retina as a result of intra- or extracellular edema or deposition of abnormal metabolic by-products in the retinal ganglion cells. The "red spot" is evident in the macular region because ganglion cells are absent or only one layer thick in this area, allowing the normal choroidal and pigmentary appearance of the fundus to be clearly visible (see Fig. 13-1). Macular hemorrhages or holes may give the appearance of a cherry-red spot but can be differentiated by comparison with the other eye, history, and the evolution of the lesion. The most typical clinical setting in which a cherry-red spot is seen in a child is a patient with a neurological disorder who has been referred to the ophthalmologist. The majority of these children have already been recognized to have an abnormality of a more general nature before they reach the ophthalmologist. *Tay–Sachs* is the most common metabolic disease causing this clinical picture; however, several other storage diseases can result in an identical appearance (Table 13-1). The

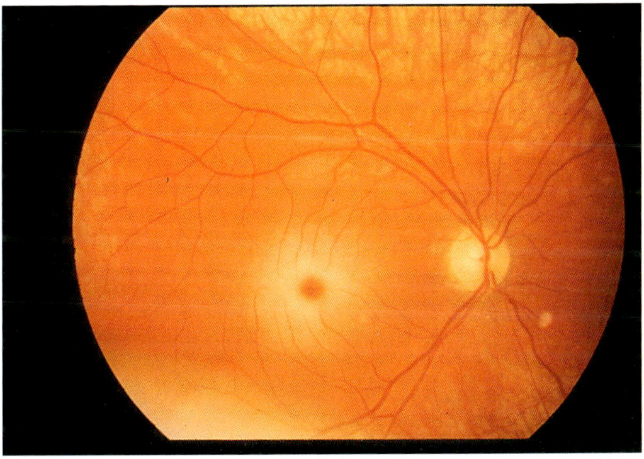

FIGURE 13-1. Cherry-red spot in sialidosis. The other eye appeared identical to this one. (Courtesy of Dr. G.F. Judisch)

TABLE 13-1. Patterns of Retinal Disease in Children.

1. Cherry-red spot
   a. Tay–Sachs disease (GM$_2$ gangliosidosis type I)
   b. Sandhoff Disease (GM$_2$ gangliosidosis type II)
   c. Niemann–Pick disease
   d. Sialidosis
   e. Farber's lipogranulomatosis
   f. Metachromatic leukodystrophy
   g. GM$_1$ gangliosidosis
   h. Central retinal artery occlusion*
   i. Trauma (retinal edema)
2. Vascular tortuosity
   a. Retinopathy of prematurity
   b. Fabry's disease
   c. Sickle cell disease
   d. Respiratory insufficiency
   e. Incontinentia pigmenti
   f. Fucosidosis
   g. Coats' disease
   h. Optociliary shunt vessels
   i. Peripapillary vascular loops
   j. Capillary hemangioma
   k. Cavernous hemangioma
   l. Diabetes mellitus*
   m. Racemose hemangioma
   n. Familial retinal arteriolar tortuosity
   o. Eales' disease*
3. Macular colobomas
   a. Typical macular coloboma
   b. Leber's congenital amaurosis
   c. North Carolina macular dystrophy
   d. Toxoplasmosis
   e. Aicardi's syndrome
   f. Idiopathic infantile hypercalcuria
   g. Pathologic myopia
   h. Down's syndrome (trisomy 21)
   i. Lymphocytic choriomeningitis virus
4. Foveal hypoplasia
   a. Albinism
   b. Aniridia
   c. Prader–Willi syndrome
   d. Isolated foveal hypoplasia
5. Retinal detachment
   a. Retinoblastoma
   b. Retinopathy of prematurity
   c. Trauma*
   d. Coats' disease
   e. Stickler's syndrome
   f. Norrie disease
   g. Retinal dysplasia
   h. Persistent hyperplastic primary vitreous (persistent fetal vasculature)
   i. Incontinentia pigmenti
   j. Familial exudative vitreoretinopathy
   k. X-linked juvenile retinoschisis
   l. Inflammatory/exudative
   m. Optic nerve pit
   n. Ehlers–Danlos VI
   o. High myopia/lattice degeneration*
   p. Spondyloepiphyseal dysplasia congenita

TABLE 13-1. (continued)

6. Angioid streaks
   a. Pseudoxanthoma elasticum
   b. Paget's disease of bone
   c. Sickle cell hemoglobinopathies
   d. Senile elastosis
   e. Thalassemia
   f. Ehlers–Danlos syndrome
   g. Abetalipoproteinemia
   h. Hereditary spherocytosis
   i. Calcinosis
   j. Acromegaly
7. Vitreoretinal dysplasia/aplasia
   a. Norrie disease
   b. Trisomy 13
   c. Incontinentia pigmenti
   d. Warburg's syndrome
   e. Autosomal recessive vitreoretinal dysplasia
8. Salt-and-pepper fundus
   a. Rubella
   b. Syphilis
   c. Alstrom syndrome
   d. Mitochondrial myopathy
   e. Fundus pulverulentus
9. Bull's-eye maculopathy
   a. Stargardt's disease
   b. Neuronal ceroid lipofuscinosis
   c. Olivopontocerebellar atrophy type III (SCA 6)
   d. Hallervorden–Spatz disease
   e. Bardet–Biedl
   f. Alstrom syndrome
   g. Cone dystrophy
   h. Mucolipidosis type IV
   i. Cone–rod dystrophy
   j. Drug toxicity (desferoxamine, chloroquine)
10. Congenital retinal disease
    a. Cytomegalovirus
    b. Herpes simplex
    c. Syphilis
    d. Toxoplasmosis
    e. Herpes zoster
    f. Rubella
    g. HIV (human immunodeficiency virus)
    h. Lymphocytic choriomeningitis virus (LCMV)
11. Geographic pigmentary disturbance
    a. Gyrate atrophy
    b. Choroideremia
    c. Pathological myopia
12. Retinal causes of leukocoria
    a. Chorioretinal coloboma
    b. Coats' disease
    c. Retinoblastoma
    d. Toxoplasmosis
    e. Toxocariasis
    f. Morning glory disc
    g. Myelinated nerve fibers
    h. Other disruptions of the retina and choroid

*Diseases that are common in adults but rare in children.

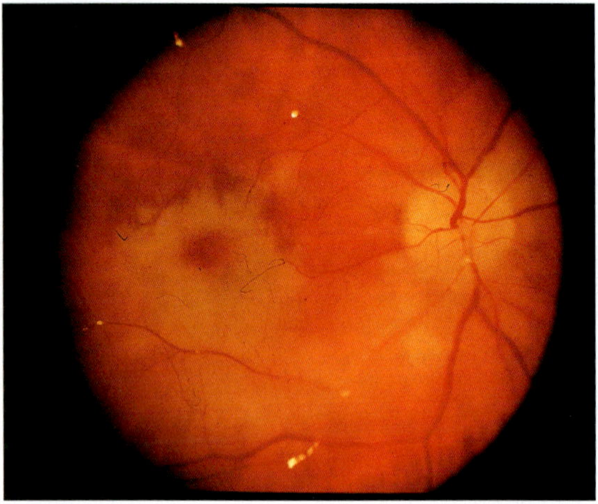

FIGURE 13-2. Cherry-red spot secondary to central retinal artery occlusion. The fellow eye was normal. Note the refractile emboli in several of the vessels. Emboli are not always seen.

cherry-red spot has been reported to disappear over time as the ganglion cells die and the material deposited there is released. Therefore, the absence of a cherry-red spot, especially in older children, does not rule out the presence of a suspected metabolic disorder.[37] Aside from metabolic disorders, retinal edema is the other likely cause of a cherry-red spot. The most common etiology is a cilioretinal or central retinal artery occlusion (Fig. 13-2), which is extremely rare in children but more common in adults. Underlying causes of thrombotic diathesis, such as *homocystinuria*, *Fabry's disease*,[71,72] blood dyscrasias, oral contraceptives, or history of radiation therapy should be suspected. Retinal artery occlusion is usually unilateral, not bilateral as is the case in metabolic disease. Trauma with resulting retinal edema must also be ruled out.

Vascular Tortuosity

Tortuosity of retinal aterioles and venules, often associated with vascular dilatation, can be a congenital or acquired condition in children. Congenitally anomalous blood vessels are seen in *Coats' disease* (Fig. 13-3), *racemose hemangioma*, *capillary and cavernous hemangiomas, familial retinal arteriolar tortuosity*, and *peripapillary vascular loops*. Coats' disease is usually sporadic, occurs more often in males, is generally unilateral, and may present with or progress to an exudative retinal detachment. Cryotherapy or laser treatment may halt progression. Capillary hemangiomas and familial retinal tortuosity can both be inherited in an autosomal dominant fashion.[27,89] Capillary hemangiomas may be the presenting sign in Von Hippel–Lindau disease (VHL), a potentially lethal autosomal dominant disorder affecting the brain, kidneys, and other organs as well as the eye.[27] Sporadic, isolated capillary hemangiomas usually occur at a later age than those associated with VHL, because the latter are caused by mutations in a gene that appears to act via a "two-hit" mutation model, similar to retinoblastoma.[10] A complete medical workup of the patient and family members, in addition to ocular examinations, should therefore be performed when capillary hemangiomas of the retina are diagnosed. Familial retinal tortuosity may be associated with hemorrhages, at times following exercise.[23] Racemose hemangioma may be associated with intracranial lesions in the *Wyburn–Mason syndrome*. Cavernous hemangioma appears as a grapelike cluster that is more

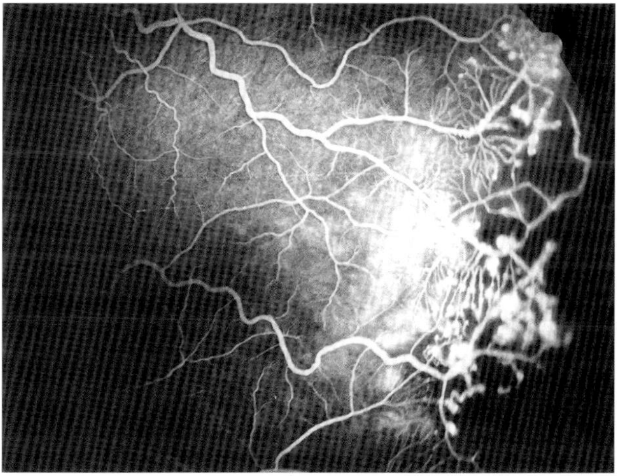

FIGURE 13-3. Fluorescein angiogram of the periphery in a female child with Coat's disease. Note the bulblike telangiectasias and the avascular area beyond the tortuosity.

likely to present in early adulthood than childhood. *Fucosidosis* is a storage disease in which retinal vascular tortuosity is associated with telangiectatic conjunctival vessels, corneal clouding, and mental retardation.

Some acquired causes of vascular tortuosity have an underlying genetic etiology that may not become manifest until later in life. The telangiectatic skin and conjunctival lesions, cornea verticillata, and peripheral neuropathy seen in *Fabry's disease* may go undiagnosed in early childhood. Retinal vascular tortuosity (Fig. 13-4), along with occlusions and beading, are seen in the second decade in this X-linked disorder.[71] Retinal ischemia induces neovascularization in sickle cell disease (lesions tend to be peripheral) and in diabetes mellitis (lesions tend to be in the posterior pole and rarely occur before the patient has had the disease for at least 10–15 years). *Retinopathy of prematurity* (ROP) exhibits dilated and tortuous anastomotic vessels at the peripheral demarcation zone between normal and avascular retina early in the disease (see Chapter 10). If the disease progresses to a "plus" stage, the arterioles in the posterior pole also become dilated, tortuous, and leaky, and iris neovascularization may occur. Some of this tortuosity may persist into childhood,

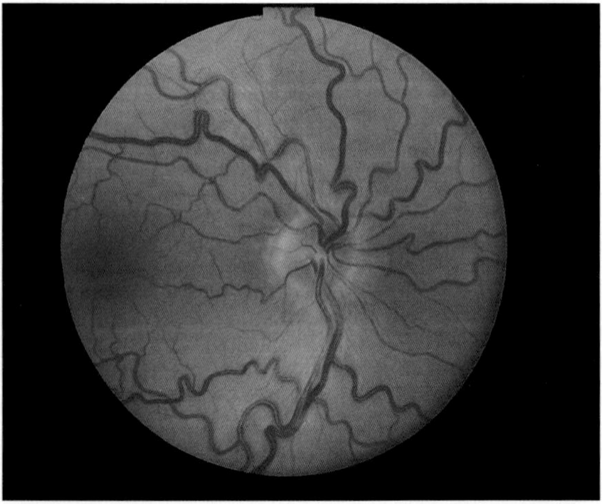

FIGURE 13-4. Retinal vascular tortuosity develops in the second decade in Fabry's disease. See Figure 13-18 for an illustration of other associated features.

even if the disease regresses, or vessels may be straightened and dragged. Children with chronic respiratory insufficiency from a variety of causes may have dilated, tortuous retinal vessels in the posterior pole;[83] this may be similar in etiology to the vascular tortuosity seen in some adults with hypoxemia and hypercapnia from chronic obstructive pulmonary disease.[77] Optociliary shunt vessels are engorged vessels on or near the disc that may occur with compressive lesions such as orbital meningiomas or gliomas and must be differentiated from benign peripapillary loops. *Incontinentia pigmenti* is a rare X-linked dominant disorder that may have peripheral vascular changes resembling ROP. Affected females may be mentally retarded and have characteristic skin changes. As in ROP, cryotherapy or laser treatment may prevent cicatricial disease and blindness.[58] Enzyme replacement therapy may be beneficial in Fabry's disease.[66]

Macular Coloboma

Macular colobomas are excavated, whitish lesions surrounded by normal retina. A typical coloboma (Fig. 13-5) is a developmental defect resulting from failure of closure of the fetal fissure in the embryonic optic cup. These colobomas may include the iris and lens as well as the retina and choroid; they are typically inferonasal and may involve the optic nerve as well as some or all of the macula. Although vision is often severely affected, it does not necessarily correlate with the severity of the lesion ophthalmoscopically. Predictions of level of vision are best delayed until the child is old enough for some form of acuity testing. Typical colobomas are often idiopathic, especially if unilateral, but they may be inherited as an autosomal dominant trait with variable expressivity, with or without other congenital anomalies.[5] Typical colobomas, especially if bilateral, may be markers of chromosomal abnormalities, or syndromes such as the CHARGE[86] association, or Goltz syndrome. Isolated colobomatous microphthalmia has been mapped to chromosome 15q12–q15.[52] Atypical colobomas, which may be congenital or acquired, are not secondary to abnormal closure of the fetal fissure but have a white excavated appearance similar to typical colobomas. Pathological myopia (Fig. 13-6), intrauterine infections such as toxoplasmosis (Fig. 13-7), lymphocytic choriomeningitis virus (LCMV), or a retinal dystrophy such as North Carolina macular dystrophy are often

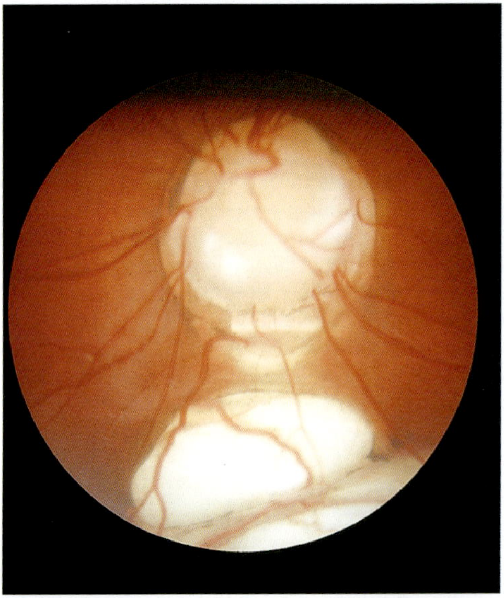

FIGURE 13-5. Typical colobomas result from failure of closure of the fetal fissure; they often involve the nerve, as seen in this patient. (Courtesy of Dr. G.F. Judisch)

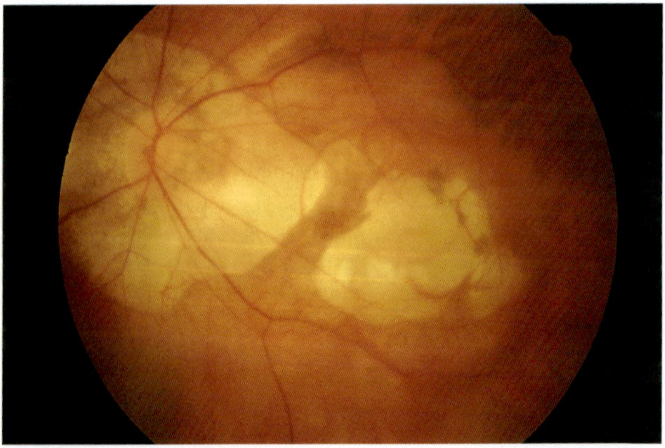

FIGURE 13-6. Coloboma-like lesions secondary to severe myopia involving the macula and peripapillary retina.

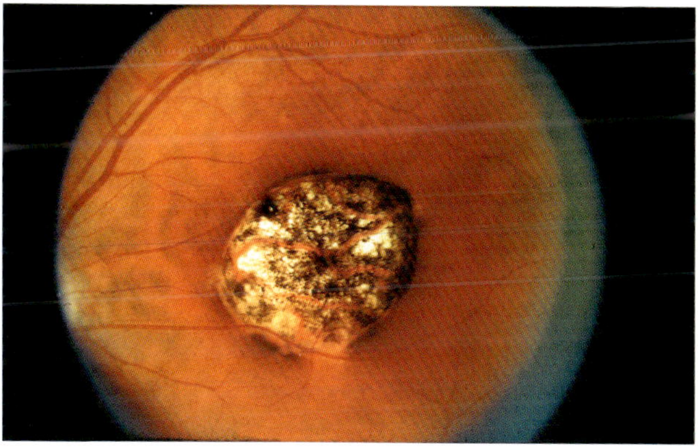

FIGURE 13-7. Toxoplasmosis may leave a colobomatous scar in the macular area. With time, these scars often develop characteristic hyperpigmentation.

the cause. Children with Aicardi's syndrome, in which females have infantile spasms, an absent corpus callosum, and chorioretinal scars, may have coloboma-like lesions in the posterior pole. Patients with trisomy 21 (Down's syndrome) may have coloboma-like lesions in the macula.[91] Development of a macular coloboma in Leber's congenital amaurosis is a poor prognostic sign for stability of vision.[29]

Foveal Hypoplasia

Foveal hypoplasia is recognized clinically as a dulled or absent foveal reflex in a child with poor vision and, usually, nystagmus. An idiopathic form has been described, which may be sporadic or autosomal dominant.[54,55] This form is the exception, however, and an underlying ocular syndrome can often be found. The most common is one of the forms of ocular or oculocutaneous (OCA) albinism. This disorder should be suspected in any child or adult presenting with congenital nystagmus. The stigmata are present at birth, but the diagnosis is often not made until much later. The hallmarks are iris transillumination defects (Fig. 13-8) and, in the oculocutaneous forms, diffuse hypopigmentation. In complete oculocutaneous albinisim, the diagnosis is obvious: the hair is white, the skin has no pigmentation, and the irides

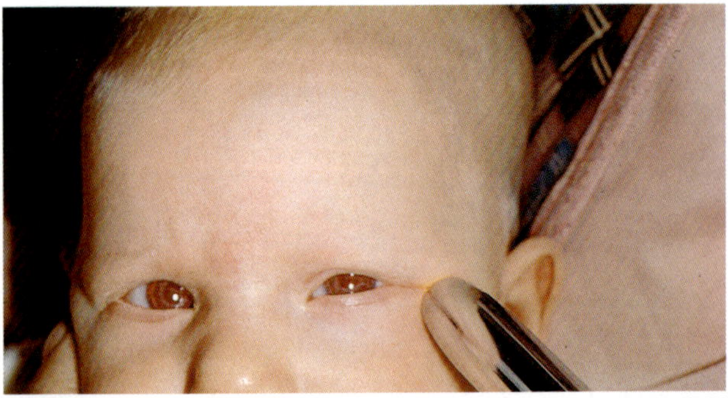

FIGURE 13-8. Searching for transillumination defects in a young child using the penlight technique. In this photograph, the red reflex from the camera flash illuminates both eyes. In clinical use, the flashlight held to the lids in a darkened room reveals iris transillumination defects beautifully, a test that is much easier to perform than a slit lamp examination in most infants. (Courtesy of Dr. G.F. Judisch)

are pink. In the various incomplete forms, and in all ocular albinism patients, the signs may be far more subtle. Pigmentation may appear normal, but may be less than expected given the patient's racial and ethnic background and the parents' pigmentation. In such patients, a careful search for iris transillumination defects and foveal abnormalities should be performed in the proband and family members.

Infants with albinism often have delayed visual responses suggesting the diagnosis of Leber's congenital amaurosis. Vision often improves with time to approximately 20/200 with even better vision at near. The optic nerves may appear gray or indistinct (Fig. 13-9), and macular hypoplasia may be so profound that retinal vessels course over the area that should include the macula.[78] A history of easy bruising or frequent infection should be sought to rule out the potentially life-threatening syndromes of *Hermansky–Pudlak* and *Chediak–Higashi*. The fundus appears blonde in all forms of albinism; however, small pigmented RPE clumps or diffuse moderate pigmentation may be seen in tyrosinase-positive incomplete OCA patients. The other disorder in which foveal hypoplasia is prominent is aniridia (Fig. 13-10). Affected infants present with poor vision, nystagmus, and hypoplasia of the iris. Most patients have some rudimentary iris tissue and may therefore appear to have widely dilated amaurotic pupils, leading to an erroneous diagnosis. The macular

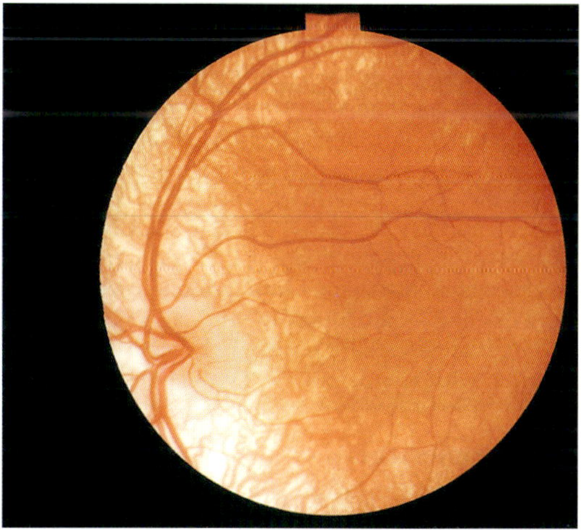

FIGURE 13-9. The optic nerves may be grayish with indistinct margins in children with albinism. Note the prominent red color of the choroid, which is evident when there is no overlying pigment. (Courtesy of Dr. G.F. Judisch)

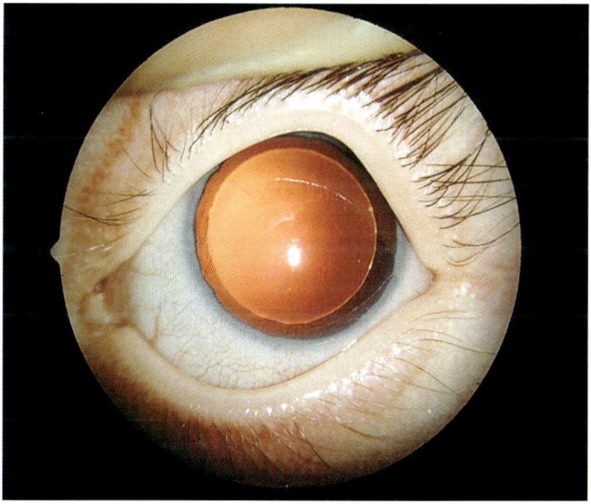

FIGURE 13-10. Some iris tissue is usually present in aniridia. Foveal hypoplasia, glaucoma, pannus, and subluxated lenses may be associated features.

reflex is blunted but the fundus pigmentation is normal for that individual. It is usually possible to see the edge of the lens, which may be easier to do with a 20 diopter (D) lens and an indirect ophthalmoscope than a slit lamp in a very young child. The diagnosis of aniridia is an important one because sporadic cases are associated with Wilm's tumor. Such children should have close follow-up by a pediatrician throughout childhood. The hereditary forms may be autosomal dominant or recessive. In some dominant pedigrees of aniridia, foveal hypoplasia is not present, there is no nystagmus, and vision is good.[16] Glaucoma often may develop in patients with *aniridia*. Congenital, developmental, and angle-closure glaucoma have also been reported in association with albinism.[9,17,43]

Retinal Detachment

Retinal detachment in infants and children is extremely rare, and this finding should lead one to suspect a specific disease, syndrome, or trauma. Nonaccidental trauma should always be considered because in these cases the child's life, as well as vision, may be at stake.

Several broad categories should be considered when a newborn or infant presents with a retinal detachment. The first is the presence of a tumor in the eye, which should be ruled out with ultrasound or CT scan. Once this potentially life-threatening diagnosis has been excluded, other causes of congenital or infantile detached retina should be considered, including *Stickler syndrome*, retinopathy of prematurity, *retinal dysplasia*, and *Norrie disease* (Fig. 13-11). The latter may be confirmed by molecular genetic techniques and is caused by mutations of the Norrie disease gene on the X chromosome.[92] Defects in this gene may also cause later onset retinal detachment as part of *familial exudative vitreoretinopathy* (FEVR).[11] Premature infants with mutations in the Norrie disease gene may be predisposed to more severe ROP and retinal detachment as well.[70]

FIGURE 13-11A,B. Sagittal (**A**) and axial (**B**) MRI of a child with Norrie disease. Note the blood density filling the globe and the detached retina anterior to it. MRI or CT may distinguish this disorder from retinoblastoma, but not from vitreous hemorrhage or persistent hyperplastic primary vitreous (PHPV). Retinal detachment in Norrie disease is usually, although not always, bilateral. (Courtesy of Dr. I. Maumenee)

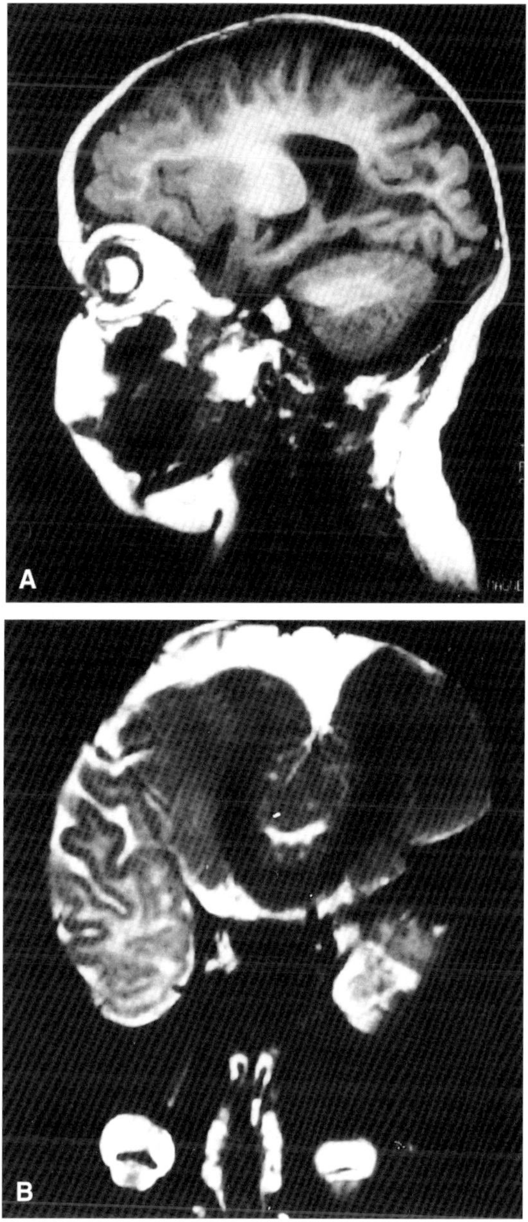
A
B

Persistent hyperplastic primary vitreous (PHPV), also called *persistent fetal vasculature* (PFV), may also present with a retinal detachment at birth; however, the associated microphthalmos and cataract often simplify the diagnosis. Bilateral PHPV may be a sign of a genetic syndrome. A complete systemic and genetic workup should be performed in these cases. In infants who are born with attached retinas that subsequently detach, a likely diagnosis is cicatricial retinopathy of prematurity. There is evidence that retinal degeneration occurs very rapidly following detachment in these immature eyes.[38] Incontinentia pigmenti may also predispose to early-onset retinal detachment. If retinal detachments occur in later infancy or childhood, underlying exudative, inflammatory, or tractional causes should be sought. The retinal detachments seen with Stickler's syndrome, *spondyloepiphyseal dysplasia congenita, X-linked juvenile retinoschisis, optic nerve pits*, and *Ehlers–Danlos VI* usually occur after infancy. In Ehlers–Danlos VI, there may be extreme fragility of the globe resulting in rupture from relatively minor injury. Safety glasses should be prescribed for these children. Some, although not all, of the latter patients have a measurable deficiency of lysyl dehydrogenase.[34] Pyridinium cross-link abnormalities in urine may help make the diagnosis of Ehlers–Danlos VI.

Angioid Streaks

Angioid streaks are seen ophthalmoscopically as subretinal lines of variable width, usually radiating out from the disc (Fig. 13-12), which represent breaks in Bruch's membrane with atrophy of the overlying RPE and eventually of the underlying choriocapillaris as well. The color of the streaks may be red or gray (recent) or yellowish (atrophic). About half the patients with angioid streaks have an underlying systemic cause.[13,73] The associated disorders (Table 13-1) are syndromes in which elastic tissue is abnormally fragile because of either an increased affinity for calcium or deposition of iron. The breaks in Bruch's membrane may be secondary to mechanical forces acting on this relatively inelastic structure.[46] Angioid streaks usually develop in the second decade of life and are associated with macular subretinal neovascular membranes, macular degeneration, and visual loss in more than 50% of eyes, often at a young age.[47]

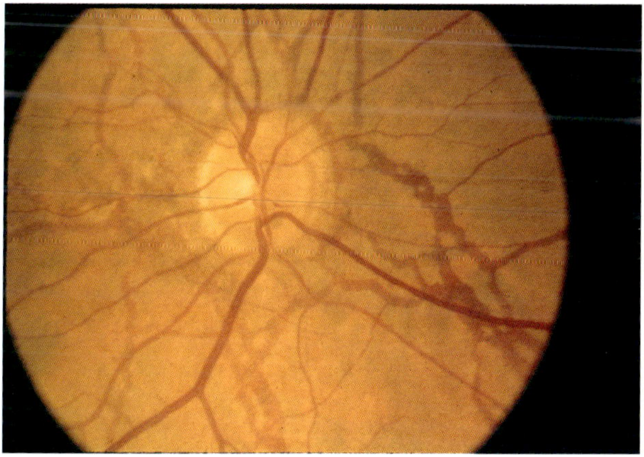

FIGURE 13-12. Fundus of a patient with angioid streaks. These linear lesions typically radiate out from the disc and represent breaks in Bruch's membrane. Fifty percent of patients with angioid streaks have an underlying systemic etiology.

Vitreoretinal Dysplasia or Aplasia

Most infants with *vitreoretinal dysplasia or aplasia* have bilateral white retrolental masses associated with nystagmus and other congenital anomalies or syndromes. Norrie disease is X-linked and thus occurs almost exclusively in males. About 25% of these children are mentally retarded and 33% have hearing loss.[56] Retinal folds and detachment are usually present at birth. Carrier females are normal, but molecular genetic techniques can be used for diagnosis in some families.[11,92] In trisomy 13, multiple systemic defects are present and the infants usually do not survive. Patients with Warburg syndrome (autosomal recessive) are mentally retarded and have hydrocephalus, agyria, and in some cases an encephalocoele.[87] Incontinentia pigmenti occurs almost exclusively in females; it is usually inherited as an X-linked dominant that is lethal in males. Isolated cases of vitreoretinal dysplasia have been presumed to be autosomal recessive.

Salt-and-Pepper Fundus

The clinical picture of a "salt-and-pepper" fundus is the result of fine pigment clumping and dispersion that is most often caused by a congenital infection which disrupts the normal embryogenesis of the RPE. A fine pigmentary change in the fundus is the most common ocular finding in the *congenital rubella syndrome* (Figs. 13-13A,B). Histologically, it corresponds

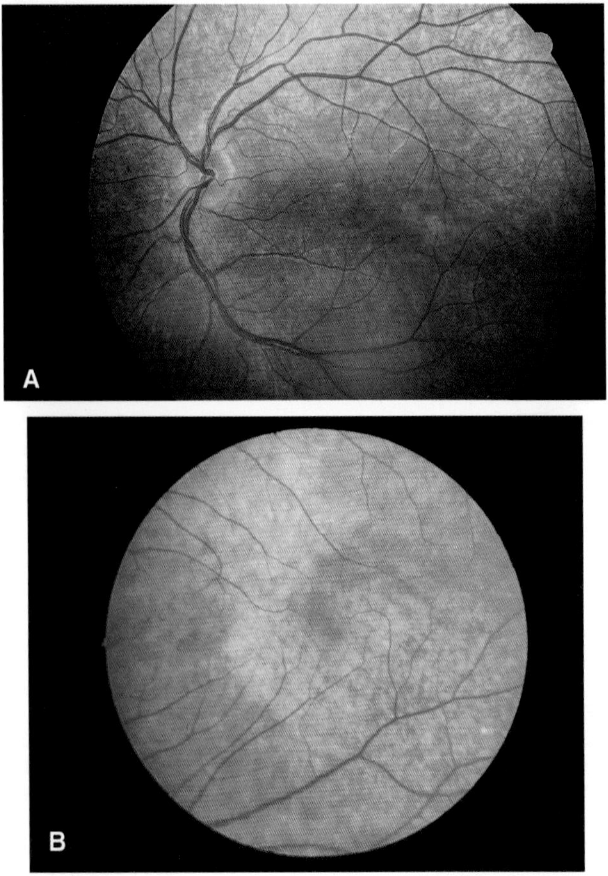

FIGURE 13-13A,B. (**A**) Diffuse salt-and-pepper pigmentary disturbance seen in a patient with congenital rubella syndrome. (**B**) Close-up of macular pigmentary changes in another child with congenital rubella. The pigmentary changes do not affect vision, but macular subretinal neovascular membranes may develop in later life.

to irregular degeneration of the RPE with adjacent pigment migration and clumping.[93] However, the vision and electro-oculogram (EOG) are usually normal, and the electroretinogram (ERG) is recordable but may be reduced.[39] In later life (after the age of 9 years in all reported patients), subretinal neovascular membranes may form. Some of these membranes resolve without disciform scarring but others reduce vision.[75] Other ocular findings may include cataract, microphthalmos, and glaucoma. Hearing loss is common, and endocrine abnormalities also develop in some patients later in life, making the appropriate diagnosis of more than academic interest.[69] Infants born with congenital rubella can shed live virus and are therefore infectious. Interestingly, they may not retain immunity from their congenital infection and are therefore susceptible to reinfection at a later time. For the same reason, negative rubella titers in a child older than 3 or 4 years do not rule out congenital infection. Although vaccination programs have all but eradicated epidemics of rubella in the United States, 10% to 20% of adults in their childbearing years remain seronegative,[76] and cases of congenital rubella continue to be reported in the United States and around the world.

Another congenital infection causing this fundus picture is syphilis. The incidence of this disease is on the rise in the United States. Babies often have rhinitis causing the "sniffles" shortly after birth. Retinitis, uveitis, interstitial keratitis, and abnormal teeth develop later. If congenital syphilis is diagnosed at any age, systemic antibiotics may be warranted. Even if treated, congenital syphilis may lead to recurrent uveitis, arthritis, progressive hearing loss, and interstitial keratitis mediated by autoimmune effects. Any child with positive syphilis serology should be evaluated for other sexually transmitted diseases such as human immunodeficiency virus (HIV), gonorrhea, and chlamydia.

Alstrom syndrome may resemble congenital rubella with deafness, pigmentary retinopathy, and diabetes mellitis. Although the fundus may have a salt-and-pepper appearance, a bull's-eye or other maculopathy is more typical. The histopathology is very different from congenital rubella, with an absence of rods and cones.[68] The ERG may initially show a cone defect but usually becomes nonrecordable over time. Mitochondrial myopathy may also be associated with salt-and-pepper retinopathy. In a series of 61 patients with mitochondrial myopathy, 36% had retinal pigmentary changes. Of these, 82% were described as "salt and pepper," usually with good vision.[53]

Bull's-Eye Maculopathy

The neuronal ceroid lipofuscinoses (NCL) are a group of autosomal recessive disorders characterized by progressive neurological deterioration, seizures, and pigmentary retinopathy. Three of the four types exhibit retinopathy. The infantile form (Haltia–Santavuori syndrome, onset between 8 and 18 months of age) and the late infantile form (Jansky–Bielschowsky syndrome, onset between 2 and 4 years of age) usually present with neurological deterioration before vision loss occurs. In the juvenile form (Batten syndrome), the onset is between 4 and 8 years of age and the visual disturbance usually precedes neurological symptoms; this form is most likely to be diagnosed by an ophthalmologist. The earliest ophthalmoscopic finding is usually a decreased foveal reflex or bull's-eye maculopathy (similar to that shown in Figs. 13-14A,B). In contrast to NCL, olivopontocerebellar atrophy type III also called SCA 6 (spinocerebellar atrophy 6) is an autosomal dominant disorder. The age of presentation is extremely variable, and patients with a younger age of onset are usually more severely affected. Visual problems may be the first symptoms, especially in older children or young adults. A bull's-eye or atrophic maculopathy may be present and with time may become diffuse. Subtle cerebellar signs should be sought because these may be present even in patients who have not yet complained about neurological problems. Older family members should be examined for maculopathy which may appear isolated.[82]

Hallervordan–Spatz syndrome is an autosomal recessive disorder with rapidly progressive neurological and retinal deterioration and death. In some patients, early symptoms may be subtle and psychological disorders are initially suspected. The retinopathy is typically of a flecked type with a bull's-eye maculopathy.[14] *Stargardt's disease* is usually an autosomal recessive disorder although autosomal dominant pedigrees have been described (see Chapter 4). The usual presentation is with gradual bilateral visual loss in the first two decades of life. The fundus picture includes a beaten bronze or bull's-eye macular appearance with or without peripheral flecks. Stargardt's and fundus flavimaculatus are probably the same disorder because both can occur in the same pedigree and have been associated with the same gene in some pedigrees. The visual disturbance may precede the pigmentary changes, leading to an erroneous diagnosis of hysterical blindness.[25] The Bardet–Biedl syndrome is an

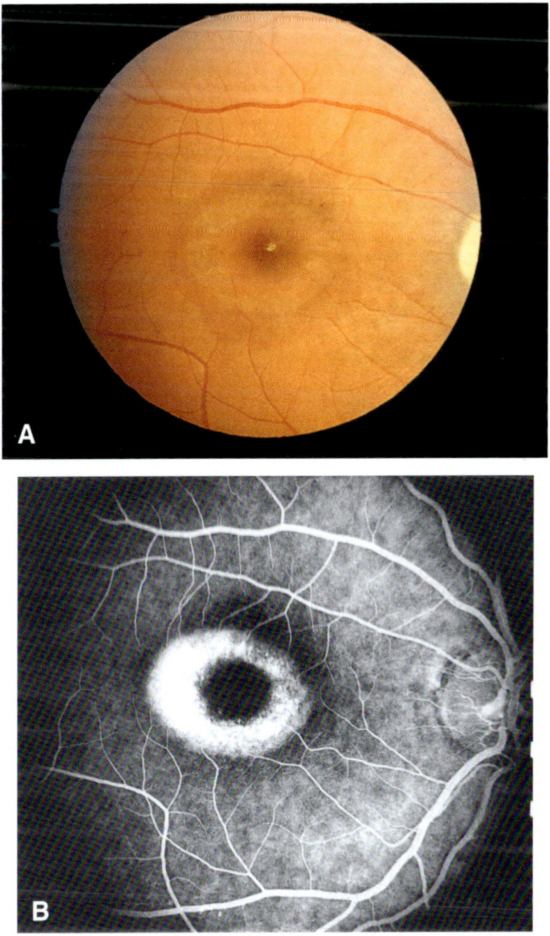

FIGURE 13-14A,B. Color fundus photograph (**A**) and fluorescein angiogram (**B**) of a patient with a cone dystrophy exhibiting a classic bull's-eye pattern in the macula. Several retinal diseases may present with this sign.

autosomal recessive disorder that has features which are evident at birth. However, diagnosis is frequently delayed until later in life. Polydactyly, obesity, hypogenitalism, and at times mild mental retardation accompany a pigmentary retinopathy that is usually apparent in the early school years along with markedly decreased vision. A bull's-eye maculopathy is often seen, although in some patients pigmentary changes may be subtle. The ERG may initially show rod dysfunction but can progress to nonrecordable. The *Lawrence–Moon syndrome* is similar to *Bardet-Biedl*, but there is no polydactyly and spastic paraplegia may be present.[65]

Some medications and toxins may cause a retinopathy that often begins as, or includes, a bull's-eye maculopathy. The iron chelator desferoxamine is commonly used in children who are transfusion dependent as a result of sickle cell disease or thalasemia. A progressive, severe retinopathy with gradual pigmenatary changes of the macula may result, with concomitant ERG changes. Rapid discontinuation of the medication may restore vision. It may be prudent to follow children on chronic desferoxamine therapy with serial ERGs. This drug can also cause optic neuropathy. Chloroquine can cause maculopathy as well.

Congenital Retinal Disease

The ophthalmologist is frequently called upon to examine the eyes of a newborn suspected to have an infection contracted in utero. The eye examination can help make a rapid diagnosis in some cases, allowing appropriate treatment to be started. Some infections can cross the blood–placenta barrier, whereas others are contracted when there is premature rupture of membranes or during the baby's passage through the birth canal. All of the *TORCH infections* (toxoplasmosis, rubella, cytomegalovirus, and herpes), as well as HIV, can cross the placenta, and antibody titers can be drawn at birth. Because IgG crosses the placenta, and therefore may be of maternal origin, IgM titers should be examined specifically. Titers drawn after the first few months of life should be interpreted with caution because exposure may have occurred postnatally. Rubella virus interferes with organogenesis. Affected children are small, and the organs actually have fewer cells than normal. For this reason, children affected later in gestation, after most of the organs have formed, have few or no defects. Live virus may persist for years in the various tissues of affected children. Varicella and cytomegalovirus may cause defects even if contracted later in pregnancy because they can attack organs that have already formed.[42] Syphilis (Fig. 13-15) and toxoplasmosis should be treated with antibiotics

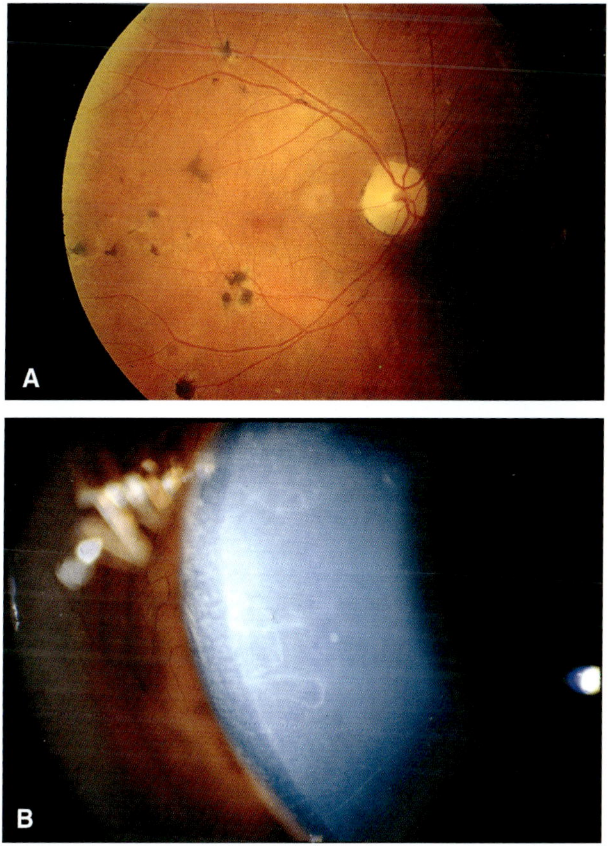

FIGURE 13-15A,B. (**A**) Congenital syphilis may present with either a fine salt-and-pepper retinopathy (see Fig. 13-13) or the fundus picture shown in this photograph in which large black retinal pigment epithelium (RPE) clumps are seen throughout the retina. (**B**) This patient also had ghost vessels from previous interstitial keratitis. In early childhood, acute interstitial keratitis may also be seen.

prenatally and postnatally if congenital infection has occurred. Combination antibiotic treatment for congenital toxoplasmosis must be continued for at least 1 full year and should be combined with systemic steroids and close monitoring if active retinal lesions are present.[48] Similarly, babies born with congenital herpes may require antiviral medication in the neonatal period.

In all these disorders the chorioretinitis appears similar, and the importance of ophthalmoscopy is not to differentiate between these infections but to identify an abnormality and stimulate an appropriate workup including CT scan of the head and serologies. It is not yet known whether congenital HIV can cause a typical chorioretinitis. Cotton wool spots may be present. Opportunistic infections must be ruled out in these infants, and whenever one sexually transmitted disease is present, the possibility of others, including chlamydia, must be excluded. Cytomegalovirus (CMV) retinitis in children may not present with the acute hemorrhagic picture seen in adults.[45] Parents of infants with quiescent toxoplasmosis lesions should be informed about the possibility of reactivation. Pregnant women should be advised to avoid undercooked meat and contact with cat feces, which may harbor the toxoplasmosis organisms. *Lymphocytic choriomeningitis virus* (LCMV) can also cross the placenta. This virus is carried by rodents such as mice, rats, and hamsters. A pigmentary retinopathy with coloboma-like lesions may result. Titers for LCMV should be drawn in suspected congenital infection cases.[51]

Geographic Pigmentary Disturbances

Several disorders occurring during childhood may present with progressive geographic pigmentary changes in the fundus. Pathological myopia (Fig. 13-16) may cause confluent areas of chorioretinal degeneration in the posterior pole. There may be excavation of the region, and the sclera can be seen. Isolated pathological myopia usually appears to be autosomal recessive or sporadic. Several connective tissue disorders with systemic features have pathological myopia as an associated finding, however, and a complete physical examination should be performed in any child with pathological myopia. *Gyrate atrophy* (Fig. 13-17) causes confluent areas of chorioretinal atrophy in the periphery that progress toward the posterior pole over time. Choroidal vessels and some pigmentation are often visible within the atrophic patches. This disorder is also autosomal

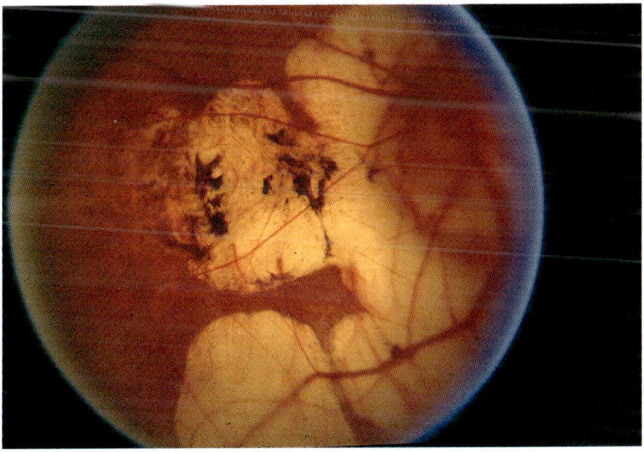

FIGURE 13-16. High degrees of myopia can cause large areas of chorioretinal atrophy in late childhood. This degree of pigmentary change is usually not seen until adolescence or early adulthood.

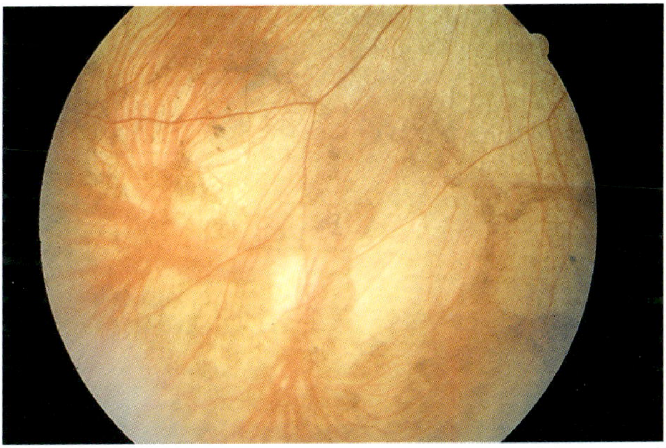

FIGURE 13-17. Gyrate atrophy is characterized by areas of chorioretinal atrophy that start in the midperiphery and progress to the posterior pole. Dietary restriction may slow the progression.

recessive and is associated with high myopia in childhood. Night blindness is also a feature. The diagnosis can be made by detecting elevated plasma *ornithine* levels. Dietary changes may halt progression. The cause is a mutation of the ornithine aminotransferase gene, leading to hyperornithinemia. Myopia, early-onset cataracts, and abnormal ERG are also found.[57] Choroideremia is X-linked recessive, and affected patients are therefore almost always male. Night blindness is present, but high myopia is not usually seen. The chorioretinal atrophy is seen first in the midperiphery and also has scalloped edges. It is caused by mutations in the RAB27A gene.[80]

Retinal Causes of Leukocoria

Leukocoria in an infant or young child may be secondary to corneal or lens pathology. Once these factors are excluded, a retinal source is likely. The first step is always to rule out *retinoblastoma*, because this is a potentially fatal condition that has a fairly good prognosis with treatment (see Chapter 9). Fundus examination, ultrasound, and CT scan all have a role in the evaluation of these patients. The child may need to be sedated to obtain an optimal examination. Many other disorders with various etiologies can cause the normal red reflex to appear whitish or yellow (Table 13-1). In general, any disorder that destroys, detaches, or changes the normal color of the retina in an area likely to be in line with the pupil (i.e., the posterior pole) can cause leukocoria.

SYSTEMIC DISORDERS ASSOCIATED WITH RETINAL ABNORMALITIES

Ichthyosis and Other Dermatological Disorders

In a child presenting with retinal disease, the first step in a general examination should be an evaluation of the skin. Ichthyosis is abnormal scaling, dryness, and tightness of the skin. Isolated ichthyosis is commonly associated with anterior segment complications, but ichthyosis in association with pigmentary retinopathy should suggest the diagnoses of *Refsum disease*[60] or *Sjogren–Larsson syndrome*[74] (see Table 13-2). *Darier's disease* is an autosomal dominant disorder characterized by scaling, papules, and dystrophic nails. Typical retinitis pigmentosa has been reported in association with this disease.[31] Other skin findings that should alert the ophthalmologist to the presence of a systemic syndrome are whorls of brown pigment, usually on the trunk, that were preceded in infancy by blister-like lesions (*incontinentia pigmenti*), atrophic changes (Flynn-Aird syndrome),[18] skin photosensitivity (*Cockayne syndrome and Allagille syndrome*), or areas of hypopigmentation (vitiligo and Vogt–Koyanagi–Harada). Petechial lesions may be seen in *Fabry's disease* (Fig. 13-18). A "plucked chicken" appearance (Fig. 13-19A) is characteristic of pseudoxanthoma elasticum. The presence of *"peau d'orange" fundus* changes (Fig. 13-19B) is essentially pathognomonic of this disorder,[49] unlike the less specific finding of angioid streaks (see Fig. 13-12).

Linear atrophic scarlike lesions on the face, neck, and upper body may be associated with retinal colobomas or Peter's anomaly in *Goltz syndrome* and *microphthalmia with linear skin defects* (MLS), respectively. Both are X-linked dominant.[94]

Deafness

A significant number of deaf children have associated retinopathy. Deaf children are often referred for ophthalmologic evaluation both to ensure optimal function of their remaining sensory input and to rule out the presence of a syndrome. These syndromes can be divided into those that typically present with deafness and those which present first with visual problems. In the former group, the most common disorder is *Usher syndrome*, types I and II. Patients with type I Usher syndrome are born with profound deafness and vestibular abnormalities. Retinopathy, night blindness, and ERG changes usually occur in the first decade of life. In type II, abnormal hearing is present at birth, but is less severe, and vestibular function is intact. Retinopathy does not begin until the teens. There are many subsets of these two types, and at least six different genetic loci have been identified.[8] Usher syndrome is autosomal recessive, and there is also a later-onset form (type III) with progressive hearing loss and retinopathy in adulthood. Infants born with congenital rubella syndrome often have hearing loss, in association with a salt-and-pepper retinopathy and, at times, cataracts.

Alport syndrome is a relatively common disorder. Hearing loss, which may be mild initially, is usually present within the first decade, along with renal disease. Approximately 30% of patients develop ocular involvement, with males predominat-

TABLE 13-2. Diseases with Systemic Signs Associated with Retinal Abnormalities.

1. Ichthyosis and other dermatological disorders
    a. Sjogren–Larsson syndrome
    b. Refsum's disease
    c. Incontinentia pigmenti
    d. Pseudoxanthoma elasticum
    e. Darier's disease
    f. Flynn–Aird syndrome
    g. Allagille syndrome
    h. Cockayne syndrome
    i. Vogt–Koyanagi–Harada
    j. Vitiligo
    k. Goltz syndrome/MLS
2. Deafness
    a. Usher's syndrome
    b. Alstrom syndrome
    c. Refsum disease
    d. Alport syndrome
    e. Congenital rubella
    f. Cockayne syndrome
    g. Peroxisomal disorders
    h. Mucopolysaccharidoses
    i. Kearns–Sayre syndrome
    j. Osteopetrosis
    k. Norrie disease
    l. Flynn–Aird syndrome
    m. Cogan's syndrome
    n. Stickler's syndrome
    o. Spondyloepiphyseal dysplasia congenita
3. Polydactyly
    a. Bardet–Biedl syndrome
    b. Jeune's syndrome
    c. Trisomy 13
4. Short stature/skeletal anomalies/facial dysmorphism
    a. Bardet–Biedl syndrome
    b. Cockayne syndrome
    c. Jeune's syndrome
    d. Osteopetrosis
    e. Spondyloepiphyseal dysplasia congenita
    f. Mucopolysaccharidosis IH, IS, II, III
    g. Stickler's syndrome
    h. Infantile phytanic acid storage disease (infantile refsum)
    i. Allagille syndrome
    j. Chorioretinopathy and pituitary dysfunction
5. Renal disease
    a. Senior–Loken syndrome
    b. Bardet–Biedl syndrome
    c. Alport's syndrome
    d. Idiopathic infantile hypercalcuria
    e. Renal dialysis
    f. Oxalosis

TABLE 13-2. (continued)

- g. Cystinosis
- h. Renal-coloboma syndrome
- i. Alstrom syndrome

6. Hepatic disease
   - a. Allagille syndrome
   - b. Zellweger's syndrome
7. Neurological/neuromuscular disorders
   - a. Neuronal ceroid lipofuscinosis
   - b. Olivopontocerebellar atrophy type III (SCA 6)
   - c. Kearns–Sayre syndrome
   - d. Myotonic dystrophy
   - e. Hallervorden–Spatz disease
   - f. Joubert syndrome
   - g. Mucolipidoses
   - h. Zellweger's syndrome
   - i. Neonatal adrenoleukodystrophy
   - j. Refsum's disease
   - k. Infantile phytanic acid storage disease
   - l. Flynn–Aird syndrome
   - m. Abetalipoproteinemia
8. Obesity
   - a. Bardet–Biedl syndrome
   - b. Alstrom syndrome

ing.[32] The most common ocular finding is anterior lenticonus, which is not present at birth but develops later in childhood or adolescence. Retinal changes, which may appear as RPE mottling or whitish dots, are also a later finding.[7,64] Alport syndrome is genetically heterogeneous, with approximately 80% of cases X-linked recessive and most of the remainder autosomal recessive; it is caused by mutations in various genes coding for basement membrane type IV collagen.[3,36] Some patients develop leiomyomas of the esophagus, tracheobronchial tree, and genitalia (in females).

The presenting sign in *Flynn–Aird syndrome* is usually hearing loss, with retinopathy and neurological changes occurring later. This rare disorder is autosomal dominant, but symptoms often do not appear until early adulthood.[18] In the congenital rubella syndrome, deafness is usually present at birth and the typical salt-and-pepper retinopathy, which is either congenital or develops within the first year, may help to make the diagnosis. Rarely, deafness may not develop until later in childhood.[69] In contrast to the preceding disorders, children with Norrie disease or Alstrom syndrome present with a visual problem and only later develop hearing loss. In several other dis-

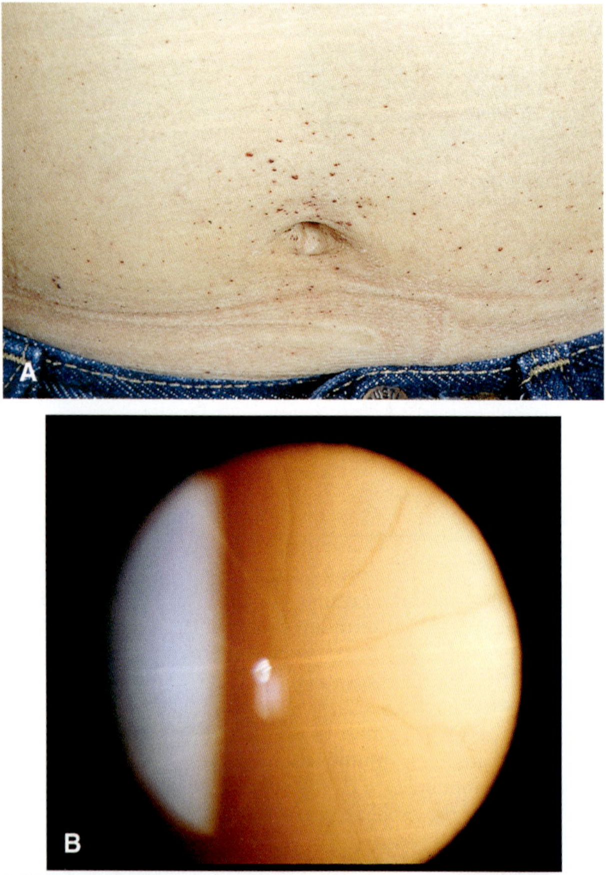

FIGURE 13-18A,B. **(A)** Characteristic skin lesions in a young man with Fabry's disease. **(B)** Another patient with Fabry's disease demonstrates characteristic spoke-like lens opacities on retroillumination. Corneal changes may also occur and have a whorled pattern.

orders, the retinal disease and deafness develop at approximately the same age. Thus, the ophthalmologist examining a child in whom hearing loss has been recently diagnosed must suspect these disorders. Similarly, children with newly diagnosed retinal disease suggestive of one of these syndromes should be

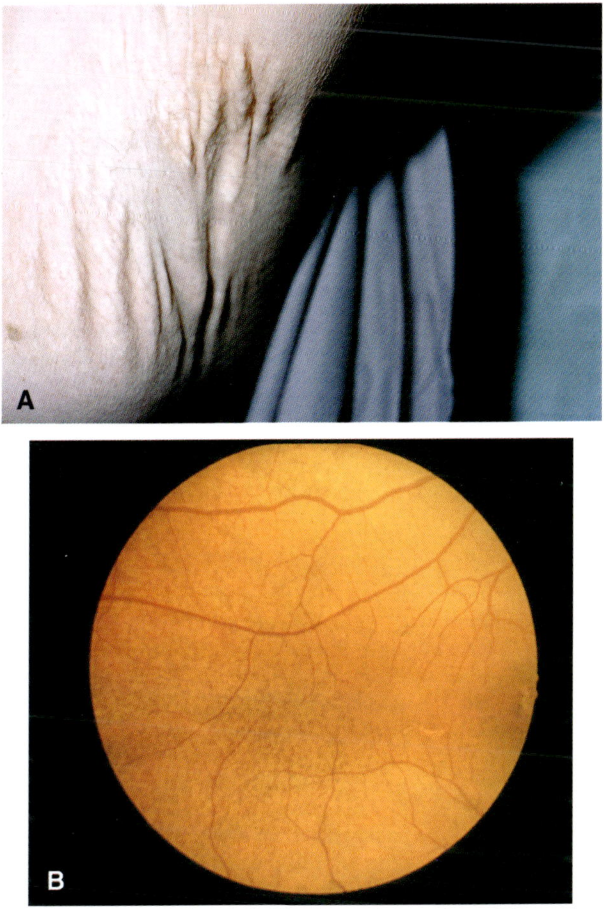

FIGURE 13-19A,B. **(A)** Typical skin changes in a patient with psuedoxanthoma elasticum. (Courtesy of Dr. M. Stone) **(B)** Peau d'orange fundus appearance in another patient with psuedoxanthoma elasticum.

referred for audiology. These diseases include neonatal adrenoleukodystrophy (apparent within the first months of life), infantile Refsum disease (presents in the first year of life), Cockayne syndrome, and mucolipidosis (MPS) II and III (present shortly after the first year of life). MPS I may present within the first 5 years of life and includes corneal clouding, hearing loss, and retinal dystrophy. Bone marrow transplantation and enzyme replacement therapy may halt or partly reverse the disease process.

Kearns–Sayre syndrome usually presents before 20 years of age. The most common initial symptom is ptosis, with hearing loss and a pigmentary retinopathy developing later. Visual loss is often not severe. Rarely, Cogan syndrome presents with acute vestibuloauditory disturbance and chorioretinitis, with or without interstitial keratitis. Prompt treatment with systemic corticosteroids may prevent permanent hearing loss and other complications.[28]

Patients with Stickler syndrome and spondyloepiphyseal dysplasia congenita may have progressive hearing loss. Patients with *Waardenburg's syndrome* have heterochromia iridis and may have a white forelock of hair. Congenital deafness is associated. The fundus ipsilateral to the lighter iris (usually bright blue) may be more blond than the contralateral fundus, but vision is usually normal. This disorder is autosomal dominant and has at least two subtypes with two different genetic loci.[44]

Polydactyly

Extra digits may be an important diagnostic clue in the evaluation of children with retinal disease. Although infants with trisomy 13 have multiple other severe anomalies, children with the *Bardet–Biedl syndrome* may go undiagnosed for many years. Children with the latter condition are obese, have hypogonadism, and may be mildly mentally retarded in addition to having extra digits and poor vision. Because supernumerary fingers are often ligated at birth, scars on the hands may be the only remaining clue (Fig. 13-20A,B). Children with *Jeune's syndrome* (*asphyxiating thoracic dysplasia*) have multiple abnormalities, including short-limbed dwarfism, thoracic dysplasia, liver abnormalities and RPE mottling with decreased vision. Polydactyly is an occasional feature. Polydactyly occurs most commonly as an isolated finding, without associated retinal disease, and may be familial.

Short Stature/Skeletal Anomalies/ Facial Dysmorphism

In a child with retinal disease, short stature for age may indicate the presence of a syndrome. A normative growth chart, or the

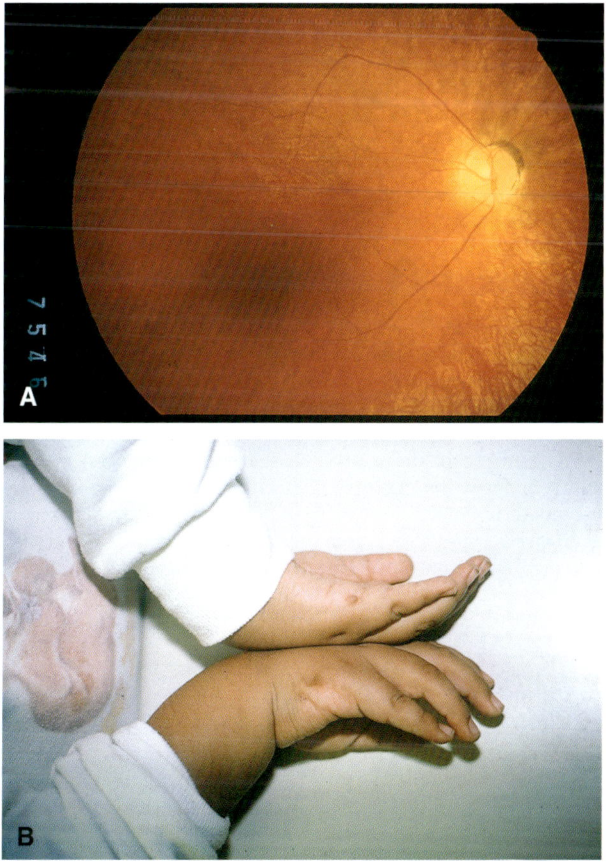

FIGURE 13-20A,B. **(A)** Children with the Bardet–Biedl syndrome are obese and have poor vision secondary to a pigmentary retinal degeneration. They may also have endocrine abnormalities and postaxial polydactyly. Retinal changes may be diffuse or may take on a bull's-eye appearance. Early changes are often subtle. **(B)** The extra digits present on this girl's hands were ligated at birth, leaving only small scars. (Courtesy of Dr. J. Horton)

child's pediatrician, should be consulted. In young adults, the height should be compared to other family members. In some disorders, short stature is accompanied by abnormal facies, for example, the coarse appearance in some of the mucopolysaccharidoses or the birdlike facies with atrophy of periorbital fat and progeria in Cockayne syndrome. In Jeune syndrome, the dwarfism is of the short-limbed type. Patients with Allagille syndrome have dysmorphic facies. In Stickler syndrome, a characteristic midface hypoplasia is present, with a flattened nasal bridge. Epiphyseal abnormalities can be seen on bone X-rays, arthropathy may develop, and a cleft palate or bifid uvula may be present. Osteopetrosis also can be diagnosed on X-ray by noting increased density of bone. Children may be small with failure to thrive, and optic atrophy may be present secondary to narrowing of the optic foraminae. A baby with infantile Refsum disease presents with dysmorphic facies, deafness, retinal disease, and often nystagmus. Elevated serum phytanic acid levels confirm the diagnosis.[67] Classical Refsum disease is more subtle and usually presents in late childhood; dysmorphic facies are not a major feature. In spondyloepiphyseal dysplasia congenita, short stature is present as well as a barrel chest and high myopia.[26] In the rare syndrome of chorioretinopathy and pituitary dysfunction, deficiency of growth hormone is associated with short stature, poor vision, and very long eyelashes.[33]

Renal Disease

Senior–Loken syndrome is an autosomal recessive condition that presents either as typical Leber's congenital amaurosis (Fig. 13-21) followed by medullary cystic kidney disease and renal failure later in life or, conversely, as a child with renal failure who develops retinal disease at an older age. All children with a diagnosis of Leber's congenital amaurosis should have serial renal function studies to rule out this disorder. Renal disease and hypertension may develop in the Bardet–Biedl syndrome and may be severe.[12] These children should also have monitoring for renal insufficiency. Alstrom syndrome predisposes to diabetes mellitis and renal dysfunction. Idiopathic hypercalcuria and oxalosis predispose patients to recurrent renal stones. *Cystinosis* may present in the first year of life with acidosis and failure to thrive, followed by renal failure in the first decade. In some cases, however, the renal insufficiency develops in the second or third decade. Retinal pigmentary mottling and deep crystals

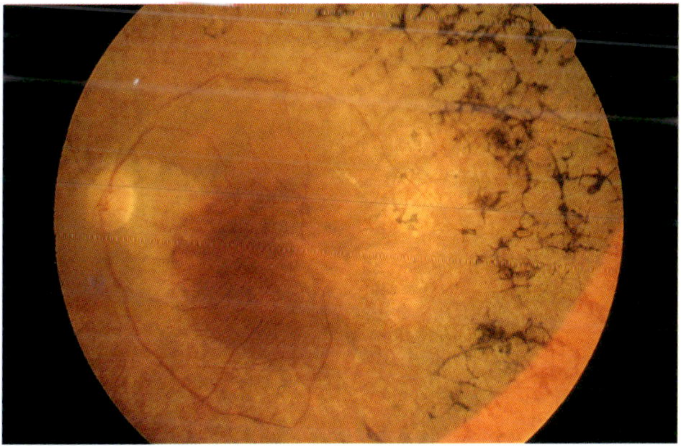

FIGURE 13-21. Leber's congenital amaurosis. The fundus may appear normal in infancy, but with time, typical bone spicules, as shown in this picture, may develop. Arteriolar narrowing, coloboma-like lesions of the macula, and other patterns of pigmentary changes have also been described.

may be seen in both types, but all patients with the infantile form have been reported to have retinal changes by 7 years of age.[15] Corneal crystals and photophobia usually occur. Cysteamine eyedrops may dissolve corneal crystals.[21,22] There is also a nonnephropathic ocular cystinosis, caused by mutations in the same gene, CTNS, that causes the nephropathic form:[1] both are autosomal recessive. Renal disease generally precedes the retinal changes in Alport syndrome but may be preceded by the acquired lenticonus.[64] Renal dialysis has also been associated with retinal pigmentary changes.[30]

In the renal-coloboma syndrome, kidney hypoplasia is associated with optic nerve colobomas; it can be transmitted as an autosomal dominant trait and is caused by mutations of the PAX2 gene.[19]

Hepatic Disease

Neonatal jaundice, failure to thrive, and subsequent pigmentary retinopathy are characteristic of Allagille syndrome (Fig. 13-22). This disorder is autosomal dominant. There is congenital hypoplasia of the interlobular bile ducts, and liver dysfunction

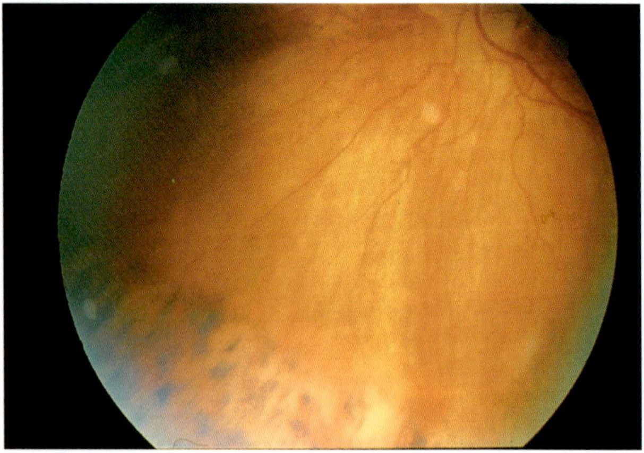

FIGURE 13-22. Peripheral retinal changes in Allagille syndrome. (Courtesy of Dr. G.F. Judisch)

is frequently mild. Prominent posterior embryotoxon may an early diagnostic clue, and optic nerve drusen are common. Conversely, infants with Zellweger syndrome, a peroxisomal disorder, have hepatic interstitial fibrosis as well as other anomalies, and usually die before 1 year of age. It is autosomal recessive.

Neurological/Neuromuscular Disorders

All children with retinal disease should have a careful history taken because many hereditary neurological disorders have retinopathy as a feature. The presence of a seizure disorder, ataxia, or developmental delay is important. Infants with retinal disease and neurological or neuromuscular abnormalities should be evaluated for infantile phytanic acid storage disease (Refsum), Zellweger's syndrome, neonatal adrenoleukodystrophy, infantile neuronal ceroid lipofuscinosis (Haltia–Santavuori syndrome), and olivopontocerebellar atrophy type III (also called SCA 6). The latter two may be differentiated by inheritance (autosomal recessive versus dominant respectively); the frequent occurrence of seizures and microcephaly in the former, but not the latter; and, in some cases, by the electron microscopic findings from biopsies. Prenatal diagnosis is possible in NCL.[59] SCA 6 results from expanded CAG repeats and exhibits anticipation. Genetic testing of the CACNL1A4 gene is available.[47a]

Infantile Refsum disease, neonatal adrenoleukodystrophy, and Zellweger's syndrome overlap clinically; these are peroxisome biogenesis disorders caused by mutations in the PEX1 gene.[85] Zellweger's is the most severe, with hypotonia, seizures, psychomotor retardation, pigmentary retinopathy, and cataracts developing early in life. Neonatal adrenoleukodystrophy is very similar, but patients have less extensive central nervous system demyelination and live slightly longer. Refsum's is the mildest. All are autosomal recessive. Joubert's syndrome is characterized by respiratory irregularity, developmental delay, oculomotor apraxia, and a retinal picture similar to Leber's congenital amaurosis.[41] In mucolipidosis IV, mental retardation, cloudy corneas, a retinal dystrophy, and athetosis develop after the first few months of life. The facies in mucolipidosis IV may be only minimally coarse. Congenital myotonic dystrophy can occur in children born to affected mothers, but the retinal changes are rarely present at birth.

If the onset of symptoms is in early childhood (roughly 2–10 years old), the late infantile (Jansky–Bielschowsky) or juvenile (Batten) forms of NCL, Refsum disease, olivopontocerebellar atrophy III (SCA 6), Kearns–Sayre syndrome, or Hallervorden–Spatz syndrome should be suspected. Abetalipoproteinemia (Bassen–Kornzweig) may also begin early in life with pigmentary retinopathy, night blindness, and progressive ataxic neuropathy. With onset in adolescence or early adulthood, the most common diagnoses are olivopontocerebellar atrophy (SCA), Kearns–Sayre, Refsum disease, myotonic dystrophy, and Flynn–Aird syndrome.

TREATABLE SYSTEMIC DISORDERS WITH ASSOCIATED RETINOPATHY

Many systemic metabolic defects affect the retina, and several of these are treatable (Table 13-3). The ophthalmologist may have the first opportunity to make the correct diagnosis and to refer the patient for treatment of the underlying systemic disorder. In some cases, treatment can halt progression of visual loss and improve the patient's overall well-being. Gyrate atrophy of the choroid and retina is an autosomal recessive disorder caused by a deficiency of the enzyme ornithine aminotransferase, with

TABLE 13-3. Some Treatable Systemic Disorders with Associated Retinopathy.

a. Gyrate atrophy of the choroid and retina
b. Cobalamin C defects (methylmalonic aciduria/homocystinuria)
c. Abetalipoproteinemia
d. Cystinosis
e. Mucopolysaccharidoses
f. Refsum's disease
g. Osteopetrosis
h. Allagille syndrome
i. Syphilis
j. Vitamin A deficiency
k. Remote effects of cancer
l. Oxalosis
m. Cogan's syndrome
n. Idiopathic infantile hypercalcuria
o. Desferoxamine retinopathy

resultant hyperornithinemia. Retinopathy has been slowed in some patients by treatment with pyridoxine,[88] proline,[79] and dietary restriction of protein and arginine.[6,84]

Homocystinuria is another recessive disorder that often has severe systemic manifestations such as mental retardation and thrombotic episodes. Patients treated with hydroxycobalamin, with or without the medication betaine, have a better outcome.[4] Metronidazole may also be helpful.[2] Abetalipoproteinemia (Bassen–Kornzweig disease) is a rare autosomal recessive disorder in which all major plasma lipids are reduced; this decreases absorption of fat-soluble vitamins from the intestine, leading to low levels of vitamin A and E. Oral supplementation with these vitamins and vitamin K is helpful.[6,24,63] Patients with classic Refsum's disease benefit from low phytol–low phytanic acid diets.[6] Plasmapheresis may be beneficial in some cases.[61] Cystinosis is a recessive condition in which progressive renal failure accompanies crystalline corneal and retinal deposits. Systemic cysteamine,[22] topical cysteamine,[35] growth hormone,[90] and carnitine[20] may be beneficial.

Bone marrow transplantation and enzyme replacement therapy are showing promise in clinical trials for some of the mucopolysaccharidoses. Bone marrow transplantation is being tried as a treatment for sickle cell and osteopetrosis. Because of the liver abnormalities in Allagille syndrome, oral supplementation of vitamins A and E and of triglycerides may be helpful. Syphilis should be treated with systemic antibiotics even in the case of congenitally acquired disease. Vitamin A supplementation may reverse the affects of vitamin A deficiency.

Remote effects of cancer may appear as a pigmentary retinopathy, but this is very rare in children. If this is suspected, a search for and treatment of the underlying cancer should be undertaken.

Oxalosis, which presents as widespread retinal crystals, often with a "black macula," may be primary or secondary; it has been reported following methoxyflurane anesthesia, tamoxifen, rhubarb ingestion, or other agents.[50,81] Recurrent renal stones may lead to kidney failure before the age of 5 years. Pyridoxine, phosphate, and magnesium have been used to reduce the precipitation of oxalic acid with calcium. Cogan's syndrome rarely includes retinopathy, but when it does it can sometimes be reversed by prompt treatment with immunosuppressants, as can the hearing loss.[28] Treatment for renal stones in patients with infantile hypercalcuria may be beneficial. If retinal toxicity from desferoxamine is suspected, it should be stopped immediately; often, vision and ERG will improve. In some cases, a lower dose of desferal may be restarted without further vision loss, but close follow-up is necessary.

Oral vitamin A may retard progression of common forms of retinitis pigmentosa.[6] However, testing in children has not been done. Cryotherapy or laser ablation benefits many patients with retinal vasculopathies.

In the future, gene therapy and medical therapies of retinal dystrophies may add to the treatment armamentarium.

Acknowledgments. Revision of this chapter was supported in part by the Georgia Lions Children's Eyecare Center at Emory University. We thank William Emerson for technical support.

References

1. Anikster Y, Lucero C, Guo J, et al. Ocular nonnephropathic cystinosis: clinical, biochemical, and molecular correlations. Pediatr Res 2000;47(1):17–23.
2. Bain MD, Jones M, Borriello SP, et al. Contribution of gut bacterial metabolism to human metabolic disease. Lancet 1988;1:1078–1079.
3. Barker DF, Hostikka SL, Zhou J, et al. Identification of mutations in the COL4A5 collagen gene in Alport syndrome. Science 1990;248:1224–1227.

4. Bartholomew DW, Allen RH, Roe CR, et al. Therapeutic approaches to Cbl-C methylmalonic acidemia and homocystinuria. J Pediatr 1988;112(1):32–39.
5. Bateman JB. Eye, microphthalmia/coloboma. In: Buyse ML (ed) Birth defects encyclopedia. London: Blackwell, 1990:660–662.
6. Berson EL. Nutrition and retinal degenerations. Int Ophthalmol Clin 2000;40(4):93–111.
7. Blasi MA, Rinaldi R, Renieri A, et al. Dot and fleck retinopathy in Alport syndrome caused by a novel mutation in the COL4A5 gene. Am J Ophthalmol 2000;130(1):130–131.
8. Bolz H, von Brederlow B, Ramirez A, et al. Mutation of CDH23, encoding a new member of the cadherin gene family, causes Usher syndrome type 1D. Nat Genet 2001;27(1):108–112.
9. Catalano RA, Nelson LB, Schaffer DB. Oculocutaneous albinism associated with congenital glaucoma. Ophthalmol Pediatr Genet 1988;9(1):5–6.
10. Chang JH, Spraul CW, Lynn ML, Drack AV, Grossniklaus HE. The two-stage mutation model in retinal hemangioblastoma. Ophthalmol Genet 1998;19(3):123–130.
11. Chen ZY, Battinelli EM, Fielder A, et al. A mutation in the Norrie disease gene (NDP) associated with X-linked familial exudative vitreoretinopathy. Nat Genet 1993;5(2):180–183.
12. Churchill DN, McManamon P, Hurley RM. Renal disease: a sixth cardinal feature of the Laurence–Moon–Biedl syndrome. Clin Nephrol 1981;16:151–154.
13. Clarkson JG, Altma RD. Angioid streaks. Surv Ophthalmol 1982;26: 235–246.
14. Dooling EC, Schoene WC, Richardson EP Jr. Hallervorden–Spatz syndrome. Arch Neurol 1974;30:70.
15. Dufier JL, Dhermy P, Gubler MC, et al. Ocular changes in long term evaluation of infantile cystinosis. Ophthalmol Paediatr Genet 1987; 8:131–137.
16. Elsas TJ, Maumenee IH, Kenyon KR, Yodar F. Familial aniridia with preserved ocular function. Am J Ophthalmol 1977;83:718–724.
17. Fivgas GD, Beck AD. Angle-closure glaucoma in a 10 year old girl. Am J Opthalmol 1997;124(2):251–253.
18. Flynn A, Aird RB. A neuroectodermal syndrome of dominant inheritance. J Neurol Sci 1965;2:161–182.
19. Ford B, Rupps R, Lirenman D, et al. Renal-coloboma syndrome: prenatal detection and clinical spectrum in a large family. Am J Med Genet 2001;99(2):137–141.
20. Gahl WA, Bernardini I, Dalakas M, et al. Oral carnitine therapy in children with cystinosis and Fanconi syndrome. J Clin Investig 1988; 81:549–560.
21. Gahl WA, Kuehl EM, Iwata F, Lindblad A, Kaiser-Kupfer MI. Corneal crystals in nephropathic cystinosis: natural history and treatment with cysteamine eyedrops. Mol Genet Metab 2000;71(1–2):100–120.

22. Gahl WA, Reed GF, Thoene JG, et al. Cysteamine therapy for children with nephropathic cystinosis. N Engl J Med 1987;316:971–977.
23. Goldberg MF, Pollack IP, Green WR. Familial retinal arteriolar tortuosity with retinal hemorrhage. Am J Ophthalmol 1972;73:183–191.
24. Gouras P, Carr RE, Kunkel RD. Retinitis pigmentosa in abetalipoproteinemia: effects of vitamin A. Investig Ophthalmol 1971;10:784.
25. Hadden BO, Gass JDM. Fundus flavimaculatus and Stargardt's disease. Am J Ophthalmol 1976;82:527–539.
26. Hamidi-Toosi S, Maumenee IH. Vitreoretinal degeneration in spondyloepiphyseal dysplasia congenita. Arch Ophthalmol 1982;100:1104–1107.
27. Hardwig P, Robertson DM. Von Hippel–Lindau disease: a familial often fatal phakomatosis. Ophthalmology 1984;91:263–270.
28. Haynes BF, Kaiser-Kupfer MI, Mason P, et al. Successful treatment of sudden hearing loss in Cogan's syndrome: studies in thirteen patients, long term followup, and a review of the literature. Medicine (Batlim) 1980;59:426–441.
29. Heher KL, Traboulsi EI, Maumenee IH. The natural history of Leber's congenital amaurosis: age-related findings in 35 patients. Ophthalmology 1992;99(2):241–245.
30. Hilton AF, Harrison JD, Lamb AM, et al. Ocular complications in haemodialysis and renal transplant patients. Austr J Ophthalmol 1982;10:247–253.
31. Itin P, Buchner SA, Gloor B. Darier's disease and retinitis pigmentosa; is there a pathogenetic relationship? Br J Dermatol 1988;119:397–402.
32. Jacobs M, Jeffrey B, Kriss A, Taylor D, Sa G, Bakratt M. Ophthalmologic assessment of young patients with Alport syndrome. Ophthalmology 1992;99:1030–1044.
33. Judisch GF, Lowry B, Hanson JW. Chorioretinopathy and pituitary dysfunction. The CPD syndrome. Arch Ophthalmol 1981;99:253–261.
34. Judisch GF, Waziri M, Krachmer JH. Ocular Ehlers Danlos syndrome with normal lysyl dehydrogenase deficiency. Arch Ophthalmol 1976;94:1489–1491.
35. Kaiser-Kupfer MI, Gazzo MA, Datiles MB, et al. A randomized placebo-controlled trial of cysteamine eyedrops in nephropathic cystinosis. Arch Ophthalmol 1990;108:689–693.
36. Kashtan CE. Alport syndrome. An inherited disorder of renal, ocular, and cochlear basement membranes. Medicine (Baltim) 1999;78(5):338–360.
37. Kivlin JD, Sanborn GE, Myers GG. The cherry red spot in Tay Sachs and other storage diseases. Ann Neurol 1985;17(4):356–360.
38. Kretzer FL, Mintz-Hittner HA. The "documented disappointment" of vitrectomy for ROP can be explained histologically. Presented at the 95th Annual Meeting of the American Academy of Ophthalmology, October 13–17, 1991.

39. Krill AE. The retinal disease of rubella. Arch Ophthalmol 1967;77: 445–449.
40. Lahav M, Albert DM, Wyand S. Clinical and histopathological classification of retinal dysplasia. Am J Ophthalmol 1973;75:648–667.
41. Lambert SR, Kriss A, Gresty M, et al. Joubert syndrome. Arch Ophthalmol 1989;107:709–713.
42. Lambert SR, Taylor D, Kriss A, et al. The ocular manifestations of the congenital varicella syndrome. Arch Ophthalmol 1989;107:52–56.
43. Larkin DF, O'Donoghue HN. Developmental glaucoma in oculocutaneous albinism. Ophthalmol Pediatr Genet 1988;9(1):1–4.
44. Liu XZ, Newton VE, Read AP. Waardenburg syndrome type II: phenotypic findings and diagnostic criteria. Am J Med Genet 1995;55(1): 95–100.
45. Lonn L. Neonatal cytomegalic inclusion disease chorioretinitis. Arch Ophthalmol 1972;88:434–438.
46. Mansour AM. Systemic associations of angioid streaks. Int Ophthalmol Clin 1991;31(3):61–68.
47. Mansour AM, Shields JA, Annesley WH, et al. Macular degeneration in angioid streads. Ophthalmologica 1988;197:36–41.
47a. Matsuyama Z, et al. Molecular features of the CAG repeats of SCA 6. Hum Molec Genet 1997;6(8):1283–1287.
48. McAuley J, Boyer KM, Patel D, et al. Early and longitudinal evaluations of treated infants and children and untreated historical patients with congenital toxoplasmosis: the Chicago collaborative treatment trial. Clin Infect Dis 1994;18:38–72.
49. McDonald HR, Schatz H, Aaberg TM. Reticular-like pigmentary patterns in pseudoxanthoma elasticum. Ophthalmology 1988;95(3): 306–311.
50. Meredith TA, Wright JD, Gammon, et al. Ocular involvement in primary hyperoxaluria. Arch Ophthalmol 1984;102:584–587.
51. Mets MB, Barton LL, Khan AS, Ksiazek TG. Lymphocytic choriomeningitis virus: an underdiagnosed cause of congenital chorioretinitis. Am J Ophthalmol 2000;130(2):209–215.
52. Morle L, Bozon M, Zech JC, et al. A locus for autosomal dominant colobomatous microphthalmia maps to chromosome 15q12–q15. Am J Hum Genet 2000;67(6):1592–1597.
53. Mullie MA, Harding AE, Petty RKH, et al. The retinal manifestations of mitochondrial myopathy. A study of 22 cases. Arch Ophthalmol 1985;105:1825–1830.
54. O'Donnell FE Jr, Pappas HR. Autosomal dominant foveal hypoplasia and pre-senile cataracts: a new syndrome. Arch Ophthalmol 1982; 100:279–281.
55. Oliver MD, Dotan SA, Chemke J, Abraham FA. Isolated foveal hypoplasia. Br J Ophthalmol 1987;71:926–930.
56. Parvin A, Warburg M. Audiological findings in Norrie's disease. Audiology 1977;16:124–131.

57. Peltola KE, Nanto-Salonen K, Heinen OJ, et al. Ophthalmologic heterogeneity in subjects with gyrate atrophy of the choroid and retina harboring the L402P mutation of ornithine aminotransferase. Ophthalmology 2001;108(4):721–729.
58. Rahi J, Hungerford J. Early diagnosis of the retinopathy of incontinentia pigmenti: successful treatment by cryotherapy. Br J Ophthalmol 1990;74:377–379.
59. Rapola J, Santavuori P, Heiska H. Placental pathology and prenatal diagnosis of infantile type of NCL. Am J Hum Genet 1988;5:990–103.
60. Refsum S. Heredopathia atactica polyneuritiformis. Phytanic acid storage disease (Refsum's disease) with particular reference to ophthalmologic disturbances. Metab Ophthalmol 1977;1:73–79.
61. Refsum S. Heredopathia atactica polyneuritiformis. Phytanic acid storage disease, Refsum's disease: a biochemically well-defined disease with a specific dietary treatment. Arch Neurol 1981;38:605–606.
62. Rodrigues MM, Ballintine EJ, Wiggert B, et al. Choroideremia: a clinical electrom microscopic and biochemical report. Ophthalmology 1984;91:873–883.
63. Runge P, Muller DPR, McAllister J, et al. Oral vitamin E can prevent the retinopathy of abetalipoproteinaemia. Br J Ophthalmol 1986;70:166–173.
64. Sabates R, Krachmer JH, Weingeist TA. Ocular findings in Alport's syndrome. Ophthalmologica 1983;186:204–210.
65. Schachat AP, Maumenee IH. Bardet–Biedl syndrome and related disorders. Arch Ophthalmol 1982;100:285–288.
66. Schiffmann R, Kopp JB, Austin HA III, et al. Enzyme replacement therapy in Fabry disease: a randomized controlled trial. JAMA 2001;285(21):2743–2749.
67. Scotto JM, Hadehouel M, Odieve M, et al. Infantile phytanic acid storage disease. A possible variant of Refsum's disease: three cases including ultrastructural studies of the liver. J Inherit Metab Dis 1982;5:83–90.
68. Sebag J, Albert DM, Craft JL. The Alstrom syndrome, ophthalmic histopathology and retinal ultrastructure. Br J Ophthalmol 1984;68:494–501.
69. Sever J, South MA, Shaver K. Delayed manifestations of congenital rubella. Rev Infect Dis Suppl 1985;7:164–169.
70. Shastry BS, Pendergast SD, Hartzer MK, Liu X, Trese MT. Identification of missense mutations in the Norrie disease gene associated with advanced retinopathy of prematurity. Arch Ophthalmol 1997;115(5):651–655.
71. Sher NA, Letson RD, Desnick RJ. The ocular manifestations in Fabry's disease. Arch Ophthalmol 1978;97:671–676.
72. Sher NA, Reiff W, Letson RD, Desnick RJ. Central retinal artery occlusion complicating Fabry's disease. Arch Ophthalmol 1978;96:815–817.

73. Shields JA, Federman JL, Tomer TL, et al. Angioid streaks: I. Ophthalmoscopic variations and diagnostic problems. Br J Ophthalmol 1975;59:257–266.
74. Sjogren T, Larsson T. A clinical and genetic study of oligophrenia in combination with congenital ichthyosis and spastic disorders. Acta Psychiatr Neurol Scand 1957;32(suppl 113):1–112.
75. Slusher MM, Tyler ME. Rubella retinopathy and subretinal neovascular membranes. Ann Ophthalmol 1982;14(3):292–294.
76. South MA, Sever JL. Teratogen update: the congenital rubella syndrome. Teratology 1985;31:297–307.
77. Spalter HF, Bruce GM. Ocular changes in pulmonary insufficiency. Trans Am Acad Ophthalmol Otolaryngol 1964;68:661–676.
78. Summers CG, Knobloch WH, Witkop CJ, King RA. Hermansky–Pudlak syndrome: ophthalmic findings. Ophthalmology 1988;95(4): 545–554.
79. Tada K, Saito T, Hayasaka S, et al. Hyperornithinemia with gyrate atrophy: pathophysiology and treatment. J Inherit Metab Dis 1983;6: 105–106.
80. Tolmachova T, Ramalho JS, Anant JS, Schultz RA, Huxley CM, Seabra MC. Cloning, mapping, and characterization of the human RAB27A gene. Gene (Amst) 1999;239(1):109–116.
81. Traboulsi EI, El-Baba F, Barakat AY, Faris BM. The retinopathy of primary hyperoxaluria. Retina 1985;5(3):151–153.
82. Traboulsi EI, Maumenee IH, Green WR, et al. Olivopontocerebellar atrophy with retinal degeneration. A clinical and ocular histopathologic study. Arch Ophthalmol 1988;106:801–806.
83. Tso AY, Sinclair SH. Respiratory insufficiency. In: Gold DH, Weingeist TA (eds) The eye in systemic disease. Philadelphia: Lippincott, 1999:491–495.
84. Valle D, Walser M, Brusilow SW, et al. Gyrate atrophy of the choroid and retina. Amino acid metabolism and correction of hyperornithinemia with an arginine deficient diet. J Clin Investig 1980;65: 371–378.
85. Walter C, Gootjes J, Mooijer PA, et al. Disorders of peroxisomal biogenesis due to mutations in PEX1: phenotypes and PEX1 protein levels. Am J Hum Genet 2001;69(1):35–48.
86. Warburg M. Ocular coloboma and multiple congenital anomalies. The CHARGE association. Ophthalmic Pediatr Genet 1983;3:189–199.
87. Warburg M. The heterogeneity of microphthalmia in the mentally retarded. Birth Defects 1971;7:136–154.
88. Weleber RG, Kennaway NG, Buist NRM. Vitamin B6 in the management of gyrate atrophy of the choroid and retina. Lancet 1978; 2(8101):1213.
89. Wells CG, Kalina RE. Progressive inherited retinal arteriolar tortuosity with spontaneous retinal hemorrhages. Ophthalmology 1985; 92:1015–1021.

90. Wilson DP, Jelley D, Stratton R, et al. Nephropathic cystinosis: improved linear growth after treatment with recombinant human growth hormone. J Pediatr 1989;115:758–761.
91. Yamaguchi K, Tamai M. Congenital macular coloboma in Down syndrome. Ann Ophthalmol 1990;22(6):222–223.
92. Zhu DP, Antonarakis SE, Schmeckpeper BJ, Diergaarde PJ, Greb AE, Maumenee IH. Microdeletion in the X chromosome and prenatal diagnosis in a family with Norrie disease. Am J Med Genet 1989; 33(4):485–488.
93. Zimmermann LE. Histopathological basis for ocular manifestations of congenital rubella syndrome. Am J Ophthalmol 1968;65(6):837–862.
94. Zvulunov A, et al. Reticulolinear aplasia cutis congenita of the face and neck: a distinctive cutaneous manifestation in several syndromes linked to Xp22. Br J Derm 1998;138(6):1046–1052.

Index